Orthopaedic Technology Innovation

A Step-by-Step Guide from Concept to Commercialization

T0200196

Orthopaedic Technology Innovation

A Step-by-Step Guide from Concept to Commercialization

Adam E.M. Eltorai, MD, PhD
The Warren Alpert Medical School of Brown University
Providence, Rhode Island

Thomas A. Zdeblick, MD
A.A. McBeath Professor and Chair
Department of Orthopedics and Rehabilitation
University of Wisconsin School of Medicine and Public Health
Madison, Wisconsin

Arnold-Peter C. Weiss, MD
R. Scot Sellers Scholar of Hand Surgery, Vice Chair and
    Professor
Department of Orthopaedic Surgery
The Warren Alpert Medical School of Brown University
Providence, Rhode Island

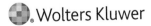 Wolters Kluwer

Philadelphia · Baltimore · New York · London
Buenos Aires · Hong Kong · Sydney · Tokyo

Acquisitions Editor: Brian Brown
Product Development Editor: Stacey Sebring
Editorial Coordinator: Blair Jackson
Marketing Manager: Julie Sikora
Production Project Manager: David Saltzberg
Design Coordinator: Teresa Mallon
Manufacturing Coordinator: Beth Welsh
Prepress Vendor: TNQ Technologies

Copyright © 2020 Wolters Kluwer.

All rights reserved. This book is protected by copyright. No part of this book may be reproduced or transmitted in any form or by any means, including as photocopies or scanned-in or other electronic copies, or utilized by any information storage and retrieval system without written permission from the copyright owner, except for brief quotations embodied in critical articles and reviews. Materials appearing in this book prepared by individuals as part of their official duties as U.S. government employees are not covered by the above-mentioned copyright. To request permission, please contact Wolters Kluwer at Two Commerce Square, 2001 Market Street, Philadelphia, PA 19103, via email at permissions@lww.com, or via our website at shop.lww.com (products and services).

9 8 7 6 5 4 3 2 1

Printed in China

Library of Congress Cataloging-in-Publication Data

ISBN-13: 978-1-4963-8436-2

Cataloging-in-Publication data available on request from the Publisher.

This work is provided "as is," and the publisher disclaims any and all warranties, express or implied, including any warranties as to accuracy, comprehensiveness, or currency of the content of this work.

This work is no substitute for individual patient assessment based upon healthcare professionals' examination of each patient and consideration of, among other things, age, weight, gender, current or prior medical conditions, medication history, laboratory data and other factors unique to the patient. The publisher does not provide medical advice or guidance and this work is merely a reference tool. Healthcare professionals, and not the publisher, are solely responsible for the use of this work including all medical judgments and for any resulting diagnosis and treatments.

Given continuous, rapid advances in medical science and health information, independent professional verification of medical diagnoses, indications, appropriate pharmaceutical selections and dosages, and treatment options should be made and healthcare professionals should consult a variety of sources. When prescribing medication, healthcare professionals are advised to consult the product information sheet (the manufacturer's package insert) accompanying each drug to verify, among other things, conditions of use, warnings and side effects and identify any changes in dosage schedule or contraindications, particularly if the medication to be administered is new, infrequently used or has a narrow therapeutic range. To the maximum extent permitted under applicable law, no responsibility is assumed by the publisher for any injury and/or damage to persons or property, as a matter of products liability, negligence law or otherwise, or from any reference to or use by any person of this work.

shop.lww.com

CCS1019

Preface

Have an idea for a new or improved device or technology?
How do you develop it?
How do you commercialize it?
What are the first steps?

Written by a team of medical, engineering, and business experts, this step-by-step guide to *Orthopaedic Technology Innovation* outlines the process of innovation from concept to commercialization. This comprehensive resource serves as a practical reference for the surgeon, the entrepreneur, the inventor, the researcher, and the innovator aiming to advance orthopaedics successfully.

Adam E.M. Eltorai, MD, PhD
Thomas A. Zdeblick, MD
Arnold-Peter C. Weiss, MD

Contributor List

Katharina Barta
Business Analytics Specialist
The Atticus Group, LLC
Portsmouth, New Hampshire

Steven L. Bokshan, MD
Resident Physician
Department of Orthopedic Surgery
Brown University
Providence, Rhode Island

Brian J. Cole, MD, MBA
Associate Chairman and Professor,
Department of Orthopedics Chairman, Department of Surgery,
Rush OPH Managing Partner,
Midwest Orthopaedics at Rush Sports Medicine and Surgery,
Shoulder, Elbow and Knee Care Section Head,
Cartilage Restoration Center at Rush
Chicago, Illinois

Jennifer A. Daudelin, MSJ
Regulatory Project Manager
M Squared Associates, Inc.
New York, New York

Paul DiCesare, BS
President
Start, LLC, Medical Product Development
Shelton, Connecticut

Roman Dimov
Research Fellow
The Taylor Collaboration
San Francisco Orthopedic Surgery Research Program
San Francisco, California

Becky Ditty, MS
Consultant, Medical Devices
Biologics Consulting
Alexandria, Virginia

Ronald L. Docie, Sr
President
Docie Development, LLC
Athens, Ohio

David J. Dykeman, JD, BS
Shareholder & Patent Attorney
Co-chair, Global Life Sciences & Medical Technology Group
Greenberg Traurig, LLP
Boston, Massachusetts

Deborah Lavoie Grayeski, JD, RAC
Senior Project Manager
M Squared Associates, Inc
New York, New York

Hani Haider, PhD
Professor, Director of Orthopaedic Biomechanics and Advanced Surgical
    Technologies Laboratory
Department of Orthopaedic Surgery and Rehabilitation
University of Nebraska Medical Center
Nebraska Medical Center
Omaha, Nebraska

Joseph E. Hale, PhD
Graduate Faculty
Technological Leadership Institute
University of Minnesota
Minneapolis, Minnesota

Joshua D. Herwig, BS, MS
Co-Founder/CTO
SOMAVAC Medical Solutions, Inc
Memphis, Tennessee

Ken Hsu, MD
Professor of Orthopedic Surgery
St. Mary's Spine Center
San Francisco, California

David Jacobs, BSME, MBA
Director, Medical Devices
Boston Engineering Corporation
Waltham, Massachusetts

Jeffrey A. Karg, PE, MSME
Managing Director
Boston Innovation
Bolton, Massachusetts

Jeremi Leasure, MSE
Director of Research
The Taylor Collaboration
San Francisco Orthopedic Surgery Research Program
San Francisco, California

Haim Mendelson, PhD
The Kleiner, Perkins, Caufield and Byers Professor of Electronic Business
    and Commerce, and Management
Graduate School of Business
Stanford University
Stanford, California

Nancy Patterson, MBA
President and CEO
Strategy Inc
Austin, Texas
Los Angeles, California
Raleigh, North Carolina

Terry Sheridan Powell, MA
Senior Project Manager
M Squared Associates, Inc
New York, New York

Robert A. Rabiner, MBA
Founder & Chief Technical Officer
IlluminOss Medical, Inc
Providence, Rhode Island

Sean Michael Ragan, BA/BS, MS
Co-Founder
Foundry Heavy Industries, LLC
Austin, Texas

Rahul Ram, BS
Senior Staff Regulatory Affairs Specialist
BD
Franklin Lakes, New Jersey

Esra Roan, PhD
Co-Founder/CEO
SOMAVAC Medical Solutions, Inc
Memphis, Tennessee

Alexander Rosinski, MS
Research Fellow
The Taylor Collaboration
San Francisco Orthopedic Surgery Research Program
San Francisco, California

Jesse Rusk, MS, MBA
Director, Medical Devices
Boston Engineering Corporation
Waltham, Massachusetts

Josh Sandberg
President and CEO
Ortho Spine Partners
Scottsdale, Arizona

Kusumal Joseph Silva, CMfgT, CMfgE
Director of Quality and Engineering
Ortho-Precision Products Inc
Hawthorne, California

Christopher K. West, MBA
President
ZeroTo510 Medical Device Accelerator
Memphis, Tennessee

Miles C. Wilson, MBA, MEd
President
Nerves & Bones, Inc
Providence, Rhode Island

Larry Yost, RPh
Founder and Managing Partner
The Atticus Group, LLC
Portsmouth, New Hampshire

Robin R. Young
CEO, Publisher and Managing Editor
RRY Publications LLC
PearlDiver, Inc. (Data Mining for Academic Research)
Lansdale, Pennsylvania

James Zucherman, MD
Professor of Orthopedic Surgery
St. Mary's Spine Center
San Francisco, California

Table of Contents

CHAPTER 1

Identifying an Unmet Need

STEVEN L. BOKSHAN, BRIAN J. COLE

ABOUT THE AUTHORS

Steven Bokshan, MD, is an orthopedic surgery resident at Brown University and a serial med-tech entrepreneur. His previous companies utilized *Google Glass* to enhance surgical teaching in the United States. With a strong background in statistics, he has also utilized time-based costing models and complex clinical simulations to perform economic analyses for various early stage companies. He has successfully fundraised as CEO of multiple companies. His current company, SmartOR, Inc., is working to disrupt the technological landscape of the modern operating room.

Brian J. Cole, MD, MBA, is a professor in the Department of Orthopedics at Rush University Medical Center. He is the Associate Chairman of Clinical Affairs for the Department of Orthopedics, the Managing Partner for Midwest Orthopedics at Rush, and the Chairman of Surgery at Rush's Oak Park Hospital. He is the Section Head of the Rush Cartilage Restoration Center and is widely known as a sports medicine expert for the treatment of complex shoulder, elbow, and knee conditions including cartilage transplantation. He has published more than 1,000 articles and 10 widely read text books in orthopedics and sports medicine. He is the head team physician for the Chicago Bulls and co-team physician for the Chicago White Sox. He can be heard regularly on his ESPN radio show, *Sports Medicine Weekly*.

Introduction: Embracing Innovation

Here, we discuss the process of identifying an unmet orthopedic need. Although entrepreneurship represents a separate discipline, a surgeon's unique skillset gives them significant potential for entrepreneurial innovation and identifying an unmet need. To better understand this, we must first consider the strengths of a surgeon. Dr. Arlen Meyers, otolaryngologist and president of the Society of Physician Entrepreneurs, discusses the unique skills that ultimately prepare physicians for entrepreneurship (Table 1.1).[1] Among the most crucial are pattern recognition, familiarity with research, and ability to collect real-time feedback. To identify an unmet need, an orthopedist must learn to utilize and leverage these strengths in an

Table 1.1 **Components of a Physician's Medical Training That Are Crucial for Identifying an Unmet Need**[1]
Common physician strengths essential for identifying an unmet need
Utilizing pattern recognition
Familiarity with research allows for proposing a hypothesis and systematically testing that hypothesis
Utilizing real-time feedback to adjust or pivot
Building judgment based on a series of previous experiences, successes, and failures
Performing internal risk and cost-benefit analyses
Having a bias toward taking action

entrepreneurial manner. Having passion for identifying gaps and inefficiencies in clinical treatment or operations required to deliver care is requisite to the forward thinking nature of true clinician-innovators.

PATTERN RECOGNITION

As we will discuss later in the chapter, the first step in identifying an unmet need is to **observe** a phenomenon that requires clinical improvement. In order to translate these observations into a defined **clinical problem**, the successful innovator must utilize **pattern recognition** in order to identify the common thread that is causing the clinical problem.[2] As notable endocrine surgeon Atul Gawande discusses at length in his novel *Better*, surgeons have a profound affinity toward pattern recognition.[3] Consider a recent orthopedic example. TMZF (titanium, molybdenum, zirconium, iron) femoral stems for total hip arthroplasty became available in the early 2000s and were touted by engineers and device vendors for their improved biomechanical profile. Shortly thereafter, arthroplasty surgeons began observing an uptick in the number of catastrophic stem failures. The resulting metal on metal corrosion ultimately caused dramatic metallosis, leaving patients with significant systemic side effects.[4] Although there were less than 100 cases of this catastrophic failure ultimately reported at the time of identification, arthroplasty surgeons quickly recognized this subtle association between TMZF alloy and stem failure.

Although the catastrophic failure of TMZF alloy represents a rather dramatic example of pattern recognition, orthopedists rely on less dramatic forms of pattern recognition to carry out their daily clinical duties. As part of their surgical training, orthopedists utilize pattern recognition to classify and distinguish injury types to form a treatment plan.

For example, which types of fracture patterns are anatomically stable versus unstable? Which types of meniscus tears are amenable to repair versus meniscectomy? Do patient characteristics or comorbidities affect which treatment is required? All of these questions require a complex series of pattern recognition in which an orthopedist considers prior experience and evidence-based literature to formulate a treatment strategy. Therefore, when utilizing pattern recognition to identify an unmet need, the orthopedist must simply learn to repurpose the skill as opposed to learning it de novo.

RESEARCH

Regardless of the setting an orthopedist works, they possess the ability to use research in order to build a successful practice. Through their medical training, physicians are taught to develop hypotheses based on their observations and to rigorously test those hypotheses. Consider that in 2017 alone, a total of 334 orthopedic clinical trials were under active status.[5] This ability to propose novel hypotheses and challenge dogma is one of the orthopedist's greatest potential strengths in innovating. Leveraging these skills, the innovator challenges **confirmation bias**, or the tendency to become rigidly attached to an innovation because it holds personal value or has remained dogma, a common issue with surgical specialties.

Consider a recent example. When *Google Glass* was first announced in 2012, author S.B. became one of the first surgeons to use it in the operating room. This futuristic prism sat in the surgeon's peripheral vision and allowed for real-time control of any digital media with a simple voice command of "OK Google, …." Prior to the device being released, *Glass* had made headlines and national news. A large following of surgeons believed that the device would revolutionize the surgical field, with applications ranging from real-time video conferencing to targeted tumor resections. Admittedly, when it was first released, confirmation bias played a large role in setting high expectations for the device. Many surgeons wanted the device to usher in a wave of real-time digital media processing in the operating room. Unfortunately, few surgeons had anticipated that, in an operating room environment where noise levels can exceed 100 decibels, *Glass* could recognize fewer than half of the commands it was given.

As *Glass* slowly faded away from the OR, it taught us an important lesson. With any innovation or new idea, inventors must first challenge themselves; in other words, the innovator must test their hypothesis that a need is unmet (i.e., avoiding a **type 1 error**). When a need is truly unmet, there is a tendency for the innovator to frequently and even spontaneously revisit the issue.

COLLECTING REAL-TIME FEEDBACK

Orthopedic surgeons use real-time feedback to enhance patient care. This is, perhaps, the most important innovation-related skill that orthopedists possess. To cite several examples: we use dynamic stress x-rays to determine the need for acute surgical intervention, we assess our patients' responses after administering medical therapies, and we modify surgical techniques based on intraoperative success and patient outcomes. This ability to modify behavior based on real-time feedback is essential to identifying an unmet need.

For example, consider a surgeon who wished to develop a novel device for internal fixation of a meniscal tear. Prior to product development, the surgeon must collect feedback from colleagues regarding the device. An optimal device would incorporate the most successful components of a competing device but exclude its disadvantages. Pilot testing is required, during which a small sample of surgeons utilize the device and make suggestions influencing further product development (this is often referred to as **focus grouping**). Through the use of real-time feedback, the innovator is able to modify the device in order to more successfully fulfill an unmet need. Product development must remain a fluid process incorporating feedback from surgeons, engineers, device companies, and patients. This fluidity, also known as **pivoting**, is a crucial part of the innovation process.

The Process of Identifying an Unmet Need

Although there is no exact formula for identifying an unmet need, the process generally follows a series of steps. These include performing mindful **observations**, translating a series of observations into a **clinical problem**, and ultimately addressing this problem with a novel **innovation**.

OBSERVATION

Orthopedists are at a unique advantage in identifying unmet clinical needs. Aside from the patient, they are the only individual to observe the entire course of a patient's care (see Figure 1.1 for description of the care process). This process begins when the patient seeks treatment for a musculoskeletal complaint and ends with the resolution of the problem. The process of delivering orthopedic care is extremely complex and involves many ancillary staff members across different environments (e.g., office, operating room). It is important to realize that an innovation can be made in any or all of these aspects of care, with the first step being careful observation.

In order to identify an unmet need, an orthopedist must make unbiased and mindful observations about the success of the orthopedic care

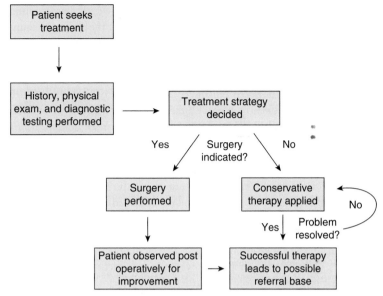

Figure 1.1 A simplified flow diagram of the orthopedic care process.

they are providing. Collecting real-time feedback is essential, with a particular emphasis on experiences that do not occur as desired or that tend to recur in a suboptimal manner. For example, a common observation in an outpatient orthopedic practice may be that patients are being seen inefficiently, with office days lasting beyond the desired expectation. Although it is entirely possible to outsource this problem to an outside consulting service, the orthopedist may be in the strongest position to translate these mindful observations into a solution.

Returning to the previous example of an inefficient office day, consider author SB's experience with using mindful observation to identify the problem. This particular practice consisted of nearly 30 different orthopedists seeing patients in the same office building, some with upwards of 60 patients in a day. By 3 PM, there was a recurring theme. Despite average surgeon-patient interaction times of approximately 8 to 10 minutes (most patients were slotted for a 15-minute visit), patient wait times began to increase. But how could this happen if the actual patient encounter was nearly half the time allotted for each encounter? On further analysis of the wait times, we found that the largest wait times occurred on days consisting of primarily postoperative visits. These wait times seemed counterintuitive, as most postoperative visits only required a brief physical exam and suture removal. Through a series of mindful observations, we ultimately found that largest factor leading to delayed wait times was not the clinical encounter, but rather a delay from the oversaturated x-ray facility. With upwards of 90% of postoperative patients requiring x-rays, we identified the source of patient delay.

After observing aforementioned the clinical problem, we utilized an office modeling program to determine the most efficient solution: deploying digital radiography in the x-ray suites. By reducing x-ray cassette reloading requirements, digital radiography allows for smaller doses of radiation and shorter patient wait times. This solution ultimately translated to higher patient satisfaction and a greater number of patients seen per day.[6]

Patient satisfaction, however, is not the only endpoint for which mindful observation can be utilized. An orthopedist can use mindful observation to identify areas of unmet needs in many different facets of patient care, such as operating room efficiency and success of resident education. In the above example, there were actually multiple suboptimal outcomes including longer patient wait times (which has been directly tied to patient satisfaction), overburdened x-ray technicians, dissatisfied ancillary staff members from a prolonged office day, and a decreased number of overall patients seen by the orthopedist.[6] It is also important to realize that, because of the complex relationships among different resources in the care setting, a proposed innovation for an unmet need may simultaneously improve one endpoint and negatively affect another, i.e., the large cost of retrofitting x-ray facilities with digital technology. Ideally, when proposing a solution for an unmet need, the innovation should positively affect all those involved.

IDENTIFYING A CLINICAL PROBLEM

As stated before, identifying a **clinical problem** is the second step in the process of identifying an unmet need. Although observations are a series of unbiased data points used to identify a suboptimal clinical endpoint, they alone do not represent a clinical problem. In order to truly represent a problem or an unmet need, there must be sufficient **scope** surrounding the observation. Sufficient scope refers to a significant clinical or economic burden that is a direct result of the suboptimal observation. It is true that scope of a clinical problem may first be measured informally through real-time patient feedback or focus grouping with colleagues. Prior to fundraising, however, it is imperative to quantify the economic burden of the problem. If the economic burden is not significant enough to offset the potential cost of a proposed innovation, it becomes very difficult to justify the scope of the innovation.

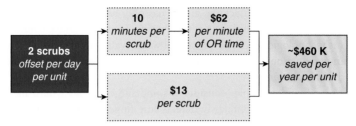

Figure 1.2 Economic burden analysis for a device that reduces breaches of surgical sterility.

For example, consider that you are developing a product that reduces breaches of sterility in the operating room. In an effort to reduce this burden, you devise a new low-footprint and ergonomic miniature fluoroscopy unit that prevents at least two accidental contaminations at a surgical center daily (based on small pilot data). As shown in Figure 1.2, the economic scope of this clinical problem must first be calculated.[7] Knowing the baseline economic scope helps to objectively value the economic advantages of the proposed innovation.

INNOVATION

Once a clinical problem of significant scope has been identified, the orthopedist may begin the process of **innovation**, or creating a solution to an unmet need. First and foremost, this process must begin with appropriate documentation. It is imperative that an innovator has a notebook for written documentation of their ideas. This written record serves a twofold utility. First, as more feedback is collected, documenting previous iterations of the product aids in telling the timeline and story of the product: a step that is crucial during initial pitch meetings. The second advantage of written documentation is to have a written record (signed, dated, and timed by the creator) of which you initially conceived the idea. This information can serve as a source of legal documentation.

Once you have begun the process of innovation, it is essential to have a complete understanding of the technological landscape surrounding the concept. Despite existence of an unmet need, it is possible that the current state of technology precludes a reasonable solution. Consider the previous example of *Google Glass* in the operating room. Upon its initial release, the state of voice recognition was very different from the present.[8] With noise levels in the operating room exceeding 100 decibels, previous voice recognition was unable to achieve command recognition rates above 50%. Recent advances in artificial intelligence algorithms allow for complex noise cancellation and vocal tracking, and it has only recently become possible to perform vocal recognition in the operating room. An understanding of what is technologically possible is crucial when evaluating the attractiveness of innovation around an unmet need; the need will remain unmet without a technical solution.

As a second example, consider a spine surgeon who would like to develop a device that wirelessly detects fine finger motions to track the rehabilitation process for a cervical cord spinal injury. Over the course of the last decade, wireless motion technology has advanced dramatically from recognizing only gross motion at larger joints to now measuring millimeter-level finger movements. Such technology would be appropriate to measure the small improvement seen in cervical cord rehabilitation.[9] Specifically, Project Soli from Google X utilizes radar waves to detect finger movements at a higher resolution than previously reported. These recent advances have made the creation of wireless finger movement detection technologically possible, a feat that was not possible in the early 2000s.

Although innovating can often be the most rewarding step in the process, successful innovation is best supported by the observation and problem identification phases; skipping these earlier, foundational phases is a common pitfall. This is particularly true as advances in technology facilitate rapid movement from idea generation to product development. This lack of **due diligence** frequently yields difficulty during the fundraising process and can be a fatal flaw in the early business lifecycle. As an example of poor due diligence, consider an orthopedist who seeks to develop a novel device to more accurately measure blood loss during surgery. With recent advances in biosensor development, one potential solution would be to outfit a suction device with an infrared sensor to measure the volume of blood passing through the suction tubing per unit of time. Although this device represents a novel solution to an important problem, it does not add any value to the current surgical landscape, as postoperative blood counts are often checked routinely following surgery. Here, it is unlikely that a clinical problem was identified prior to the device development, as the clinical and economic scope of this potential innovation would not justify the cost of product development.

Conclusion

Orthopedists are uniquely situated to identify areas of unmet needs. With a training that fosters many of the core strengths of entrepreneurship, orthopedists can translate these abilities to identify unmet clinical needs. An innovation is best received when an unmet need has sufficient scope and the technological landscape provides a cost-effective solution. Although there any many pitfalls that may occur during the innovation process, a disciplined approach supported by due diligence is much more likely to result in a successful outcome. Perseverance is essential, as the vast majority of innovations will require significant evaluation, modification, and reevaluation to achieve a successful result.

KEY TAKEAWAY POINTS

- ▶ Orthopedists' training provides them with many strengths that should be utilized when identifying an unmet need. These include pattern recognition, familiarity with research, and the ability to collect real-time feedback.

- ▶ The process of identifying an unmet need includes observation, defining a clinical problem, and innovating.

- ▶ An observation is the process of mentally or physically recording an aspect of the patient care process, frequently one that occurs in a suboptimal manner.

- ▶ A clinical problem has been observed multiple times and represents an inefficient or suboptimal delivery of care.

- ▶ It is essential to avoid bias and common pitfalls during the process of innovation.

REFERENCES AND RESOURCES

1. AMeyers. 10 Reasons Why Doctors Make Great Entrepreneurs | The MIT Entrepreneurship Review; 2013. [online] Miter.mit.edu. Available at http://miter.mit.edu/10-reasons-why-doctors-make-great-entrepreneurs/. Accessed October 15, 2017.
2. Baron R. Opportunity recognition as pattern recognition: how entrepreneurs "connect the dots" to identify new business opportunities. *Acad Manag Perspect.* 2006;20(1):104-119.
3. Gawande A. *Better.* New York: Metropolitan; 2007.
4. Walker P, Campbell D, Della Torre P, et al. Trunnion corrosion and early failure in monolithic metal-on-polyethylene TMZF femoral components: a case series. *Reconstr Rev.* 2016;6(3).
5. Search of: Orthopedic | Active, Not Recruiting Studies – List Results –Clinicaltrials. Gov. Clinicaltrials.gov. Accessed October 15, 2017.
6. Huang XM. Patient attitude towards waiting in an outpatient clinic and its applications. *Health Serv Manag Res.* 1994;7:2-8.
7. Gurnea TP, Frye WP, Althausen PL. Operating room supply costs in orthopaedic trauma: cost containment opportunities. *J Orthop Trauma.* 2016;30(1):S21-S26.

8. Norris DJ. *Introduction to Artificial Intelligence. Beginning Artificial Intelligence with the Raspberry Pi.* Apress; 2017:1-15.
9. Lien J, Gillian N, Karagozler ME, et al. Soli: ubiquitous gesture sensing with millimeter wave radar. *ACM Trans Graph.* 2016;35(4):142.

CHAPTER 2

Market Analysis—Determining Market Size

NANCY PATTERSON

ABOUT THE AUTHOR

Nancy Patterson, MBA, is a Venture Analyst and the President and CEO of Strategy Inc., www.strategyinc.net, a life science market and financial due diligence company founded in 2000. Strategy Inc. provides market and business analysis services for emerging life science technology entities to inform the probability for successful commercialization. Clients include emerging entrepreneurs, enterprise companies, and financiers with technologies in all product lifecycle stages; however, over half of the innovations where clients seek Strategy Inc. insight are preclinical. Global Reach: Nearly 46% of entities seeking Strategy Inc. services over the last 10 years have been international from Europe (especially France, Spain, and Germany), Israel, Asia, and South America.

Overview

A market analysis is a multistep, qualitative, and quantitative iterative process to determine the probability of successful technology commercialization within a specific market. Orthopedic innovators have a learned understanding of unmet clinical needs, however require a business perspective of the market to be able to accurately project the successful commercialization of their technology. This chapter focuses on methods to determine market size, market opportunity, and approaches to benchmark technology against competitive offerings.

The orthopedic market landscape is the total market of all solutions to promote healing in orthopedics. Orthopedic devices and technologies are designed to deliver improved clinical status of the skeletal structure, joint movement, spinal stability and motion preservation, soft-tissue damage and trauma or other deformities of the musculoskeletal structure, and bone growth. These technologies provide clinical support, are inserted or implanted surgically through open or minimally invasive procedures, or are externally attached. The US orthopedic devices market, valued at >$20B

USD in 2016, is anticipated to exceed $25B in 2024[1] and includes companies that develop, manufacture, and market technology for joint reconstruction and arthroscopy, trauma repair and fixation, spinal fixation and fusion, soft-tissue repair and reconstruction, orthopedic bracing, orthobiologics, orthopedic accessories, orthopedic prosthetics, and others.

US national annual health spending, which includes spending by federal and state governments, the private sector, and individuals, rose from just 5% as a share of the economy in 1960 to 17.9% in 2016 and is projected to rise to 19.9% by 2025, according to the most recent data from the Centers for Medicare and Medicaid Services.[2] In addition, a detailed analysis of health care spending in the United States and 10 other high-income, predominantly European, countries found that the United States spends approximately twice as much on medical care per capita.[3] Such escalation exerts significant pressure on technology innovators, as most institutions, outpatient services, group practices, and individual practitioners are driven to seek the most cost-effective, improved clinical outcomes. Economic pressures mean that innovation must deliver evidence-based and value-driven clinical results to ensure adoption. In a 2017 report about cost-effectiveness and the introduction of new surgical techniques and technologies in orthopedic surgery, Jeremy Burnham, MD from UPMC Center for Sports Medicine states, "As the pace of technological innovation advances in lockstep with an increased focus on value, orthopedic surgeons will need to have a working knowledge of value-based healthcare decision-making. Value-based healthcare and cost-effectiveness analyses can aid orthopedic surgeons in making ethical and fiscally responsible treatment choices for their patients."[4]

One of the critical earliest stage activities, before development work initiates, is to determine the probability of commercial viability of an orthopedic innovation. Assuming that the innovation can deliver cost-effective clinical outcomes as designed, a market analysis is instrumental to confirm that a positive return on an investment is achievable. Although identification of an unmet need, as previously discussed, is an area where the surgical training, clinical observation skills, and experience of the orthopedic surgeon deliver valuable insight, the validation of potential commercial viability is required to prioritize developmental funding and resource allocation. Based on the economic pressures facing health care, early-stage market analysis is critical to provide insight into the potential market for a technology in the earliest stage of development, before a prototype is developed, prior to animal testing, and before the significant expenditures and time of clinical testing. The question is: What are the steps of market analysis, and how are they best executed?

Market analysis is a multistep, iterative process that delivers increased understanding of the probability of commercial success for a technology within a specific market. Developing a market plan framework ensures that the entrepreneur can initially identify and assess the total potential market landscape and then work toward increasing depth to the specific address-able market size for the innovation under consideration for development. A broader-scope approach is often the most effective initial step, adding specific market detail, as additional information is available to inform the market segments with the highest value.

Market research can be performed by company employees through field interaction or by dedicated in-house research teams to provide the insight on product/service/company offerings. Such frequent, cost-effective close to the customer efforts can identify and clarify potential customer needs, and ensure that customers are heard. Third party market research is most often perceived as more objective and thus more influential to drive investments. It is often possible to determine anticipated adoption, reduce business risk with deeper probing where customers may be more prone to provide expanded insight to addressing objectives. Third party market research has been shown to shape strategies that reach new markets, recognize emerging trends, benchmark your business against competitors and enact initiatives to acquire the desired target customer.

Market Analysis Process: Segment, Score, and Select

The three critical elements of the market analysis are Segment, Score, and Select (Table 2.1). Each will be covered as it pertains to development of orthopedic innovation to provide an introductory roadmap to determining the potential for commercial viability. **Segment** includes the market segmentation to highlight defined market segments and align clinical segments with technology that provides related solutions. **Score** outlines the methods to determine market size and market opportunity and the procedure volumes for specific procedures. **Select** outlines analytical methods to determine projected adoption and clarify market opportunity.

Table 2.1 Segment, Score, and Select Market Analysis		
Segment	**Score**	**Select**
• Segment market • Identify market landscape • Competitive analysis	• Incidence and prevalence • Procedure volumes • Market trends	• Determine projected adoption • Identify market opportunity • Target market value

THE SEGMENT STAGE

The initial step of the market analysis, the **Segment** stage, fully defines the market sectors. As an orthopedist developing an innovative orthopedic technology, it is important to classify a device into the correct category. This step ensures that an innovation is correctly aligned with similar technologies and has these six (or more) important benefits:

1. Ensure that companies and investors clearly understand the market landscape where a technology is positioned. This is especially important with paradigm-changing technology,
2. Positively highlight and influence investment speed and levels of funding in segments where significant returns have flourished,
3. Identify and benchmark potential merger, acquisition, and exit timelines,
4. Emphasize areas with existing reimbursement coding, coverage, and payment,
5. Outline a projected adoption trajectory of aligned innovation,
6. Spotlight markets where advances in materials or processes are driving new clinical capabilities in health care advancements. These market segments are continually expanding and changing, as new innovations emerge.

Figure 2.1 highlights the 2016 to 2017 estimated annual revenue of the seven US orthopedic markets.

Expanded Descriptions of the Orthopedics Market Segments

Joint Reconstruction and Repair

Joint reconstruction and repair devices and accessories include technology for full or partial replacement or repair of the shoulder, ankle, hip, knee, elbow, or digits.

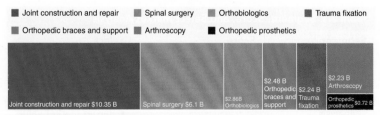

US Orthopedic Market Sizes

■ Joint construction and repair ■ Spinal surgery ■ Orthobiologics ■ Trauma fixation
■ Orthopedic braces and support ■ Arthroscopy ■ Orthopedic prosthetics

Joint construction and repair $10.35 B | Spinal surgery $6.1 B | $2.86B Orthobiologics | $2.48 B Orthopedic braces and support | $2.24 B Trauma fixation | $2.23 B Arthroscopy | Orthopedic prosthetics $0.72 B

Figure 2.1 US orthopedic market sizes.

Spinal Surgery

The spinal surgery market includes surgical devices and implants for fusion, fixation, vertebral compression fractures, decompression, and motion preservation. Devices include products for thoracic, lumbar and cervical fusion, vertebral compression fracture treatment, spine bone stimulators, nonfusion and spinal decompression devices, and spine biologics. Based on the type of surgery, spinal implants and spinal surgical devices are divided into open and minimally invasive surgery.

Trauma Fixation

Fixation of physical trauma from application of external force or violence is divided into internal and external fixation devices. Internal devices, which are increasing in adoption, include plates and bone screws, pins, rods, intramedullary nails, and compression hip screws. External fixation devices are used for marked soft-tissue loss and instability where tension and compression forces to the bone are applied to stimulate bone growth. External fixation is divided into unilateral, circular, and hybrid fixation devices.

Orthobiologics

Orthobiologics are implants composed of cells and proteins naturally found in human body that provide accelerated healing by stimulating efficient regrowth of musculoskeletal tissues. These technologies include bone grafts, stem cells, autologous blood, autologous conditioned serum, platelet-rich plasma, and growth factors.

Arthroscopy

Minimally invasive technology to visualize, diagnose, and repair hip, knee, shoulder, spine, ankle, wrist, and elbow joints. Examples include torn joint cartilage, anterior cruciate ligament (ACL) repair, and sports-related joint injuries. Hip and knee arthroscopy are the most common arthroscopic procedures and most often performed on athletes and older patients. Arthroscopic procedures can avoid or delay total or partial joint replacement or repair. Innovation in this market segment includes smart and customized implants and has enjoyed increased adoption, thus investments in development.

Orthopedic Braces and Support

Orthopedic brace systems to protect, support, and strengthen the joints and muscles are used in injury prevention, injury rehabilitation, postoperative care, and osteoarthritic care. Based on the application, orthopedic braces and support systems are classified as spinal orthoses, ankle, knee, wrist, and upper extremity braces and supports.

Orthopedic Prosthetics

Orthopedic prosthetics are artificial devices that replace a missing body part that may have been lost through trauma or disease leading to surgical removal. The devices are classified into upper extremity prosthetics (hand, elbow, shoulder) and lower extremity prosthetics (foot and ankle, knee, and hip). By technology, they are divided by manual, electric-powered, and hybrid prosthetics.

To provide selected examples of procedures and technology categories, along with innovative technology examples within each category, Table 2.2 includes reference examples with hyperlinked examples available in the online version. This table provides expanded understanding of the market segments to correctly position an innovation.

Segment: Identify the Specific Market Landscape

An initial landscape map creates an important preliminary market framework. Each landscape includes many variables that influence clinical adoption. One effective method, developed by this chapter author, is to combine and weigh the variables, to capture the competitors to your planned technology with graphic representation, realizing that a new solution must deliver value in the critical areas against which competitors are measured. Each market landscape is individual to the specific technology and can be adjusted based on market dynamics.

An orthopedic innovator understands the clinical metrics most influential around an innovation, as well as expanded metrics such as utilization, cost, and relative effectiveness. At this stage it is not necessary to be exact with each variable but rather to generally position the different aspects that influence the market. The following example highlights a **landscape map for** therapeutic procedures for degenerative disc disease. This landscape map has a US perspective and was reviewed by US physicians. It is targeted at motion preservation, to outline the prospective landscape "gap," identify a need statement, and develop an expanded needs specification. It is important to note that although recent literature has shown improved outcomes using robotic and computer-assisted navigation for pedicle screw and spacer placements, such improvements have not been incorporated into this landscape map.

Included in the market landscape map are:

1. Posterior lumbar interbody fusion (PLIF)
2. Anterior lumbar interbody fusion (ALIF)
3. Lateral lumbar interbody fusion (LLIF/XLIF)

Table 2.2 Examples of Orthopedic Markets, Procedures, and Innovative Technologies

Orthopedic Device Market Segments	Procedures (Selected Examples)	Technology Categories (Selected Examples)	Example Technologies
Joint reconstruction	**Partial and total joint replacement:** Hip, knee, ankle, shoulder, elbow, wrist	Total/partial knee joint replacement system Total/partial hip joint replacement system Anatomic shoulder system Total wrist replacement system	**Aesculap Implant Systems**—Vega System for Knee Arthroplasty **Wright Medical**—Latitude EV Total Elbow Arthroplasty **Zimmer Biomet**—Anatomical Shoulder Domelock System
Spine	Discectomy Kyphoplasty Laminectomy Spinal disc replacement Spine fusion Vertebroplasty	Implants/instrumentation Pedicle screws, rods, hooks, plates, cages, interspinous process spacers Motion preservation systems/dynamic stabilization Spinal stimulators	**Mighty Oak Medical**—X-Caliber Porous Pedicle Screw **SIGNUS Medizintechnik GmbH**—ROTAIO (Cervical disc prosthesis—implantable like a cage, moves like a disc) **TranS1**—Pylon MIS Posterolateral Graft Delivery System is a reusable spinal instrument **VersaSpine LLC**—VersaSpine Dual-Ended Minimally Invasive Pedicle Screw System **ZygoFix Ltd.**—ZLOCK Facet Fusion System
Trauma fixation	External fixation Intramedullary nailing Open reduction and internal fixation	**Internal trauma fixators** Plates, screws, rods, wires and pins, and fusion nails **External trauma fixators** Circular, unilateral, hybrid	**Acumed**—Ulna Rod **DePuy Synthes**—3.5 mm VA LCP Proximal Tibia Plate **OrthoXel**—Apex Tibial Nailing System with micromotion locking mode

Continued

Table 2.2 Examples of Orthopedic Markets, Procedures, and Innovative Technologies—Cont'd

Orthopedic Device Market Segments	Procedures (Selected Examples)	Technology Categories (Selected Examples)	Example Technologies
Orthobiologics	Hip preservation surgery Orthobiologic injection for nonsurgical treatment of musculoskeletal conditions Spinal fusion Trauma fracture repair	Allograft Bone morphogenetic protein (BMP) Demineralized bone matrix (DBM) Viscosupplementation	**Amniox**—Respina Restorative Spine Matrix **Bioventus**—Signafuse **Regenexx**—Regenexx Orthopedic Stem Cell **RTI Biologics**—Elemax PLIF Allograft
Soft tissue/ arthroscopic	ACL reconstruction Carpal tunnel release Rotator cuff repair Removal of the loose bone or cartilage in the knee, shoulder, elbow, ankle, wrist	ACL soft-tissue graft fixation Endoscopic carpel tunnel release systems Knotless anchors Radio-frequency probes	**Arthrex**—PushLock Anchor for Arthroscopic Glenohumeral Joint Instability Repair **MicroAire**—SmartRelease Endoscopic Carpal Tunnel Release System **Zimmer Biomet**—ToggleLoc Device with ZipLoop for ACL Reconstruction **Stryker**—SERFAS Radio-Frequency Probes
Orthopedic braces, accessories	Injury rehabilitation Osteoarthritic care	Brace and supports Orthopedic prosthestics Spinal orthoses	**FLA Orthopedics**—FlexLite Sport Hinged Ankle Brace **Moyarta 2**—The Stand and Deliver, Brace Solutions for Scoliosis
Orthopedic prosthetics	Amputation	Prosthetic leg—above or below the knee Upper-limb prosthesis	**Ottobock**—X3 Prosthetic Leg **Össur**—Proprio Foot **Touch Bionics (Össur)**—i-limb ultra **Motion Control**—Utah Arm 3+

Created by Strategy Inc. www.strategyinc.net.

4. Transforaminal lumbar interbody fusion (TLIF)
5. Disk prosthesis
6. Anterior cervical decompression fusion (ACDF)
7. Posterior interspinous distractors
8. Pedicle-based dynamic rod devices
9. Posterior dynamic stabilization systems

The x-axis in this graphic represents procedural complexity (Table 2.3), which combines metric weightings for a range of clinical processes versus procedural outcomes on the y-axis. Bubble sizes are an outcome metric, where bubble size is equal to reversibility. There may be additional factors to ensure that no important source of differentiation is omitted.

The weighting metrics outline the probable variables, and a scoring for each metric is shown in Table 2.4. Each innovator can select and weigh the different metrics that surround their innovation and adjust as desired and then plot different variables against each other.

The 2 × 2 graphic can provide a directional sense of where high-value opportunities exist. As the landscape becomes more defined, innovators can better project the level of effectiveness that a new solution would have to deliver to provide value for the target market. A new technology can address a subset of the total population, which can be highlighted by the landscape map.

Table 2.3 Degenerative Disc Disease Market Landscape

Lumbar Degenerative Disc Disease Market Landscape

x-axis	Surgical complexity	Computed metric to include surgical approach, bony decompression, surgical time, inpatient/outpatient, minimally invasive, hospital LOS
y-axis	Outcomes Metric	Computed metric to include blood loss, preserved anatomy, risk of adjacent levels degeneration, efficacy, implant-related complications
Bubbles	Product Categories	Spinal fusion, lumbar disk prosthesis, posterior interspinous distractors, pedicle-based dynamic rod devices, posterior dynamic stabilization systems
Bubble Size	Reversibility	Level of bony anchorage

LOS, length of stay.

Table 2.4 Complexity Scaling Metric

Surgical Complexity Scaling Metric					
Surgical Approach	Bony Decompression	Surgical Time	Inpatient vs. Outpatient	Minimally Invasive	Hospital Length of Stay
5	7	9	5	5	7
1 = Posterior approach 3 = Lateral approach 5 = Anterior approach	0 = No bony decompression 1 = Hemilaminectomy 2 = Facetectomy 5 = Discectomy 5 = Laminectomy 7 = Combination of multiple	1 = <1 h 3 = 1-2 h 5 = 2-3 h 7 = 3-4 h 9 = >5 h	1 = Outpatient 5 = Inpatient	1 = Minimally invasive 3 = Half MIS/half open 5 = Open procedure	0 = Outpatient 1 = 1 d 3 = 2-3 d 5 = 3-4 d 7 = >4 d

Created by Strategy Inc. www.strategyinc.net

Procedure Outcomes Scaling Metric				
Blood Loss	Preserved Anatomy	Risk of Degeneration of Adjacent Levels	Efficacy	Implant Risk–Related Complications
6	5	7	13	16
1 = Very low 2 = Low 4 = Moderate 6 = Extensive	1 = Preserved 3 = Partially preserved 5 = Not preserved	1 = None 3 = Minimal 5 = Moderate 7 = Significant	1 = 95%+ 3 = 90%-94% 5 = 85%-89% 7 = 80%-84% 9 = 75%-79% 11 = 70%-74% 13 = <70%	Add two pts for each: Risk as patient presents • Dural leak • Great vessel damage/venous injury • Implant migration/dislocation • Misaligned screw • Muscle retraction • Nerve damage • Pseudo-arthrodesis • Spinous process fractures

Scale: Lower number = More highly desired outcome. Higher number = less desired outcome. MIS, minimally invasive surgery.

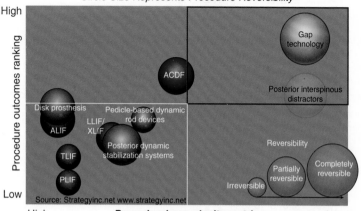

Procedure Complexity versus Anticipated Outcomes
Circle Size Represents Procedure Reversibility

Segment: Competitive Analysis

A comprehensive competitive landscape analysis ensures that an entrepreneur can accurately benchmark their technology against other solutions available to the target market, which yields a perspective to optimize business decisions. Competitive analysis is not just market research but an increasingly essential element to ensure that development decisions are prioritized based on market preferences and trends. In recent years, health care facilities and group purchasing organizations have added value analysis teams to the purchasing process to compare the features and cost-effectiveness of any new product being considered for inclusion. Members of these diverse, professional, and experienced teams execute this rigorous analysis as a component of the purchasing cycle. Understanding that a health care facility value analysis team will audit an innovation as a component of the technology assessment process confirms the importance of competitive analysis in the product development market analysis process.

To achieve strategic competitiveness with an emerging technology, an objective market assessment must include both direct and indirect competitors currently available and, as discernible, innovation in development at competitive companies, universities, think tanks, or technology accelerators. To be effective, the process must be dynamic, not static, as new market entrants and enhancements of existing products to address market needs are continually emerging.

In addition, competition can include new indirect markets or product features available with the emergence of innovative biomaterials or processes.

THE SCORE STAGE

This stage of market analysis includes several components: incidence, prevalence, and procedure volumes to determine patient numbers with the disease or condition applicable for an innovation and current numbers of procedures being performed. Disease incidence and prevalence, as defined below, provides the overall target population, which can then be segmented to the most applicable subgroup.[5]

- **Incidence:** Occurrence rate of a disease or condition within a population, over a given time, usually annually
- **Prevalence:** Burden of disease within a population at a given location within a specific period, usually expressed as a percentage of the population

Incidence and prevalence disease rate variances across geographic regions may be significant for specific diseases based on epidemiological differences. Sources for obtaining current data are available from medical records databases, government and clinical society references, and journal publications. Examples compiled from 20 different sources, with links (available in the online version), are included for incidence, prevalence, and procedure volumes (Table 2.5).

An example of an incidence and prevalence calculation shown below exemplifies the variability of data and the importance of inclusion of a range of sources. Data averaged from a minimum of five reputable sources will most often be acceptable to investors. It is important to select peer-reviewed rather than corporate or popular media sources for accuracy. In the following tables, the numbers denoted in bold refer to referenced data. Numbers are rounded to reasonable significant figures. Current population data are often segmented by gender and age-appropriate populations, when applicable to a specific innovation. As shown in Table 2.6, the average annual US incidence of ACL tears is estimated to be 190,000.

Incidence of ACL Tears

The US prevalence of adolescent idiopathic scoliosis is calculated at an estimated 9,100,000 (Table 2.7). Note one outlying data point from the *Cochrane Database of Systematic Reviews* (CDSR); however it was included since CDSR is considered one of the leading resources for systematic reviews in health care. This one data point motivated the increase in data sources to seven to manage the statistics.

Table 2.5 Incidence, Prevalence, and Procedure Volume Resources

Medical Records Databases	Government/Society References	Published Journal Databases
HCUP: The Healthcare Cost and Utilization Project includes a collection of longitudinal hospital care data in the United States.	North American Spine Society—NASS International Society for the Advancement of Spine Surgery American Association of Orthopedic Surgeons American Joint Replacement Registry outcomes of >860,000 US joint procedures from 654 institutions and 4755 surgeons CDC—Centers for Disease Control and Prevention ClinicalTrials.gov—a database of privately and publicly funded clinical studies conducted around the world United States Census Bureau World Health Organization—WHO Kaiser Family Foundation	**PubMed,** >28 million citations for biomedical literature from MEDLINE, life science journals, and online books
MEPS: The Medical Expenditure Panel Survey data from surveys of families, individuals, medical providers, and employers across the United States.		**Embase,** a global, multipurpose, and up-to-date biomedical database with literature dating back to 1947
NAMCS/NHAMCS: The National Ambulatory Medical Care Survey data of the use of ambulatory medical care services in the United States. The **National Hospital Ambulatory Medical Care Survey** data on the utilization of ambulatory care services in hospital emergency and outpatient departments and ambulatory surgery locations.		**Cochrane collection** This collection is an essential source of high-quality health care data, not only useful for providers and patients but also for those responsible for researching, teaching, funding, and administrating at all levels of the medical profession
SEER Incidence Data: From population-based cancer registries covering the United States on patient demographics, primary tumor site, tumor morphology, stage at diagnosis, and first course of treatment, and follow-up for vital status.		**MEDLINE** A database of full-text for biomedical and health journals, indexed in MEDLINE. Many are available to doctors, nurses, health professionals, and researchers
SCISM: The National Spinal Cord Injury Model Systems Database captures data from an estimated 6% of new spinal cord injury cases in the United States and operates through the National Spinal Cord Injury Statistical Center.		**Google Scholar** A web search engine that indexes scholarly literature across an array of publishing formats and disciplines

Table 2.6 Incidence of anterior cruciate ligament Tears[23-28]

US Population	Incidence	Incidence Rate	Source
308,745,538	211,800	**0.000686**	*American Journal of Sports Medicine*
	120,000	0.000389	*Clinics in Sports Medicine*
	250,000	0.000810	CDC—University of North Carolina Injury Prevention Research Center
	166,700	**0.000540**	*Orthopaedic Journal of Sports Medicine*
	200,000	0.000648	*Orthopedic Research Online Journal*
Average	189,700		

Procedures Volumes

Procedure volumes have much higher variability from year to year, between countries, and even within a single country compared with incidence and prevalence data. Procedure volumes are influenced by market trends in adoption of new procedures, clinical trial results, published literature,

Table 2.7 Prevalence of Adolescent Idiopathic Scoliosis[29-34]

US Population	Prevalence	Prevalence Rate	Source
308,745,538	7,718,600	**0.025000**	American Association of Neurological Surgeons
	7,718,600	**0.025000**	National Scoliosis Foundation
	7,718,600	**0.025000**	Scoliosis
	6,174,900	**0.020000**	*Journal of the American Medical Association*
	5,880,000	0.019045	United States Bone and Joint Initiative
	19,914,100	**0.064500**	*Cochrane Database of Systematic Reviews*
	8,644,900	**0.028000**	*International Journal of Epidemiology*
Average	9,109,957		

adverse events, reimbursement levels and availability of new reimbursement codes, and even significant marketing programs. Frequent monitoring and iterative research into procedure volumes is critical for market size projections. For emerging change in the standard of technology, determination of procedure volumes is more challenging and usually requires the assistance of a market research professional.

The orthopedic resource table for incidence, prevalence, and procedure volumes includes data sources from medical records databases, government and clinical society references, and journal publications and is provided for reference. The URLs are accessible in the online version (see Table 2.5 Incidence, Prevalence, and Procedure Volume Resources).

Market Trends Influencing Emerging Technology Innovation

Market trends, both positive and negative, influence the potential for an emerging innovation to realize successful commercialization. Figure 2.2 highlights the influencing forces in orthopedic innovation. Positive influencers include the aging population with the requisite increase in degenerative disease prevalence juxtaposed with an increasing interest in an

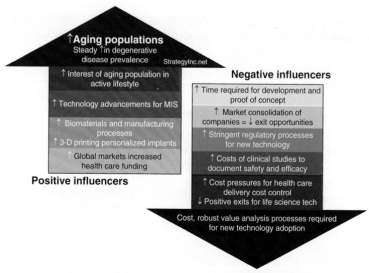

Figure 2.2 Market trends influencing orthopedic innovation. MIS, minimally invasive surgery.

active lifestyle in the later decades of life. There is an increasing demand for minimally invasive surgeries, and fortunately biomaterials and manufacturing processes support advances in innovative orthopedic technology including, for example, the emergence of 3-D printing for personalized implants. The biomedical advances positively influence orthopedic innovation development.

Negative influencers for orthopedic innovation development are mostly financial. Health care delivery cost pressures mean that new technology must pass the highly regulated comparative value analysis processes before it will be available in facilities. Development costs and time for orthopedic innovation include regulatory review and clinical trials. Furthermore, exit levels for orthopedic technology have fluctuated because of consolidation. Such hurdles mean that it is critical to ensure a technology market size is verified and interest level of a target market is confirmed.

SELECT

The final stage of market analysis is to determine projected market revenue and number of anticipated units sold to aid in selection of the technology and the specific features that will drive the highest probability of successful commercialization. This analysis includes confirming the total addressable market versus the market opportunity. The total addressable market refers to the current size and market growth of the market segment. This differs from the market opportunity, which is the potential market segment anticipated to be captured by the technology over time. The penetration rate within the projected market opportunity is the most critical to the investment community. A first-time entrepreneur's pitfall is segmenting the full market as the anticipated potential, rather than a segment applicable for the emerging technology.

Rotator Cuff Repair Market Opportunity

Market size can be calculated from either a top-down or a bottom-up method or a combination of both. A top-down method begins with the overall disease revenue and then divides the total spend into segments based on segment percentages. This process delivers more of a market overview but can be an efficient method in the early stages of market sizing. The bottom-up method segments the applicable number of patients and then calculates the market revenue on a per-patient basis with determined pricing data, segmented by severity or other market delimiters. This method yields a more defensible total market size. Comparison of market adoption of competitive technology within the market segment of an innovation will be best received by financiers (Figure 2.3).

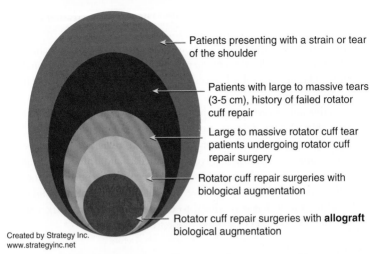

Patients presenting with a strain or tear of the shoulder

Patients with large to massive tears (3-5 cm), history of failed rotator cuff repair

Large to massive rotator cuff tear patients undergoing rotator cuff repair surgery

Rotator cuff repair surgeries with biological augmentation

Rotator cuff repair surgeries with **allograft** biological augmentation

Created by Strategy Inc.
www.strategyinc.net

Figure 2.3 Rotator cuff repair market opportunity.[6-10]

Lumbar Spinal Stenosis Market Size Versus Total Market Opportunity

The final stage is the determination of the projected adoption for an emerging technology, which requires objective projections influenced by four stakeholders:

1. Patients
2. Health care providers (clinicians and ancillary health care staff)
3. Facilities
4. Third-party payors

Needs of stakeholders may compete, and it is the innovator's responsibility to balance requirements. Each party's anticipated willingness to pay for innovation is affected by peer-reviewed clinical outcomes, value analysis data, price of current technology solution including bundling with other products, competitive dynamics, procedure volumes, sales channel purchasing relationships, acquisition sales cycle, and more (Figure 2.4).

Primary Market Data

Realistic defensible high, moderate, and low revenue projection at 6 years post launch will provide the range of potential revenue and will be both expected and appreciated by financiers. Average market adoption for paradigm-changing technology should be included for the target market for innovation able to deliver consistent cost-effective clinical outcomes. Defensible market projections are based on market preference data

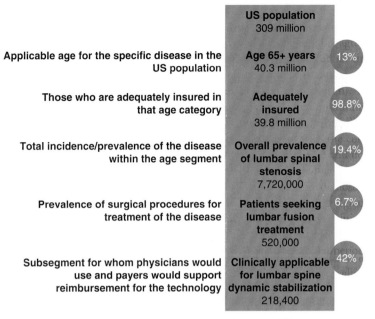

Figure 2.4 Market size based on population.[11-22]

obtained through direct data collection of prospective end users, prioritizing and weighting needs. Such market preferences are obtained based on an objective discussion able to capture forced ranking of key market influences.

KEY TAKEAWAY POINTS

- ▶ Early-stage market analysis is critical to provide insight into the potential market for a technology in the earliest stage of development, before a prototype is developed, prior to animal testing, and before the significant expenditures and time of clinical testing.

- ▶ Innovation must deliver evidence-based and value-driven clinical results to ensure adoption. The increased emphasis in value analysis–driven product purchasing is driven by the escalation of cost pressures for all health care delivery systems including institutions, outpatient services, group practices, and individual practitioners alike.

- ▶ Understanding the market landscape where technology is positioned is especially critical with paradigm-changing technology to ensure the space of the market need is accurately confirmed.

- ▶ Benchmarking both the total market size and the projected addressable market opportunity for an innovation ensures that accurate market projections will be defensible for investment scrutiny.

- ▶ Properly segmenting the market can positively influence investment speed and levels of funding in segments where significant returns have flourished; identify and benchmark potential merger, acquisition, and exit timelines; emphasize areas with existing reimbursement coding, coverage, and payment; and spotlight markets where advances in materials or processes are driving new clinical capabilities in health care advancements.

- ▶ Strategic competitiveness with an emerging technology benefits from an objective, dynamic market assessment that includes both direct and indirect competitors of technology currently available and in development.

- ▶ Market trends, both positive and negative, influence the potential for an emerging innovation to realize successful commercialization.

- ▶ Market opportunity shows the potential market segment anticipated to be captured by the technology over time. A first-time entrepreneur's pitfall is segmenting the full market as the anticipated potential, rather than a segment applicable for the emerging technology.

REFERENCES AND RESOURCES

1. Satarupa D. *U.S. Orthopedic Devices Market to Witness Massive Growth Over 2017-2024.* ODTMag.com; May 9, 2018.
2. *2016-2025 Projections of National Health Expenditures Data.* CMS.gov; February 2017.
3. Emanuel EJ. The real cost of the US health care system. *JAMA.* 2018;319(10):983-985.
4. Burnham JM, Meta F, Lizzio V, Makhni EC, Bozic KJ. Technology assessment and cost-effectiveness in orthopedics: how to measure outcomes and deliver value in a constantly changing healthcare environment. *Curr Rev Musculoskelet Med.* 2017;10(2):233-239.
5. Saleh A, Cornell CN. The prevalence of disabling musculoskeletal conditions and the demand for orthopedic surgery in the twenty-first century. In: MacKenzie CR, Cornell CN, Memtsoudis SG, eds. *Perioperative Care of the Orthopedic Patient.* New York: Springer; 2014:13-24.
6. McCormack RA, Shreve M, Strauss EJ. Biologic augmentation in rotator cuff repair: should we do it, who should get it, and has it worked? *Bull Hosp Jt Dis.* 2014;72(1):89-96.
7. Gilot GJ, Attia AK, Alvarez AM. Arthroscopic repair of rotator cuff tears using extracellular matrix graft. *Arthrosc Tech.* 2014;3(4):e487-e489.
8. Sears BW, Choo A, Yu A, Greis A, Lazarus M. Clinical outcomes in patients undergoing revision rotator cuff repair with extracellular matrix augmentation. *Orthopedics.* 2015;38(4):e292-e296.
9. Varvitsiotis D, Papaspiliopoulos A, Antipa E, Papacharalampous X, Flevarakis G, Feroussis J. Results of reconstruction of massive irreparable rotator cuff tears using a fascia lata allograft. *Indian J Orthop.* 2015;49(3):304-311.
10. Cheung EV, Silverio L, Sperling JW. Strategies in biologic augmentation of rotator cuff repair: a review. *Clin Orthop Relat Res.* 2010;468(6):1476-1484.

11. *Spinal Intervention: Markets for Surgical, Replacement and Neurostimulation Technologies*. BCC Research. Report, Region: Global; January 2017:181.
12. *2017 US Population Estimates*. Census.gov. 2010.
13. Barnett JC, Berchick ER. *Health Insurance Coverage in the United States: 2016*. Census.gov. September 2010.
14. Ravindra VM, Senglaub SS, Rattani A, et al. Degenerative lumbar spine disease: estimating global incidence and worldwide volume. *Glob Spine J*. 2018;8(8):784-794.
15. Yavin D, Casha S, Wiebe S, et al. Lumbar fusion for degenerative disease: a systematic review and meta-analysis. *Neurosurgery*. 2017;80(5):701-715.
16. Rajaee SS, Bae HW, Kanim LE, Delamarter RB. Spinal fusion in the United States: analysis of trends from 1998 to 2008. *Spine*. 2012;37(1):67-76.
17. Andersson G, Watkins-Castillo SI. *Spine Procedures*. boneandjointburden.org; 2014.
18. Dobran M, Nasi D, Esposito DP, Gladi M, Scerrati M, Iacoangeli M. The incidence of adjacent segment degeneration after the use of a versatile dynamic hybrid stabilization device in lumbar stenosis: results of a 5-8-year follow-up. *Asian Spine J*. 2018;12(2):263-271.
19. *Medtronic Announces Launch of X-Stop® Peek IPD® System for U.S. Patients Suffering from Symptoms of Lumbar Spinal Stenosis*. Medtronic.com. Newsroom; October 14, 2008.
20. *Total Number of Medicare Beneficiaries*. kff.org. State Health Facts; 2015.
21. Ploumis A, Christodoulou P, Kapoutsis D, Gelalis I, Vraggalas V, Beris A. Surgical treatment of lumbar spinal stenosis with microdecompression and interspinous distraction device insertion. A case series. *J Orthop Surg Res*. 2012;7:35.
22. Kalichman L, Cole R, Kim DH, et al. Spinal stenosis prevalence and association with symptoms: the Framingham Study. *Spine J*. 2009;9(7):545-550.
23. Friedberg RP. *Anterior cruciate ligament injury*. UpToDate.com, August 4, 2017.
24. Sanders TL, Maradit Kremers H, Bryan AJ, et al. Incidence of anterior cruciate ligament tears and reconstruction: A 21-year population-based study. *Am J Sports Med*. 2016;44(6):1502-1507.
25. Runyan C. *Funded Injury Control Research Centers (ICRCs): UNC Injury Prevention Research Center*. CDC.gov; August 2009.
26. Gans I, Retzky JS, Jones LC, Tanaka MJ. Epidemiology of recurrent anterior cruciate ligament injuries in national collegiate athletic association sports: the injury surveillance program, 2004-2014. *Orthop J Sports Med*. 2018;6(6):2325967118777823.
27. Singh N. International epidemiology of anterior cruciate ligament injuries. *Ortho Res Online J*. 2018:1(5):1-3.
28. Kaeding CC, Léger-St-Jean B, Magnussen RA. Epidemiology and diagnosis of anterior cruciate ligament injuries. *Clin Sports Med*. 2017;36(1):1-8.
29. *Scoliosis*. National Scoliosis Foundation; June 2017.
30. Correa A, Watkins-Castillo SI. *Prevalence of Adult Scoliosis*. boneandjointburden.org; 2014.
31. Konieczny MR, Senyurt H, Krauspe R. Epidemiology of adolescent idiopathic scoliosis. *J Child Orthop*. 2013;7(1):3-9.
32. Asher MA, Burton DC. Adolescent idiopathic scoliosis: natural history and long term treatment effects. *Scoliosis*. 2006;1(1):2.
33. Kebaish KM, Neubauer PR, Voros GD, Khoshnevisan MA, Skolasky RL. Scoliosis in adults aged forty years and older: prevalence and relationship to age, race, and gender. *Spine (Phila Pa 1976)*. 2011;36(9):731-736.
34. Dunn J, Henrikson NB, Morrison CC, Blasi PR, Nguyen M, Lin JS. Screening for adolescent idiopathic scoliosis: evidence report and systematic review for the US preventive services. *JAMA*. 2018;319(2);173-187.

CHAPTER 3

Competitive Analysis: Understanding Your Unique Market Position

RONALD L. DOCIE, Sr

ABOUT THE AUTHOR

Ronald L Docie Sr, Founder and President of Docie Development LLC, conceived his first invention at age 20, driving a hearse while serving his apprenticeship to become a National Board Funeral Director and Embalmer. Using the primary market research techniques (taught in this chapter) that he learned from listening to key executive mentors, he had his invention funded, manufactured, and on the international market within 3 years. His "blind spot mirror" for vehicles has sold over 40 million units worldwide. He built a four-decade successful career of helping independent inventors and small companies market and license their inventions. Mr. Docie negotiated over 100 licenses and other business deals internationally, including with General Motors and others.

Docie codeveloped Johnson & Johnson, Ethicon Endo-Surgical Division's original award-winning website for the submission of invention ideas from doctors and others. He authored The Inventor's Bible, How to Market and License Your Brilliant Ideas, Fourth Edition, 2015, Ten Speed Press imprint of Penguin Random House. Mr. Docie produced and copresented over 50 unique live CLE (continuing legal education) classes to thousands of patent attorneys on the subject of intellectual property (IP) commercialization and communication ethics, through Thomson Reuters, WLE Division.

Ronald Docie is a public speaker and trainer, including at the US Patent and Trademark Office annual conference, and US Department of Energy, National Innovation Workshops. He is testified in Congress for inventor rights and is a three-term past President of the Ohio Inventor's Association. He still helps inventors with the marketing, licensing, and negotiation of their inventions. Ron enjoys flying airplanes and helicopters and is building a primitive serenity retreat on his wilderness estate.

Introduction

When you have successfully completed the market research required to do a competitive analysis, you will have learned more about the following:

- the makeup of your market,
- methods of distribution,
- manufacturing sources,
- resources available,
- candidates for licensing or acquisition of your invention,
- potential competitors,
- perceived value of your invention,
- best options for business models,
- intellectual property strategy, and more.

The answers to all these are limited only by the amount of market research information you are able to collect.

Further objectives are to determine who makes up the customer base, how many potential customers are there, where are they, how do you reach them, who else reaches them, and how much will they pay?

During the market research and interviewing process described in this chapter, you will learn affordable and "do-it-yourself" techniques to acquire surprisingly in-depth information, so you and your team will be better informed to make the many decisions that face an inventor or new-product developer.

Market Position[1]

Market position is everything. In any given market, there are seldom more than one to two manufacturing companies whose market position is that of your invention. There is normally an unspoken and undefined line that separates the companies. The market position distinction is not something that you will find in a catalog, directory, or on the internet. However, the information required to identify the market position of companies in your industry is known by insiders.

When you think about the tools that you use in your profession or trade, and specifically for the exact use or application you are thinking about, which manufacturer comes to mind? Maybe one to three at the most may come to mind. These are the companies who have established the premier market positions for that type of product.

Factors distinguishing the market position differences between manufacturers may be the product categories, general price range of products, disposable versus durable, the types of doctors or consumers being targeted, methods of distribution, types of training procedures and expertise required, the geographic regions into which they sell, and so forth. By the time you check the boxes as to which companies match up with your invention in the categories in common, it starts to become a finite group of qualified candidates that will match the specific market position of your invention/technology.

Market Research/Competitive Analysis Protocol[2]

To perform a competitive analysis requires a keen understanding of your market. The method described herein to learn about the market primarily utilizes the process of interviewing individuals and key executives in your industry. It is a form of primary market research.

A unique value of this research technique is that the research results may be used for many scenarios, no matter whether you intend to license your invention, form your own company, or otherwise.

This method may also be utilized regardless of your stage of development. This is because part or all of the activity may be done without revealing any patentable subject matter, trade secrets, know-how, and other proprietary information. How this is achieved is described later.

An effective way to examine the market for your invention is by following potential distribution channels. This process begins by backtracking through the channels of distribution, starting with the end user. The following techniques will help you recognize manufacturers activities in your product category, learn the distribution channels, and get referrals for your next level research.

You will:

- Identify similar, complimentary, and/or competitive technologies/products to your invention.
- Identify the current market: size, volume, distribution channels, and alternative methods for reaching the market.
- Identify and get referrals to key individuals—distributors, sales representatives, consultants, and other experts who can advise you about the market for your invention.
- Identify potential manufacturers. Learn about their market position, size, resources, and reputation.

SECOND LEVEL: INTERVIEWING EXPERTS

The next step in your research is to interview distributors, manufacturer reps, sales people, and other industry experts.

Your objectives will be to:

- Discover industry trends.
- Explore alternative applications for your invention.

- Define the features of your invention most preferred by the industry.
- Uncover barriers to introducing a product/technology in your category.
- Learn more about the manufacturers and their market positions.
- Learn about potential competitors and/or potential licensees.

What Are You Looking for?

It is not enough to just find a company willing to license, manufacture, or market your invention. Lots of failing and incompetent companies hastily look for new products for their salvation. The key is to identify those companies that may do the most effective job of introducing your invention to the marketplace. In the event your objective is to license your invention; you must determine which of these companies will work with outside inventors like you.

As you delve deeper into the distribution channel for your product, the people you interview will know more about the nitty-gritty details of your industry, as well as the people and companies that influence the industry. If your initial interviews provide you with a long list of potential manufacturers for your invention, this next series of interviews will help narrow your search. You will be seeking to obtain more details about the market positions of the different companies, company strengths and weaknesses, their resources, and other important information. All this will influence your decision about which manufacturers to approach first, in what manner, and in choosing the business model that may be most appropriate for you to use to commercialize your invention.

THIRD LEVEL: QUALIFYING MANUFACTURERS

In this level of market research, you will obtain more detailed background information about the potential manufacturers/licensees and further judge which of these may be the best candidate to manufacturer/license/market your invention. Even if you are not sure whether you want to license your invention or start your own company, what you find out at this stage should help you in making a decision. In the event that you ultimately choose to start your own entrepreneurial effort, the information gathered here may be invaluable for the marketing and competitive analysis section of your business plan.

Bear in mind that throughout this process, you need not necessarily reveal the trade secrets about your invention in order to gain valuable market information. Although this level of market research involves contacting manufacturers directly for the first time, you are not necessarily offering your invention for sale to them. You are still doing market research and asking the questions necessary to determine to whom you may ultimately want to share more detailed proprietary information, license or offer your invention, and how you should go about doing it.

Your objectives at this stage are to:

- Obtain catalogs, annual reports, Securities and Exchange Commission (SEC) 10-K's, and other information about perspective manufacturers/licensees.
- Identify manufacturers whose methods of producing products, and their resources, best compliment the requirements of your invention.
- Identify companies whose product line will be best complemented by your product/technology.
- Identify companies that have a market position that best aligns with your mutual objectives.
- If appropriate, determine their procedure for the submission of outside ideas, their criteria for invention submission, disclosure agreements, the manufacturer's review process, and the people in the company involved in it.

What to Share

Short answer; nothing more than necessary and certainly not anything that may be a trade secret, proprietary know-how, patentable subject matter, etc. There are ways to describe the features, benefits, and advantages of your invention that enable you to obtain the competitive analysis information effectively and not even need to necessarily have any confidentiality agreements in place. This phenomenon alone provides exceptional flexibility in being able to gather a substantive amount of information during your market research that otherwise would be stymied both in time, quality, and quantity. This is particularly so if you would otherwise have to go through the process of having legal documents reviewed. Not to mention the inherent risk of breach of corporate information security from disclosing proprietary information, even with a confidential disclosure agreement in place.

In order to facilitate preliminary discussions without a confidential disclosure and with some possible degree of safety, it is necessary to develop a way to describe the features, advantages, and benefits of your invention without saying how it does it. There may be a few instances when this is not possible, and in my experience I found it rare to have a circumstance in which you cannot accomplish this method. You need to only describe your invention's objectives adequately enough to acquire the information that ends up being helpful and gets you to the next step.

Let's say I am investigating the potential market interest in my new product, whose features include provision of more efficiency with 50% less procedure time, new ergonomic shape with less stress on the surgeon, 30% more effectiveness at controlling "blank," may minimize recovery time for the patient by up to 70%, cost estimated at 30% less than existing products, and so forth. How accurately do you think anyone would be able to guess exactly what I built, what it looks like, or how it works? Yet, this would not necessarily stop them from salivating over the notion of gaining those features, benefits, and advantages.

It is important to remember that the purpose of doing a competitive analysis is not necessarily to share with others how your invention works or how great it is. It is strictly an information-gathering process, and you may be well served to share no more than is necessary to get the information that you need to support your market research efforts.

The Value Proposition

Another important factor to ascertain is whether you have a solution looking for a problem? This is all too common in the development of new products, because although they may work better and be better in every respect, they are not necessarily sellable. It is an interesting phenomenon.

The nice thing about this information-gathering process is that you are able to give the interviewee enough information about what the value proposition is for your new product/invention to get a response from them as to whether they believe that there is any kind of desire to have the enhancements that your product/invention provides. This is sometimes referred to as the "WOW" factor. It has been my experience that the initial WOW factor can be a surprisingly reliable indicator of the potential interest and eventual market success of a new product.

The WOW factor is the energetic response you receive after presenting the value proposition. Importantly, it is an expression of energy. If your interviewee knows of a problem that already exists and then you present the notion that there may actually be a solution for it, the degree of WOW may help indicate how important your solution really is to them. This holds true whether the initial WOW response is coming from a surgeon or from the president of a manufacturing company.

If you present the value proposition and the interviewee starts to ask questions about how your invention works, how effective it can be, and other substantive questions, this is a very positive indicator that there is an interest in the solution you are providing. Stay in touch with this WOW factor response throughout your entire interviewing process. It can provide wonderful positive reinforcement and encouragement for you to proceed in your project, the confidence and effect of which may be noticed on some level by potential investors and your team.

Market Research Techniques[3]

I would normally interview at least half a dozen to a dozen key people on each level of distribution. I continue to interview different people until I start to receive nearly the same answers from each new person that I interview. I do not move to the next step until I have heard from a representation of all the various product applications and markets and/or if I believe I received enough substantive and useful nuggets.

One of the key questions on all levels in this interviewing process is "From whom would you normally expect to receive a product like this?" The answer to this question, in the minds of your interviewee, identifies the companies that perceptively assume the market position for your invention. They are the manufacturers who are identified foremost in your product category and perceived as progressive enough to introduce new products to your market. You can begin to understand how the interviewee feels about the performance of a given manufacturer's products, what the end user may be willing to pay or currently pays for something similar, recognize the types of product features that are important to them, and so forth.

This helps you establish the actual value of your invention in the eyes of the consumer and at each level of distribution. The value perceived by the end user may be different from that of the manufacturer who supplies them. This end user value translates into the manufacturer's sales, gross profit margins, market share, and other factors that support their market position. The overall value proposition begins to expand. Recognizing the wholistic value proposition is important because if you find yourself stuck in negotiation, moving the focus to the value already established by the parties at all levels along a distribution channel is a way to ground the negotiations and move it forward in a positive manner.

Using this method of primary market research is fascinating because there is generally a very positive and receptive willingness for interviewees, even executives, to share with you. The reason for this is, as you backtrack through the distribution channel, you are referred to people "up" the distribution chain who are being "fed" by the people with whom you just spoke. In other words, it is the customers of the people with whom you are about to speak that referred you to them. Therefore, when your referral comes from their customer, there is usually already an acceptance or "positive energy" around the notion of speaking with you.

On the third level of market research, you may interview companies/manufacturers that are potential candidates for acquiring your invention in some fashion. There is somewhat of a "carrot" dangling because most companies want to be on the forefront of introducing the next best product in their product category. They are as anxious as you to prequalify whether your product supports their market position. If it does not, they are typically very willing to refer you to companies that are more appropriate.

By the time you end up interviewing your industry's most experienced people, you will likely be the world's foremost expert on marketing into their product category because it is unlikely anyone else in the industry will have just concluded this type of in-depth primary market research on all levels of distribution in real time. You may even discover current industry information that the top executives do not know.

Therefore, when you can talk with them about substantive issues concerning the industry, and your product category that they understand, and they know that you understand, you earn credibility, respect, and set the stage for the formation of a friendlier business relationship. You may gain a valuable human resource and potentially an important influential champion in the company. Seldom have I known of a substantive, successful, and sustainable deal being concluded without a key internal champion in your candidate company.

Integrating Your Strategic Business and Intellectual Property Positions

Enhancing your patent portfolio may make all the difference in the world as to whether you ultimately control and benefit from the creation of your invention. If you worked tirelessly to develop your invention, invested much time and money, and then saw other companies profit from it without you making a penny, you would not be the first inventor to experience this. Sometimes patents help to "protect" the IP, and sometimes they do not.

The amount of money you spend on IP is not always a direct relationship to how effective your IP "protection" really is. In any given product development project, your IP budget could be less than $30,000 or $300,000 plus. How do you know when to hold them and when to fold them, i.e. how much to spend and for what? Will a "bluff" even work in your industry, i.e., is the notion of potentially asserting your IP rights even financially practical?

Secondly, the type of business arrangements you make, and with whom, may make more difference than any "protection" you perceptively have from IP. For example, if you end up licensing the manufacturer who controls 80+% of the market in your product category (and, sometimes this is the case), then your selection of partners/licensees may form your winning hand, i.e., their market position and moxie in the industry alone is your "protection."

Third, which aspect(s) of the "claims" of your patent is most critical to potentially "protect" you from possible plagiarism in the marketplace? All too often, the patent professionals who represent you are not informed, nor have an understanding, of the competitive market in which you operate. You may be using all your resources to patent a "straight," and then when you get deep into the market experience, you learn that it takes a "flush" to get the job done. In other words, when the patent attorney asks you which claims strategy choices may benefit you most in the market, what are you going to tell them? This is when market research results are particularly valuable. In fact, it may make a difference as to whether you take home the "pot."

This underscores the value of connecting with and learning from key executives and sages in your product category/market position. They already have a keen understanding of what works, what does not work, and other important market factors learned from their business experience. Essentially, this interviewing process allows you to "leverage" the existing expertise of industry professionals.

The information learned helps you make informed decisions in multiple disciplines, including product development, marketing, business, financing, and IP! These disciplines are integral, and they are all ultimately reliant on the influence of the market. The end-user market is the "hand that feeds" all others up the distribution chain.

Your market is further influenced by the competitors/potential partners in your market position. Understanding your product category and common market position is their lifeblood. Would not it be a good idea to get to know them? Even if they do not show their hand, others will tell you what they are holding.

KEY TAKEAWAY POINTS

- ▶ There are many diverse disciplines involved in commercializing intellectual property.

- ▶ Learning about the potential market position of your invention is critical to commercialization success. (For more information about market positioning reference: Ries A, Trout J. *Positioning: The Battle for Your Mind.* McGraw-Hill Education; 2001.)

- ▶ Understanding what information to collect, from whom, and selecting the more effective ways of acquiring it will support you in making informed decisions. (To access printable forms and reference some of the many tools you can use for interviewing key executives, reference the Workbook in the Appendix of: Docie R. *The Inventor's Bible: How to Market and License Your Brilliant Ideas.* Penguin Random House; 2015.)

- ▶ You can perform market research and prepare a competitive analysis at any stage of product development, even before patenting, and potentially without the need for disclosure agreements.

- ▶ You cannot do market research/competitive analysis too early, but you can do it too late.

- ▶ The information you need to make informed decisions regarding commercialization is limited only by the amount of market research information you acquire.

- ▶ Direct contact with people, either in-person or at least verbally, helps facilitate both success with research and may lead to the building of relationships that results in concluding successful business arrangements.

Disclaimer: The author of this chapter is not an attorney and no part of this chapter is meant to give, offer or infer legal or patenting advice or opinion.

REFERENCES AND RESOURCES

1. Ries A, Trout J. *Positioning: The Battle for Your Mind.* McGraw-Hill Education; 2001. For more information about Market Positioning.
2. Docie R. *The Inventor's Bible: How to Market and License Your Brilliant Ideas.* 4th ed.: Penguin/Random House; 2015.
3. *For a Complete List of the Types of Questions Which May be Appropriate for Use with This Method of Market Research, and Detailed How-to Methods, Please See the Workbook in the Appendix of the Inventor's Bible: How to Market and License Your Brilliant Ideas.* 4th ed., by Ronald Louis D Sr. TenSpeed Press imprint of Penguin/Random House; 2015.

CHAPTER 4

Forming a Solution: Defining Product Requirements Before Concept Development

JEFFREY A. KARG

ABOUT THE AUTHOR

Jeffrey A. Karg, Managing Director, Boston Innovation.

Jeff is a 30-year veteran of medical device development. He has over 23 patents ranging from drug delivery and discovery to clinical devices in technology areas including mechanics, fluidics, and electromechanics. He is a Master of Science in Mechanical Engineering, graduate of Stanford University. His company, Boston Innovation, proactively assists doctor/surgeon inventors and develops their ideas into products. By combining passion and planning, Jeff and his team plan, resource, and lead product development programs within budgetary and timeline limitations. He and his team ensure start-up funding is not jeopardized by incomplete product development progress. As CEO, his start-up, nAscent Biosciences, a maker of disposable drug discovery tools, was acquired by Thermo Fisher Scientific in 2008. Jeff's interests lie in the ongoing development of his living and work space in Bolton, MA, cooking for life and wife, and his two dogs, Flora and Maisy.

Introduction

In a preceding chapter, *Identifying the Unmet Need*, Dr. Bokshan and Dr. Cole prepare the surgeon to "embrace innovation" by employing skills natural to their thought process and daily activities. Concepts such as unbiased and mindful observation, gap identification, pattern recognition, research fundamentals, and the ability to collect real-time feedback are just some of the qualities of the entrepreneurial surgeon. Using these skills, the clinician/inventor must formalize documentation beyond notes, napkin sketches, and general descriptions. It becomes paramount to develop a contextual and organized set of requirements. These thoughts are usually organized into a "product requirements document" (PRD) and serve as the foundation for product development from a user, functional, safety, and regulatory perspective.

Product requirement documents have a wide range of formats. Per Wikipedia, "the product requirements document (PRD) is a document containing all the requirements to a certain product. It is written to allow people to understand what a product should do." Some PRDs carry this definition to the extreme and include business and marketing requirements; however, from the perspective of managing a product development process, we will develop a PRD from only the four descriptors: user, functional, safety, and regulatory. This allows the development team to focus on the product and leave the other topics to groups more geared to handling them.

What Are the Key Components of the Product Requirements Document?

By now, you have thought extensively about your idea, probably talked with a great number of close associates, and made notes, diagrams, and other documenting activities. You may have engaged an attorney to do patent work, and you may have built and partially tested prototypes to support your thinking. However, formal product description and development start with a PRD.

A well-formed PRD will:

- provide a thorough and contextual understanding of the problem,
- decrease development time and cost of the design process,
- provide referenceable documentation among project team members, keeping everyone on the same page,
- provide the requirements traceability foundation, easing regulatory compliance, and
- in the end, provide a quality product that meets the stakeholder's needs and is user-friendly, functional, and safe.

Although there are many PRD formats and templates to choose from, the basic parts of a product centric PRD are:

INTRODUCTION

A contextual description of the device or system (product) including what it will do and what are the major components. There will be plenty of opportunity to provide more detail in additional sections below, so conciseness and brevity are valued here. Often less than 150 words.

EXECUTIVE SUMMARY

This section adds more detail to the system description, use scenarios, general technology implementation, and where used. In both the "Introduction" and "Executive Summary," there is great latitude in what is included. In contrast, the next four sections are very precise and become part of the "traceability" activities throughout product development. Often less than 250 words.

STAKEHOLDER IDENTIFICATION

A precise and complete list of all the stakeholders who will be affected by the new product. This is the list of folks you will need to talk with to get a full list of requirements. Often less than 250 words.

INTENDED USE STATEMENT

Intended use is what you say this device is to be used for. It is important not to describe indications, which describe under what conditions the product should be used. Often less than 200 words.

REGULATORY REQUIREMENTS

Describes the regulatory path the product will take such as 510K or premarket approval (PMA). It often defines the markets the product will be offered in, such as the United States, Europe, or China as regulatory requirements may be different. Often less than 200 words.

SPECIFIC DEVICE REQUIREMENTS

This is where all the hard work goes. The specific product requirements are a list of things the product shall do and cover every aspect of the product. Often a product could have well over 100 requirements, particularly if there is software involved.

STAKEHOLDER IDENTIFICATION AND TEAM SELECTION

It is important to assemble a great team for the PRD writing process. Mistakes will cause confusion and delays. Obviously yourself as a primary reference for functionality, but others from within the industry or product segment you are addressing are highly recommended. It will help to define the stakeholder groups to assist in selecting team members.

The stakeholders identified in Table 4.1 are an example derived from a complex surgical product. It should be noted that not all products will utilize the same set of stakeholders described in this table. Each product will generate its own set of stakeholders, but this is not a bad start for an orthopedic surgical product.

From here, you can select team members to represent the various stakeholders. Not all stakeholders become development team members and may be represented by select individuals on an advisory board.

Table 4.1 Possible Stakeholder's Table and Team Member Description

Stakeholder Group	Description	Type of Person for Team
Patient	Subjects on which product will be used	Various possible patients. Can be clinicians familiar with the procedure and the patients outcomes
Surgeon	Primary user of the product. Responsible for the use of this device throughout the procedure	Likely yourself, but must add others within same profession, sometimes key opinion leaders can add insight and gravity to the work
Surgeon assistant	Secondary user of the product. Will require a surgeon to review and approve all plans prior to procedure start	Team members you currently work with, however, good also to choose someone who will not carry any bias
Engineering staff	Installs product at hospitals and other appropriate sites. Verifies compliance with safety requirements and other equipment	Current hospital engineering staff leaders. Great if you can attract the innovative staff who is always looking to do things better
Sales staff	Performs product demos at hospitals/clinics	Today's industry sales staff is often very knowledgeable and can lend very insightful direction
Service technician	Company or third-party staff maintains the product	Use individuals who work on similar product classification
Insurance providers	Determine the extent to which the device procedures are reimbursed	This role may be filled by a consultant as opposed to a permanent team role
Hospital/clinic administration	Purchasers of the product	Senior leadership to identify pathways and obstacles to your product being used within the hospital

Writing the Introduction

There are always a few statements in the introduction that are part of a pattern.

One should always prepare a document purpose statement, which also describes what the requirements are meant to provide. An example is "The purpose of this document is to describe the design requirements for the product. The design requirements, derived from stakeholder needs, will be used as inputs for the product specification document. Each requirement is written as a testable entity to be conducted during design validation."

There could be a few lines about the market you will go after as that drives regulatory activities and also a couple of sentences or so on about what the product is designed to do. If there are major components to the system, you could list them here, such as system console, sensor systems, and/or disposable components.

Think about telling a story with all these sections in the PRD. By the time one has read the document, they have a good understanding of what you are trying to do. They would not know all the product details or how to build the product yet, but they will understand it well.

You may have noticed that the design requirements lead to the product specification document. Product specifications are derived from design requirements and are needed by the product development resources such as engineers and designers so that they know specifically what to develop. This is often a confusing difference. Product requirements state generally what is needed; specifications state specifically how the performance must be. For example, the requirement, "The product must provide for easy visual monitoring of the procedure" may have a number of associated specifications. The corresponding specifications may be "The monitor must be a 23-inch OLED color display" and "The font on the display screen must be readable when monitor is 72 inch away from the surgeon" Typically, requirements are general descriptions, and specifications have defined numbers to drive engineering and design details.

Writing the Executive Summary

Here is where you get to describe the product a bit more and talk about benefits to the patient. As you may guess, there are many approaches to this. However, some topics you might address are:
- Where your product is to be used
- How your product integrates with current surgical suite or other clinical environments including existing equipment

- What procedures are your product aimed at
- How your product integrates with current medical record systems
- How your product makes the procedure safer, less costly, easier, or more intuitive
- What are some of the special technologies that enable safer, less-costly procedures, and are more user intuitive
- What are the specific benefits of your product

This is the part of the PRD that starts to bring the technology closer to the readers understanding.

Writing the Stakeholder's Section

The stakeholder's section can be something on the order in the Table 4.2. You do not need a lot of verbosity here. However, you can add a column as shown here for comments to help clarify your thoughts in the first two columns. Where the table states product, you may insert your product actual name and/or component of the product that the stakeholder engages with.

Writing the Intended Use Statement

Preparing to write the intended use statement requires you have a clear understanding of what you want to do. You will benefit from all your thinking, note-taking, and discussions along the way, and it is highly recommended that appropriate team members are engaged when devising the precise wording.

It sets the tone for regulatory activities, reimbursement classification, and outlines the specific use of the product. If the intended use statement is inadequate, the FDA, Conformité Européenne (CE), or other regulatory body reviewer cannot determine if the device has been evaluated properly for safety and efficacy. This highlights the importance of a thorough and concise description of the device. Without it, a substantive review of the submission cannot be performed, and the approval process may be slowed. In addition, to eliminate confusion, it is critical that any additional descriptions of the device be consistent within any given submission.

As an example, "The Acme 2000 trocar is intended for use by health care professionals as a port during laparoscopic surgery. The device enables access to the thoracic body cavity for various surgical procedures as deemed necessary by the clinical use requirements including organ dissection and removal." Although this statement appears to be clear, the phrase "clinical use requirements" may need clarification by incorporating the types or categories of procedures to be considered.

Table 4.2 Example Stakeholders Table

Stakeholder Group	Description	Comments
Patient	Subjects on which product will be used	Stakeholders comprised clinicians, patients who have already had a similar procedure, and patients who are preparing for the procedure
Surgeon	Primary user of the product. Responsible for the use of this device throughout the procedure	Surgeons from various geographical locations and hospital sizes
Surgeon assistant	Secondary user of the product. Will require a surgeon to review and approve all plans prior to procedure start	Surgeon assistants from various geographical locations and hospital sizes
Engineering staff	Installs product at hospitals and other appropriate sites. Verifies compliance with safety requirements and other equipment	Large and small hospital staff
Sales staff	Performs product demos at hospitals/clinics	Independent sales staff from suppliers of this type of a product
Service technician	Company or third-party staff maintains the product	
Insurance providers	Determine the extent to which the device procedures are reimbursed	Independent consultants were used for this topic
Hospital/clinic administration	Purchasers of the product	Senior leadership from various geographical locations and hospital sizes

Writing the Regulatory Section

This section can be relatively short and should include a description of the regulatory path—510K, PMA, de novo, etc. A brief restatement of the indications for use and what the product enables helps to set additional detail and context.

Writing Specific Product Requirements

The previous sections have described the product in ways that allow the reader to understand its use contextually, specifically, in a regulatory framework and whom the product will be used on, etc. Now that the stage has been set; it is time to write specific product requirements, but first some basics on the requirement format to allow professional and substantive requirement documentation.

Product Requirement Concepts

Requirements have been documented for products since the beginning of time. Alexander Graham Bell may have said, "I want this device to allow me to talk with someone without being able to see or hear them." That statement may capture the heart of his goal. Of course, there were many other requirements as well. He may have made statements such as:

- The product must allow people to talk to each other from greater than 10 miles away (functional)
- The product must be safe and not electrocute the user (safety and regulatory)
- The product must be able to be held close to the user's mouth and ear(s) (user)
- The product must be able to be installed in residential housing (functional)
- Other statements supporting the needs of stakeholders (F, S, R, U)

Notice that the structure of a requirement statement is clear and concise. The table below is one way to list requirements. Although requirements are very specific to any product under development, the wording in Table 4.3 is rather generic. For a sense of scale, if this product described a new surgical instrument including hardware, software, user interface, mechanical components, and disposables, the number of requirements could range from 75 to 150.

The requirements in Table 4.3 are very random requirements that relate to disparate parts of the system and are provided for reference only. It is paramount that you have team members who are expert in assembling this document.

Table 4.3 Example Requirements Format

DR ID	Design Requirement	Source
DR-001	The system shall enable preoperative planning of the surgical procedure.	Functional
DR-002	The system shall enable positioning of the laparoscopic tool during intraoperative procedures.	Functional
DR-003	The system shall provide for easy visual monitoring of procedure.	User
DR-004	The system shall enable laparoscopic procedures.	Functional
DR-005	The system shall comply with all applicable standards required for offering the device for sale in the specified country.	Regulatory
DR-006	System shall allow the system to be configured so that the patient's anatomy and the laparoscopic portion of the device are colocated.	Functional
DR-007	System shall be initially set up by trained personnel.	Safety
DR-009	Power cable shall be of sufficient length to access hospital power outlet.	Functional
DR-XXX	Additional requirements as the team deems necessary…	F, S, R, U

Preparing for Requirement Writing Meetings

By now, you have selected team members based on the stakeholder table guidance. You have shared the product mission with everyone and likely disseminated information such as preliminary intended use statements, product notes and descriptions, and other product concept work and its development progress. Information sharing may come in the form of prototype demonstrations, videos, and perhaps early informal stakeholder interviews. You likely have preliminary feedback from other surgeons and have kept all team members in the loop so that each can contribute contextually to the requirement writing process.

Requirement Writing Meeting Agenda

The importance of preparing an agenda, Table 4.4, prior to requirement writing meetings is to get all team members on the same page and to let them be prepared enough so that substantive progress is made. It is unfortunately very easy to hold requirement writing meetings where little progress is made, so team guidance is paramount. In an example case, a lot of prework was completed prior to a 2-day meeting that brought experts together from various parts of the country, so efficiency was necessary.

Team Member Activities during Meeting

Now you may think the requirements were all actually written during this meeting, but that is not generally the case, though any number of specific requirements might be publishable. During the meeting, interviews are recorded, copious notes are taken, and general requirement categories are defined. Requirements are generally formalized in a document following the meeting. But now you have the information to actually write them! It is common that a complex product might require multiple rewrites and 6 to 8 weeks to complete. So this exercise is not for the faint of heart.

KEY TAKEAWAY POINTS

If you drive through to a professionally written and scoped product requirements document, you are well on your way to facilitating a well-managed product development process. Keep in mind:

Document your product thoughts along the way.

- ▶ Talk with peers, possible patients, industry experts, and anyone who can provide insight into your product and its uses.

- ▶ Do not take shortcuts as it will cost time and money above your expectations.

- ▶ Engage a professional requirements writing team to ensure the process is followed.

- ▶ And above all, be prepared for your product to be scrutinized in every detail. Have no biases as you must work to get your entire team motivated by the same mission and ultimately, get your product through the FDA approval process.

Table 4.4 Sample 2-Day Agenda for Requirement Writing Conference		
Day 1	**Date**	**Presenter or Stakeholder**
8:00-8:30	Meet, greet, and introductions	
8:30-12:00	Information gathering • Team roles explained and recorded, project charter • History and status of project to date • Inventor's background • Product demonstration or video review • Product description • Patent map • FDA regulatory map • Reimbursement strategy	Appropriate team member participation
12:00-1:00	Lunch and continued conversation	
1:00-2:00	• Open discussion of issues, thoughts, and concerns the product team has experienced • Discussion on expected level of FDA scrutiny • Discuss known risks and areas for risk investigation	All
2:00-2:30	PRD format presentation and discussion • Stakeholder table discussion • Complete the stakeholders list • Requirements category discussion	Team leader
2:30-3:30	Patient requirements discussion	Stakeholders
3:30-5:00	Begin stakeholder interviews	Stakeholder—Topic one
5:00-7:00	Dinner! Time loved by all...	
Day 2	**Date**	**Presenter or Stakeholder**
8:30-5:30	Stakeholder interviews—may be in person or by phone, but the days of interviews should reflect specific scheduled time	Team interviews stakeholders for details around requirements

BIBLIOGRAPHY

1. www.fda.gov.
2. ISO 13485, Medical Devices – Quality Management Systems – Requirements for Regulatory Purposes.
3. ISO 62366–1:2015, Medical Devices – Part 1: Application of Usability Engineering to Medical Devices.

CHAPTER 5

Vetting the Concept

JOSEPH E. HALE

"Innovation comes from long-term thinking and iterative execution"

REID HOFFMAN, AMERICAN ENTREPRENEUR, VENTURE CAPITALIST AND AUTHOR

ABOUT THE AUTHOR

Joseph Hale is an innovator, educator, and leader in the medical device space. He received his doctoral degree in Biomedical Engineering with an emphasis in Orthopedic Biomechanics from The University of Iowa and has held positions in both academia and industry. Joseph is an alumnus and former director of the Innovation Fellows program at the University of Minnesota (UMN), Earl E. Bakken Medical Devices Center and currently serves on the graduate faculty for the UMN Technological Leadership Institute's master's degree program in Medical Device Innovation.

Innovation is a nonlinear and iterative process that is fraught with risk. At any point during that process, new information or insights may be discovered that lead to new questions, changes in strategy, or perhaps even a decision to abandon the project. The vetting process is an ongoing effort to identify and minimize the risks and reasons not to move forward.

Vetting is the careful and critical examination, investigation, or evaluation of *something* (Figure 5.1). In the present context, that *something* is the concept. And what exactly is the concept? In general terms, the concept comprises a set of ideas that capture the vision and passion of the founder. A concept is more than just the idea for a device or product that addresses the unmet need; it is also the outline of the business plan and strategy for how that idea can be commercialized. Founders need to recognize that the initial concept is a work in progress and may not bear much resemblance to the final commercialized product. That transformation of the initial concept is driven by vetting.

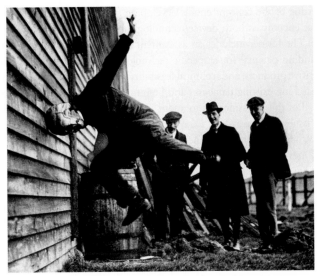

Figure 5.1 Vetting the concept, circa 1912. (Copyright © Flight Global, 1912. Reprinted with permission from Rare Historical Photos, https://rarehistoricalphotos.com.)

The risks/rewards associated with innovation are often characterized in terms of the following:

REAL: Is the opportunity real? Is there an unmet need?

WIN: Can we win? Does the technology exist? Does the concept address the need?

WORTH: Is the cost to commercialize the concept worth it? How large is the market? Will customers use/buy our solution?[1]

During the initial phase of the innovation process, vetting is used to minimize risks associated with the first group of questions and establish that an unmet need worth addressing actually exists (i.e., vetting the need). Similarly, a thorough vetting is subsequently performed to minimize the risks associated with the questions of "win" and "worth" and demonstrate that the proposed solution satisfactorily addresses the need and is likely to be adopted (i.e., vetting the concept). Vetting of the concept specifically aims to minimize risks related to technical feasibility, customer/market adoption, intellectual property (IP), and competitive products.

Vetting of the concept entails developing and testing a series of hypotheses that encompass both device/technological and customer-/market-related aspects. The former includes an assessment of the prior art (including issued and pending patents) for a specific technology known as the IP landscape, competitive products, and technical feasibility that can typically be investigated by researching existing databases and literature and/or by conducting testing. The goal of this assessment is to attain an in-depth understanding of device-related issues such as:

- What is the product concept?
- Does the technology exist?
- Can it be built?
- Does a viable solution already exist?

Examination of the latter (i.e., customer- and market-related aspects) specifically addresses questions regarding marketing and distribution and relies almost exclusively on customer interviews.

- How and to what degree are you impacted by the problem?
- How much would you pay to solve the problem?
- What product features are essential to solving the problem?
- How would you prefer to access the product?

Intellectual Property

To be commercializable, a concept must have value that can be protected as IP, usually in the form of an issued patent. A patent is a right granted by the US Patent and Trademark Office (or similar agency in other countries) that excludes others from manufacturing, selling, or importing an invention without the permission of the patent holder. To obtain patent protection, an invention must meet three criteria—it must be novel, nonobvious, and useful. The novelty of a concept should be assessed as part of the vetting process by performing a preliminary search to identify patents or other prior art that discloses the same or similar knowledge, the existence of which could represent a barrier to commercialization. Enlisting the services of a qualified attorney to make the final determination of patentability and freedom to operate is recommended. Additional information on IP protection and prior art searches is discussed in Chapters 6 and 9.

Competitive Products

The existence of other commercially available solutions to the problem (i.e., competitive products) should also be considered in the vetting process. Standard online search methods (e.g., Google) are generally sufficient to identify competitive products and their advantages and disadvantages. The concept being vetted will need to provide meaningful benefits over the competition in terms of ease of use, cost, outcomes, and/or other in order to capture a significant share of the market and present a viable opportunity. Competition analysis is addressed in detail in Chapter 3.

PROTOTYPING

Vetting of the concept is generally facilitated by the development of a physical prototype. Prototypes are useful in assessing both technical feasibility and customer/market requirements. Even low resolution (think Lego, modeling clay, cardboard and tape, etc.), three-dimensional prototypes are generally more effective than verbal descriptions or two-dimensional drawings in conveying a concept and eliciting customer feedback. As the concept evolves, a more refined, higher-resolution prototype can be developed with the goal of defining a minimal viable product. A minimum viable product (MVP) is one that embodies the concept with just enough features to satisfy early adopters. Additional features are designed and developed in response to feedback from the initial users. The ability to create prototypes at all resolutions has been greatly simplified by the ubiquity of 3-D printing (i.e., additive manufacturing) and other rapid prototyping techniques.

Technical Feasibility

Initial testing is focused on establishing feasibility of the concept and often involves preproduction versions of the device (i.e., prototypes). Results of these tests provide the basis for further concept development and prototype refinement.

The determination of which tests to perform is based on a number of factors, including regulatory requirements, reimbursement, and market adoption.
- Preclinical testing
  - Bench testing/Computational modeling
  - Animal testing
- Clinical testing

Bench testing, involving tissue analogs or in vitro animal/cadaveric specimens, is generally an easier and less-expensive means to demonstrate proof of concept and potentially minimizes the number of iterations required during subsequent animal and/or human testing.

Computational modeling and simulation plays an increasingly important role in understanding biological systems, engineered mechanisms, and the interactions between them.[2] In many instances, it is possible to create computer models to simulate the intended function of a mechanism, rapidly evaluate multiple parameters, and refine the concept based on the results before ever creating a physical prototype. Initiatives such as the Medical Device Innovation Consortium, a public-private partnership

Table 5.1 Examples of Consensus Standards for Orthopedic Testing

ASTM Standards

ASTM F384—Standard Specifications and Test Methods for Metallic Angled Orthopedic Fracture Fixation Devices

ASTM F732—Standard Test Method for Wear Testing of Polymeric Materials Used in Total Joint Prostheses

ASTM F2502—Standard Specification and Test Methods for Absorbable Plates and Screws for Internal Fixation Implants

ASTM F2267—Evaluating Spinal Intervertebral Body Fusion Devices Under Axial Compression

ISO Standards

ISO 8319-2—Orthopedic instruments—Drive connections— Part 2: Screwdrivers for single slot head screws, screws with cruciate slot and cross-recessed head screws

ISO 14242-1—Implants for surgery—Wear of total hip-joint prostheses—Part 1: Loading and displacement parameters for wear-testing machines and corresponding environmental conditions for test

ISO 9714-1—Orthopedic drilling instruments—Part 1: Drill bits, taps and countersink cutters

ISO 9585—Implants for surgery—Determination of bending strength and stiffness of bone plates

ISO 10993-1—Biological evaluation of medical devices—Part 1: Evaluation and testing within a risk management process

between FDA, NIH, CMS, industry, and patient organizations, are working to develop new computational tools that will provide more realistic simulations and reduce, or possibly even replace, the need for clinical trials.[3]

Predicate devices (i.e., devices that have been cleared/approved by the FDA for the same intended use) can help to establish the appropriate regulatory classification/pathway and provide a template of the testing that was necessary to satisfy regulatory requirements. Whenever possible, existing regulations, guidelines, and standards (e.g., ASTM, ISO, FDA guidance documents) should be used as applicable or as the basis for modifications specific to the concept/device being tested.[4-8] (Table 5.1) If a suitable predicate device (with an accepted test protocol) and/or existing standards cannot be identified, it may be necessary to develop and provide justification for new test protocols.

Decisions regarding the adoption of new technologies into clinical practice are increasingly evidence-based. Results from aforementioned testing can provide quantitative answers to questions that may arise regarding mechanical integrity, biocompatibility, clinical outcomes, comparative efficacy, etc. Ultimately, clinical trials may be needed to establish clinical efficacy and/or comparative clinical outcomes. A more in-depth discussion of concept prototyping, testing, and selection is presented in Chapters 7 and 8.

Customer Discovery

Vetting of the concept with regard to customer and market aspects primarily involves talking with and listening to as many potential customers and stakeholders as possible to learn in detail about their problems, needs, and wants with respect to your concept. Resist the temptation to think that you understand a priori what your customer actually needs or wants.

"You've got to start with the customer experience and work back toward the technology – not the other way around."

STEVE JOBS, AMERICAN ENTREPRENEUR, INVENTOR, AND COFOUNDER OF APPLE, INC.

WHO IS YOUR CUSTOMER?

It is important to understand who your customer is and how the concept/device will be used. Who the customer is may seem obvious, but depending on the particular concept/device, there is likely to be multiple customers or stakeholders with differing perspectives and responsibilities that will influence market adoption.

- Who will deliver care using the device?
- Who will make the decision to purchase?
- Who will pay for the device?
- Who is the end user?

Once you know who your customer is, talk to as many of them as possible. Vetting should include feedback from all of the customers and stakeholders including health care providers (e.g., physicians, nurses, and therapists), patients, hospital value analysis committees, purchasing organizations, insurance providers, etc. In some instances, it may be useful to further segment customers by factors such as point of care, therapeutic specialty, patient demographics, etc. Identifying and targeting a specific customer segment(s) may help define features that would be more or less desirable.

HOW WILL THE CONCEPT BE USED?

Gathering information and insights into how the customer will interact with the concept/device is an important part of the customer discovery process. Ethnography or ethnographic research is the study of people in their own environment through direct observation and face-to-face interviewing and provides a systematic approach to gathering such information.[9]

The process of customer discovery should be hypotheses-driven. In formulating hypotheses, try to avoid those that confirm what you already know or at least think is true, known as confirmational bias. Hypotheses that are easily proved tend to be less insightful. On the other hand, wrong assumptions (i.e., disproved hypotheses) can lead to changes in strategy or pivots with regard to the problem(s) being solved, features needed to solve them, and/or the target customer. Hypotheses that are disproved can then be revised based on the insights gained from customer feedback and retested.

Customer discovery occurs in two phases.[10] The initial phase focuses on the customer's perception of the problem and the need to solve it. To avoid leading the customer down a particular path, Phase 1 does not include discussion of possible solutions or presentation of prototypes. The goal is to determine if the problem or need is significant enough that customers want a solution and are willing to pay for it.

Customer Discovery Phase 1

- Does the need significantly impact the customer and how?
- Who is the customer/customer archetype?
- How badly do they want/need a solution?
- How much are they willing to pay for it?

In the second phase, the target customers (based on Phase 1 findings) are shown the concept/product (usually MVP at this point) and their enthusiasm is assessed.

Customer Discovery Phase 2

- How well does the concept satisfy the customer's needs?
- Is this something they want and would buy?
- Through what medium would they prefer to access the solution?

In both phases, customer discovery is best accomplished through face-to-face interviews and observations. Although time-consuming, individual interviews provide a better opportunity to collect in-depth information and insights. Focus groups, on the other hand, tend to encourage group-thinking, discourage participation by more introverted, less vocal members of the group, and generally provide less useful information.

Although observations of concept/device use in the clinical setting are essential, simulated procedures with clinicians using a surrogate material (e.g., Sawbones), cadaveric tissue, or other models can also be used to provide feedback on design, function, usability, procedure, etc. In conducting these studies, consideration should be given to the setting in which the provider practices (i.e., urban vs. rural, community vs. academic, primary vs. referral), level of training/years of experience, and other factors that may provide additional context to the observations.

Involving recognized experts, also known as key opinion leaders, throughout the vetting process can provide valuable feedback as well as encourage buy-in and support for the concept that can influence later adopters.

A note of caution—although discussions of your concept are an essential part of the vetting process, it is imperative that any IP related to the concept is protected legally. A nondisclosure or mutual disclosure confidentiality agreement should be signed before engaging in detailed conversations about the concept with anyone. If a public presentation of the concept is anticipated (e.g., journal publication, conference poster, or podium presentation), IP should first be protected by the filing of a provisional patent. At a minimum, until IP protection is in place, care should be taken in any interactions not to disclose the "secret sauce" or enabling information associated with the concept. Because the priority for a patent is determined by "first to file" and not "first to invent," failing to protect IP adequately leaves you vulnerable to someone else staking a claim to your concept. In addition, public disclosure of the concept before filing a patent application marks the start of a grace period (6 months in Japan, Russia, and others; 12 months in the United States, Canada, and others) during which an application must be filed before being considered "prior art." In countries that do not have a grace period, disclosure may jeopardize your ability to file for a patent altogether.

Being passionate about your ideas is great—passion inspires the persistence necessary to overcome many challenges along the road to commercialization—but it is also important not to be so in love with your idea that you disregard potential red flags. Although sometimes difficult to accept, negative feedback regarding your concept should be invited and seen as an opportunity to critically (re)evaluate the concept and alter the strategy as needed. If you are not receiving any negative feedback, it may be that you are not talking to the right customers and/or not asking the right questions. The consequences of avoiding or ignoring negative feedback are even more difficult to accept and may include lost time and money and ultimately, a failed attempt to commercialize your concept.

As noted at the outset, vetting the concept is an ongoing effort aimed at identifying risks and reasons not to move forward with commercialization. Insights obtained through the vetting process serve to minimize those risks and provide the basis for concept enhancements. Those enhancements, in turn, also require vetting. Like the innovation process itself, vetting should be viewed as an iterative undertaking that needs to be performed not just once but rather at intervals in response to concept refinement and may arguably never be complete.

KEY TAKEAWAY POINTS

- ▶ Innovation is a nonlinear, iterative process.
- ▶ Vetting is an ongoing effort to identify and minimize the risks and reasons not to move forward.

- ▶ A concept is more than just the idea for a device or product that addresses the unmet need; it is also the outline of the business plan/strategy for how that idea can be commercialized.

- ▶ The process of customer discovery is essential to understanding the problem and the relevance of the concept to the customers' need/desire for a solution.

- ▶ Insights obtained from disproved hypotheses and negative customer feedback inform concept enhancements.

REFERENCES AND RESOURCES

1. Day GS. "Is it real? Can we win? Is it worth doing? Managing risk and reward in an innovation portfolio." *Harv Bus Rev.* 2007;85(12):110-120, 146. https://hbr.org/2007/12/is-it-real-can-we-win-is-it-worth-doing-managing-risk-and-reward-in-an-innovation-portfolio.
2. Brodland WG. "How computational models can help unlock biological systems." *Semin Cell Dev Biol.* 2015;47–48:62-73. http://www.sciencedirect.com/science/article/pii/S1084952115001287.
3. Medical Device Innovation Consortium (MDIC). Computational Modeling and Simulation. http://mdic.org/computer-modeling/.
4. American Society for Testing and Materials (ASTM International). Standards & Publications. https://www.astm.org/Standard/standards-and-publications.html.
5. International Organization for Standardization (ISO). Standards. https://www.iso.org/standards.html.
6. U.S. Food & Drug Administration (FDA). Search for FDA Guidance Documents. https://www.fda.gov/RegulatoryInformation/Guidances/default.htm.
7. U.S. Food & Drug Administration (FDA). Guidance for Industry and FDA Staff – Recognition and Use of Consensus Standards. https://www.fda.gov/MedicalDevices/DeviceRegulationandGuidance/GuidanceDocuments/ucm077274.htm.
8. U.S. Food & Drug Administration (FDA). Recognized Consensus Standards. https://www.accessdata.fda.gov/scripts/cdrh/cfdocs/cfStandards/search.cfm.
9. National Park Service. Park Ethnography Program. https://www.nps.gov/ethnography/aah/aaheritage/ERCb.htm.
10. Blank S, Dorf B. *The Startup Owner's Manual: The Step-by-Step Guide for Building a Great Company.* 1st ed.: K&S Ranch, Inc; 2012:21-26, 51-273.

CHAPTER 6

Prior Art Search: Can Your Solution Be Patented?

DAVID J. DYKEMAN, ROBERT A. RABINER

ABOUT THE AUTHORS

David J. Dykeman is a registered patent attorney with over 20 years of experience in patent and intellectual property law and cochair of Greenberg Traurig's global Life Sciences & Medical Technology Group and intellectual property group in Boston. David's practice focuses on securing worldwide intellectual property protection and related business strategy for high-tech clients, with particular experience in orthopedics, medical devices, life sciences, and information technology. David has been named one of the top 250 patent and technology licensing practitioners in the world by *Intellectual Asset Management* magazine and is the founding chair of the ABA's Medical Devices Committee. David can be reached at dykemand@gtlaw.com or (617) 310-6009.

Robert A. Rabiner is a medical device entrepreneur and the Founder & Chief Technical Officer of IlluminOss Medical, Inc. located in East Providence, RI. Bob has led successful product and corporate enterprise launches, acquired and integrated new technologies, and directed external partnerships at a number of medical device companies. Prior to founding IlluminOss, he was the president of Selva Medical (sold to W.L. Gore in 2006), and was the founder, president, and CEO of OmniSonics Medical Technologies. He has also held executive-level positions at American Cyanamid, United States Healthcare, and Hospital Products Ltd, Australia. Bob has been a member of the World Economic Forum's Technology Pioneers Program since 2003 and is one of Fast Company's "Fast 50 Champions of Innovation" for his medical technologies. He is the named inventor on over 60 US-issued patents and over 125 issued patents worldwide, and has many additional patent applications pending.

Introduction

A strategic patent portfolio is crucial to an orthopedic company's growth and survival because it can provide numerous business advantages. Although patents are extremely important for orthopedic companies of all sizes, patents make up a significantly greater portion of enterprise value for early-stage orthopedic companies. Patent portfolios are often the only way for investors to place a value on an early-stage company's technology, as sales often cannot begin until after receiving regulatory approval.

Why Patents Are Important

Broad patent protection can be used both offensively to block competitors from the marketplace and defensively to serve as a bargaining chip against potential patent infringement suits. Patents should be filed to cover all aspects of the core technology, including the entire device, key components, methods of use or methods of manufacture, incremental improvements, and other aspects of the invention. As the technology evolves, incremental improvements should be patented to form a "picket fence" of patent protection around the core technology to prevent competitors from copying it.

The picket fence patent strategy, by the same token, may be valuable to some emerging orthopedic companies when looking to license a competitor's patent. By "fencing-in" in the competitor's business opportunities and limiting the competitor's future mobility, the emerging orthopedic company can leverage cross-licensing opportunities and reduce the terms of the license from the competitor. To do this, the orthopedic company can file numerous patent applications around a competitor's core patent(s) in areas, known as "white space," not already covered by the competitor's patents. Because the competitor then cannot expand out due to the picket fence of patent applications owned by the emerging orthopedic company, the competitor must license these patent applications.

Orthopedic companies can use this tool as a way to innovate or expand into new markets where they do not own the key technology. Additionally, a picket fence of patent protection can be a critical business tool for companies that are entering a market late in the game compared with their competitors. To do this effectively, a company needs to anticipate future market demand for a new feature or modification and then patent that feature or enhancement to leverage a cross-license with a more dominant competitor.

However, the picket fence patent strategy can be costly for emerging companies with modest patent budgets. They often lack the resources needed to develop patents around a competitor's patents. A picket fence patent strategy can encourage collaboration among competitors where both companies benefit from each other's patent portfolio. Ultimately, patentors will benefit from the competition, more innovations, and lower prices.

Patenting "White Space"

Patenting orthopedic inventions often requires some maneuvering around third-party patents, covering similar products because of the large number of medical technology patents already issued, but it is worth the work it takes to get strategically valuable patents.

Determining which patent strategy is most effective is largely determined by the amount of "white space" existing in the patent landscape. The amount of "white space" measures how crowded a particular area is with patents and patent applications. If a technology area is saturated with patents, there is little "white space" and less room for new patent applications. Alternatively, if the patent landscape is relatively clear, there is more "white space" to secure broad and meaningful patent claims. Developing a strategy for patenting "white space" is fruitful for orthopedic companies wishing to solidify a competitive edge in the marketplace.

By filing patent applications in areas with large "white space", companies can stake broad claims to potentially valuable patent turf. Analyzing how saturated with patents a particular technology area is allows a company to forecast what technologies will be in common use 10 to 15 years in the future. "White space" becomes problematic when a competitor develops a product that is so technologically close to a company's own product that it impedes upon the company's commercial area, essentially blocking a company from practicing its own patents or preventing it from expanding its existing product base.

Finding Freedom to Operate

To determine whether a product can be produced without infringing patents owned by third parties, a company should undertake a freedom to operate search and analysis, which determines whether the company's product avoids third-party patents. Freedom to operate searches can confirm the ability, or "clearance," to make, use, sell, or import a product or process without infringing on another's patent. After conducting thorough searches of patent databases and scientific literature databases, a company should develop a strategy to avoid third-party patents while maximizing its patent presence within that particular commercial area. It can accomplish this by identifying potential patent design-around opportunities that a competitor might use to avoid infringing the company's patent coverage for its products and seeking new patents or modifying its current patent applications to assure the broadest possible coverage for its products. By expanding its presence in the marketplace, an orthopedic company will have the ability to not only assert its patent rights against a potential infringer, but it will also have the option of granting a license to a competitor.

Record Keeping Is Important

One of the first steps in applying for a patent is to make a record of the invention. Preferably, written records should be made contemporaneously with conception of the invention and during any experiments performed related to the invention. Such record keeping should become a standard business practice for innovators. Although record keeping may appear tedious, records are important for proving when a particular invention was made and by whom it was made. Usually the records are not needed for proof until enforcement of a subsequently issued patent is attempted or until a dispute about inventorship develops. Thus, accurate and contemporaneous record keeping is essential.

No particular form of record is necessary. The preferred record, often called an "invention disclosure," includes a written description that explains the invention and includes sketches or drawings illustrating the invention. The records should be witnessed and corroborated by someone, other than the inventor, who understands the invention. A disclosure should include the name of the inventor, the date that the record is being made, and signatures and dates of signing of one or more witnesses.

The witness may use words such as "read and understood by me" or "seen and understood by me" next to his or her signature. Witnesses other than the inventor may be essential for corroborating conception of an invention and the date of completion of the invention or reduction to practice.

The records should be readable. Above all, the records should not have been altered. Any later-made alterations may make records of invention suspect.

Statutory Requirements for Patentability

Before diving into the mechanics of how to conduct a patentability search and ultimately file a patent application, it is beneficial to understand the statutory requirements for patentability. There are four main requirements of statutory patentability in the United States: (1) eligible subject matter; (2) utility; (3) novelty; and (4) nonobviousness. All four of these elements are constricted further by a statutory one-year bar in the United States.

ELIGIBLE SUBJECT MATTER

Patent protection is available for processes, machines, manufactures, compositions of matter, improvements thereof, and asexually reproduced plants (35 U.S.C. §§ 101, 161). These types of inventions are referred to as "eligible subject matter" or "patentable subject matter." Patent protection is not available for abstract ideas, phenomena of nature, basic mathematical and physical relationships, music, photographs, or mental processes.

In addition, although everything from new medical devices to new drugs can be patented, it is important to note that the United States does not offer patent protection for surgical methods and techniques. Therefore, physicians do not have to pay royalties every time they use a procedure while examining or operating on a patient.

The question of patentable subject matter sometimes arises with regard to computer programs. Data structures and computer programs are not patentable in the abstract. However, physical structures (such as a memory circuit) that represent a practical application of a data structure are patentable, as are processes that are implemented using computer programs.

UTILITY

Every patented invention (not only "utility" patent inventions) must have utility. That is, the invention must be useful (35 U.S.C. § 101). The statutory requirement of utility of an invention most frequently comes into question in patent applications having claims directed to a new composition of matter, such as a compound or pharmaceutical, that has no known or established use.

NOVELTY

In order to qualify for patent protection, an invention must have been invented by the applicant and the invention must be "new" or "novel" (35 U.S.C. § 102).

An invention is considered "novel" unless

(1) the claimed invention was patented, described in a printed publication, or in public use, on sale, or otherwise available to the public before the effective filing date of the claimed invention; or
(2) the claimed invention was described in a patent issued under section 151 or in an application for patent published or deemed published under section 122(b), in which the patent or application, as the case may be, names another inventor and was effectively filed before the effective filing date of the claimed invention (35 U.S.C. § 102(a)).

NONOBVIOUSNESS

Even though an invention may be "new" or "novel" as defined in 35 U.S.C. § 102, a patent will not be granted if it represents a trivial or "obvious" modification of the existing state of the art:

if the differences between the claimed invention and the prior art are such that the claimed invention as a whole would have been obvious before the effective filing date of the claimed invention to a person having ordinary skill in the art to which the claimed invention pertains. Patentability shall not be negated by the manner in which the invention was made (35 U.S.C. § 103).

"Prior art" refers to publicly available information before the filing date of the patent application. Prior art can come from a publication, an article, another patent, a trade show presentation, a meeting with a third party, or an offer for sale.

THE ONE-YEAR STATUTORY BAR

In addition, 35 U.S.C. § 102 provides that an inventor is barred from obtaining a patent if, more than 1 year before the US patent application is filed, the invention was:

1. patented or described in a printed publication anywhere in the world,
2. in public use in the United States,
3. "on sale" in the United States, or
4. otherwise available to the public.

These restrictions are referred to as "statutory bars," and they often arise because of acts of the inventor(s) in attempting to commercialize the product before applying for patent protection.

In general, it is advisable to file a patent application before the invention is first published, disclosed, used, or offered for sale. Although in the United States a patent application may be filed within a year of the first public disclosure, for foreign patent coverage, the patent application must be filed before *any* disclosure. Failure to file a patent application prior to public disclosure will result in the loss of potential foreign patent rights. To ensure both US and foreign patent coverage, a patent application should be filed before any public disclosure.

Complete Written Invention Disclosure Form

Given the statutory requirements to achieve patentability, it will be beneficial to complete a written invention disclosure form. It may be useful to look back on inventive records to complete this step.

A written record of an invention should be made to provide evidence of ownership of the invention. The record should:

1. disclose the invention by a written description and sketches or photographs or other evidence such as purchase orders of parts to build a unit, etc.
2. identify the inventor(s)
3. establish important dates such as conception and/or reduction to practice of the invention.

The record should describe and show the invention with sufficient clarity so that it can be understood by a person familiar with similar devices, systems, or processes. The record should include the signature of the inventor(s) and the date the record was made. In addition, the record should be signed and dated by at least two witnesses who understand the invention. Invention disclosure forms can be provided for this purpose.

The following is an example of specific information and drawings often including in an invention disclosure form.

Invention disclosure form is to be completed by the inventor(s) of the invention. Please describe the invention in excruciating detail and refer to the drawings and flowcharts. Please provide as much detail as possible as this is the best way to document the invention. Please complete the invention disclosure as a word document, adding additional pages for description and drawings.

Please add multiple pages to the invention disclosure to describe the following:

1. The background problem that your invention is trying to solve
2. Previous (prior art) attempts to solve this problem
3. Abstract—please provide a one paragraph summary of the invention
4. Detailed CAD drawings of various views
5. A flowchart showing the overall process
6. More detailed flowcharts for more key decisions and processes
7. Each step of the flowcharts with a paragraph describing what is being accomplished
8. Detailed step-by-step description of steps for using the invention
9. Three-five sentences summarizing the novelty of the invention (i.e., the essence of the invention)

The invention disclosure form is a useful tool to organize the inventor's thoughts about the invention, identify elements of the invention, and narrow down key terms and phrases for patent searching. This will ultimately help the inventor and patent attorney conduct a prudent patentability search. Additionally, because most patent attorneys charge an hourly rate, the more detailed the invention disclosure, the easier (and less expensive) it will eventually be to draft and file a patent application.

Conduct a Patentability Search

Before an application is filed in the United States Patent and Trademark Office (USPTO), an investigation of any relevant prior patents or prior art should be conducted. This investigation is called a preliminary patentability search. The cost of a preliminary search can range upwardly from $1,000 and increases in cost with search difficulty. Searches on electrical, chemical, mechanical, or more complicated medical inventions, where close reading of the reference patents is required or where the field of search is not obvious, take more time and, therefore, cost more. Patent searches are sometimes made by the USPTO but are usually made by professionally trained patent searchers. The search reports and opinions as to patentability are often written by a patent attorney after a review of the search findings. Patent searches can also be performed using electronic or internet patent databases by the inventors or the patent attorney.

The patents found in the search will be of value to try to determine (1) if there is an opportunity to obtain worthwhile patent protection, (2) if the invention is covered by an unexpired patent, (3) engineering information related to the invention, and (4) if an issued patent covering the invention may be available for purchase or license.

PATENT SEARCH OPTIONS

By the Inventor

Inventors should be careful about relying on their own patent search, as it is common for an inventor to do a patent search and find nothing even when there is prior art available that could be found by a skilled professional searcher. Nevertheless, conducting an internet patent search is a wise first move and may be helpful for the inventor to understand the prior art of the inventive field. If an inventor does find something on their own that is too close to their own invention, they will be able to save time and money while moving on to the next project.

A good place to start is with simple internet search engines. Conduct an internet search to make sure that the invention is not being sold or marketed by another company already. After determining that the product is not in the marketplace, there are numerous free tools available for patent searching.

Many websites offer free patent searching by entering key words. The following search engines are great free tools for inventors:

- USPTO Patent Full-Text Databases (http://patft.uspto.gov/)
- Google Patent Search (https://patents.google.com/)
- Free Patents Online (http://www.freepatentsonline.com/)

The USPTO patent database searches US patents and publications using resources from the USPTO and its bilateral partner EPO (European Patent Office). The USPTO website provides seven very helpful steps in a preliminary search of US Patents and Published Patent Applications guide.[1] It can be very helpful in understanding the Cooperative Patent Classification and classification schedules that the USPTO uses. Always remember that

---

[1] https://www.uspto.gov/learning-and-resources/support-centers/patent-and-trademark-resource-centers-ptrc/resources/seven.

although the classification system is helpful, patents are classified as the USPTO sees fit.

In the USPTO patent search database, the left side (PatFT or Patents Full-Text and Image) is for searching issued patents. The right side (AppFT or Applications Full-Text and Image) is for searching published patent applications. Search both sides using key words for Quick Search and/or Advanced Search, keeping track of any patent numbers that are closest to the invention.

While searching, aim to refine the search terms and search strategy to return more meaningful results. It is essential to try a variety of different key words in the patent searches. Increasing the number of search terms to describe a feature will lead to better search results. As a rule of thumb, inventors should spend 1 to 2 hours performing keyword patent searches for an initial impression of the patent landscape.

Patent Search Firms in the United States or Foreign Countries

Professional patent searchers and patent search firms conduct patent searches for a living and therefore are more familiar with the classification system than any inventor or even many patent attorneys. In addition to searching US patents, patent search firms can search international patent applications filed through the World Intellectual Property Organization/Patent Cooperation Treaty (PCT) and foreign patent offices including Europe, Japan, Korea, and many other countries. They may also have strategies to uncover prior art (including journal articles, Ph.D. theses, trade show posters, etc.) that are missed through Boolean key words and classification searching.

Ultimately, a report generated from a patent search firm can be useful in revealing trends in a certain technology area and may even be helpful to uncover expired patents. Although not without costs, these patent search firms may provide valuable peace of mind for inventors and patent attorneys in making sure that the expenses incurred while filing a patent are not in vain.

Law Firm

Particularly in cases where both searches by inventors and searches by patent search firms reveal extensive prior art, it can be helpful to work with a patent attorney to determine the relevance of the prior art in patenting the invention. Though not without its costs, an analysis provided by a patent attorney can be helpful in determining the patentability of the invention. It is important to work with the correct patent attorney with a relevant technical background and field of expertise in mechanical and biomedical engineering, so that the inventor can effectively work with the patent attorney to analyze prior art, and to make sure that the patentability analysis focuses on all aspects of the invention.

The USPTO maintains a roster of patent attorneys who are registered to practice before the USPTO and file patent applications. No patent attorney specializes in all fields, so inventors should hire a patent attorney with an orthopedic background to both analyze prior art and prepare and file the patent application. For example, there are patent attorneys who have orthopedic experience and undergraduate degrees in science, including mechanical and biomedical engineering.

When the inventor is new to a technology field, a patentability assessment by a patent attorney can save a great deal of time and money. Often, the inventor does not realize the extensive prior work that has been done in a field and therefore has false expectations of the amount of patent protection available. The patentability assessment can give the inventor and the patent attorney more realistic expectations before investing resources in preparing a patent application. If the patentability assessment shows that meaningful patent protection can be obtained on the invention, the inventor must then decide whether to pursue protection through the filing of a patent application.

Despite best efforts, patent searching only provides a snap shot for a moment in time as new patent applications are publishing and new patents are issuing each week. Prior art searches are not an exact science, and it is not uncommon that a piece of prior art is found at a later date, which was not uncovered during the search and which may be critical to the invention that is desired to patent.

Applying for a Patent

If the patent search indicates that meaningful patent protection can be obtained on the invention, the inventor must then decide whether or not to pursue protection through the filing of a patent application. If an inventor has the resources to do so, the inventor should hire a patent attorney to draft, file, and prosecute the patent application.

If an inventor does not have the financial resources to hire a patent attorney but can cover the government filing fees, the inventor can attempt to draft the patent application without the assistance of a patent attorney. Patenting an invention without a patent attorney is not impossible, but it is neither easy nor advisable. The inventor should spend a significant amount of time studying the process of patent application drafting, technical drawing, and patent claim writing.

FILING A PATENT APPLICATION

A patent application is an extensive legal document that requires careful preparation of the text and drawings. The cost of preparing and filing a patent application varies with the complexity of the invention. The inventor can either file a provisional patent application or a nonprovisional patent application. A provisional application is less formal than a nonprovisional patent application and thus costs less.

FILING A PROVISIONAL PATENT APPLICATION

A provisional application has a pendency lasting only 12 months from the date the provisional application is filed. Thus, the provisional patent application expires 12 months from the filing date. To obtain patent protection based on the priority of the provisional patent application, it will be necessary to file a nonprovisional US patent application, as well as any foreign patent applications, within 1 year of the filing date of the provisional patent application. The filing costs for provisional applications vary depending on the complexity and required attorney time but with inventor cooperation can typically range from about $5,000 to about $7,500, with a $140 USPTO government filing fee.

FILING AND PROSECUTING A UNITED STATES PATENT APPLICATION

To obtain patent protection based on the priority of the provisional patent application, it is necessary to file a nonprovisional US patent application, as well as any foreign patent applications, within 1 year of the filing date of the provisional patent application. Filing a nonprovisional application starts the official examination process with the USPTO to determine if the invention is patentable.

For nonprovisional patent applications covering medical inventions, the filing costs usually vary between about $6,500 and about $12,500. This includes preparation of the written description and abstract, drafting of claims defining the invention, the drawings, and the USPTO government filing fee. This USPTO government filing fee is a minimum of $785 for "small entities" (including individual inventors, small businesses, and nonprofit organizations) and a minimum of $1,720 for "large entities."

The additional cost of prosecuting the patent application through the USPTO is not included in the above range and might well equal the cost of the application. The cost of prosecuting the patent application will be spread over a period of about 2 or 3 years, an average time period to prosecute a patent application through the USPTO.

The patent examiner to whom the application is assigned will usually send a first office action within 12 to 24 months from the filing date. In the office action, the patent examiner will typically reject at least some of the broader claims made for the invention and will cite and send copies of the prior art patents or articles on which the rejection is based. Patent attorneys help analyze the office action and suggest whether to amend the claims to overcome the rejections, argue that the examiner has overreached in rejecting, or both. Patent attorneys draft arguments and claim amendments, and charge for it will be based on the time in working with the inventor and in preparing and filing the arguments and amendments. This process of working with the patent examiner may go through several rounds. If and when the patent application is allowed, there is a final USPTO government issue fee of at least $500 for small entities and twice that for large entities that must be paid for a patent to issue.

Each patent granted in the United States is subject to maintenance fees payable 3½, 7½, and 11½ years after the patent is granted to keep the patent in force. These fees currently are $800, $1,800, and $3,700, respectively, for small entities and twice that for large entities. Failure to pay a maintenance fee results in the patent going abandoned. Paying the three maintenance fees will keep the US patent in force for 20 years from its filing date.

Inventors should not rush into a patent application unless they have considered how to recapture or justify these expenses. If the product has a good market potential, the cost of filing a patent application may be justified for the right to mark the invention as "patent pending" or "patent applied for." Although this does not offer any legal protection, it sometimes does have a certain amount of scare or psychological value in that it does put a competitor on notice of patent interest in the invention. It is illegal to mark a product as "patent pending" or "patent applied for" when there is no patent application filed in the USPTO.

FOREIGN PATENTS

Filing international patent applications further strengthens a patent portfolio and extends a company's presence in the global marketplace. While foreign patent applications can be expensive, filing in strategic countries can be critical to the commercial success of an orthopedic product. A company should consider filing in specific countries with a large target market for the product, countries where competitors' manufacturing facilities are located, and countries that export medical products to other regions through distribution channels. Although the United States, Europe, and Japan have historically been top patent filing countries for medical inventions, China and Brazil are rising up the list.

Importance of Filing Patent Application Promptly

The US patent law permits the patent application to be filed at any time within 1 year of the first publication, offer for sale, sale, or other public use of an invention. After this 1 year is past, if a patent application is not on file, the invention has become public property and a valid US patent cannot be obtained. Some inventors feel out the market for several months before making a decision as to whether or not a patent application should be filed. This should not be done if major European countries or certain other countries are good potential markets for the invention, because there is typically no grace period in foreign countries. In the event that the inventor intends to license someone to manufacture or sell the invention, it probably would be necessary to file a patent application to serve as a basis for the license. Also, the patent application can be used as a means to disclose the invention to prospective manufacturers.

Orthopedic Patents Case Study: IlluminOss Medical, Inc.

IlluminOss Medical, Inc. (https://illuminoss.com/) is a venture-backed medical device company pioneering new frontiers in orthopedic surgery. From the company's formation in 2007, IlluminOss has worked with international law firm Greenberg Traurig to study the intellectual property landscape and develop a strong patent portfolio, directed to the company's unique designs and processes. Greenberg Traurig has developed the company's strategic worldwide patent portfolio for its revolutionary orthopedic systems for minimally invasive stabilization and treatment of broken bones. The patent portfolio has helped the company protect its innovative products and raise over $50 million in venture capital funding.

Serial entrepreneur and inventor Robert Rabiner conceived of the IlluminOss Photodynamic Bone Stabilization System while brainstorming about better ways to fix broken bones after his mother broke her hip. After much iteration, the core idea of a system using glue to fix the broken bones from the inside out seemed promising. Seeing no such devices in the market, the inventor conducted some initial patent searches on the internet and then engaged the medical device patent attorney David Dykeman to conduct a patent landscape search.

After finding "white space" in the patent landscape, the inventor and patent attorney filed strategic patent applications that targeted the open "white space" in the patent landscape. Now, a decade later, IlluminOss has over 100 issued patents in 17 countries around the world protecting its innovative products.

IlluminOss' worldwide patent portfolio includes patents covering the IlluminOss Photodynamic Bone Stabilization System, which is a revolutionary orthopedic system for minimally invasive stabilization and treatment of fractured bones from the inside out. IlluminOss patents cover all aspects of the products including the entire system, catheters, balloons, light sources, treatment kits, methods of treatment, improvements, and alternative designs, to form a picket fence of patent protection around the innovative technology. For example, US Patent No. 7,879,041 is entitled "Systems and methods for internal bone fixation" and contains 20 claims covering the IlluminOss Photodynamic Bone Stabilization System with a side fire optical fiber, as well as a method for repairing a fractured bone using the system. The device includes a delivery catheter; a conformable member releasably engaging the distal end of the delivery catheter; and an optical fiber that disperses light energy at a terminating face and along a length of the optical fiber. US Patent No. 7,879,041 is part of a large patent family having over 40 patents and patent applications in 17 different countries including: 6 US patents, over 25 foreign patents, 2 pending US patent applications, 2 PCT international applications, and 7 foreign patent applications.

Conducting thorough patent searches early provided the inventor and IlluminOss with information on existing products and an idea of patent "white space" the company could try to claim. By aggressively staking claims in the patent landscape, IlluminOss has created a strong worldwide patent portfolio of over 100 patents that provides a picket fence of patent protection around its innovative core technology, improvements, potential alternative designs, and future innovations. The patent portfolio supports the company's mission to improve the treatment of broken bones.

KEY TAKEAWAY POINTS

- ▶ Patenting orthopedic inventions often requires some maneuvering around third-party patents covering similar products because of the large number of medical technology patents already issued.

- ▶ Patent searching only provides a snap shot for a moment in time as new patent applications are publishing and new patents are issuing each week. Prior art searches are not an exact science, and it is not uncommon that a piece of prior art is found at a later date.

- ▶ The patents found in a patent search will be of value to try to determine (1) if there is an opportunity to obtain worthwhile patent protection, (2) if the invention is covered by an unexpired patent, (3) engineering information related to the invention, and (4) if an issued patent covering the invention may be available for purchase or license.

- ▶ Patent applications should be filed to cover all aspects of the core technology, including the entire device, key components, methods of use, methods of manufacture, incremental improvements, and other aspects of the invention.

- ▶ Patent portfolios are often the only way for investors to place a value on an early-stage company's technology as sales often cannot begin until after regulatory approval.

- ▶ There are four requirements for statutory patentability; (1) eligible subject matter, (2) utility, (3) novelty, and (4) nonobviousness. All four of these elements are restricted by a statutory one-year bar in the United States.

- ▶ To obtain patent protection based on the priority of the provisional patent application, it is necessary to file a nonprovisional US patent application, as well as any foreign patent applications, within 1 year of the filing date of the provisional patent application.

- ▶ The cost of prosecuting the patent application will be spread over a period of about 2 or 3 years, an average time period to prosecute a patent application through the USPTO.

- ▶ Each patent granted in the United States is subject to maintenance fees payable 3½, 7½, and 11½ years after the patent is granted to keep the patent in force for its 20-year term.

Acknowledgments

The authors wish to acknowledge and thank Brittany Schoenick for her contributions to this chapter.

BIBLIOGRAPHY

1. USPTO Patent Full-Text Databases. http://patft.uspto.gov/.
2. The Seven Steps in a Preliminary Search of U.S. Patents and Published Patent Applications. https://www.uspto.gov/learning-and-resources/support-centers/patent-and-trademark-resource-centers-ptrc/resources/seven.
3. Google Patent Search. https://patents.google.com/.
4. Free Patents Online. http://www.freepatentsonline.com/.

CHAPTER 7

Concept Development, Selection, and Testing— Passion and Planning Go Hand-in-Hand

JEFFREY A. KARG, PAUL DICESARE

ABOUT THE AUTHORS

Jeffrey A. Karg, Managing Director, Boston Innovation. Jeff is a 30-year veteran of medical device development. He has over 23 patents ranging from drug delivery and discovery to clinical devices in technology areas including mechanics, fluidics, and electromechanics. He is a Master of Science in Mechanical Engineering, graduate of Stanford University. His company, Boston Innovation, proactively assists doctor/surgeon inventors develop their ideas into products. By combining passion and planning, Jeff and his team plan, resource, and lead product development programs within budgetary and timeline limitations. He and his team ensure start-up funding is not jeopardized by incomplete product development progress. As CEO, his start-up, nAscent Biosciences, a maker of disposable drug discovery tools, was acquired by Thermo Fisher Scientific in 2008. Jeff's interests lie in the ongoing development of his living and work space in Bolton, MA, cooking for life and wife, and his two dogs, Flora and Maisy.

Paul DiCesare is the founder and President of Start LLC, a medical device development company based in Connecticut. Paul is a veteran of the medical device industry with more than 30 years of diverse medical product design experience and over 60 US patents. He has a Bachelor of Science degree in Industrial Design from the University of Bridgeport. His company, Start LLC, combines a very creative approach to product design with experienced engineering, prototyping, and designing for manufacturing capabilities. Since the company's inception, Start LLC has supported the market launch of more than 20 medical device products.

Introduction—Fun and Risk, When Passion and Planning Go Hand-in-Hand

Developing and testing concepts can be one of the most fun parts of bringing your idea to life. This is the time when you get to see your thoughts materialize into an actual useable device. And without proper planning, it is also the time where a lot of time and money can be spent without completing concept development. This chapter guides you through the concept development process to ensure you do not miss any important steps, incur prohibitive risk, or unnecessarily spend financial resources.

As a guide to where concept development fits within the product development lifecycle:

1. Requirements development—Chapter 4
2. Concept development, selection, and test—this chapter
3. Formal product development under design controls—Chapter 9
4. Commercialization

Steps 2 and 3 are where you will spend the most money. It is harder than you might think to successfully pass through steps 2 and 3 before you run out of money and/or other precious resources. In particular, you are encouraged to minimize risk and follow the recommendations in the preceding chapters on:

- Identifying the unmet need
- Market analysis
- Competition analysis
- Forming a solution
- Vetting the concept
- Prior art search

By addressing each of the above chapter references at some level as go/no-go decisions, you reduce the risk of expending significant product development resources without achieving the primary goal of starting a business and making money. In practice, each of the preceding chapters needs to be addressed at enough of a level to provide confidence to continue.

Concept Development Outline

An effective, tried, and true concept development method is based on passing through gating milestones. Each milestone is designed to minimize risk of wasted resources.

Five steps to a successful concept development process:

1. Documenting the Unmet Need—reference Chapter 4, Forming a Solution
2. Generating concepts and preliminary pro/con analysis

3. Concept specification and down selection
4. Design formalization and "concepting to scale"
5. Proof of concept

Substeps break down each milestone into manageable activities. Table 7.1 diagrams the milestones with substeps for easy process navigation. However, each substep may contain some complex activities, particularly if your product idea has electronic (HW), firmware (FW), and software (SW) components. If your product requires any of these engineering disciplines and you do not have these skills yourself, you may have to seek out help early on.

Milestones

DOCUMENTING THE UNMET NEED

Staying focused on the unmet need is important to managing risk. Writing a clear product requirements document based on Chapter 8, "Forming a Solution," is one of the most effective ways to manage risk and conserve resources. Intuitively, if you keep the ship focused on the specific destination, you will get there in as straight a line as possible. All project participants should read or have significant exposure to the product requirements document to ensure the team is well-directed.

An important outcome of this milestone is a Concept Development Plan. At a minimum, you will define who else you need on your team such as engineering, regulatory, marketing, etc. as they all will have a stake in the final product. Other possible sections of a Concept Development Plan are timeline for completion, approximate cost, and any other appropriate details. The Concept Development Plan is the roadmap for creating successful design concepts from an idea.

Deliverables

- Product requirements document
- Concept Development Plan

GENERATING CONCEPTS AND PRELIMINARY PRO/CON ANALYSIS

Generating design concepts does not require sophisticated equipment or software. For starters, a pencil and paper are still one of the best design tools available today. The point here is to generate as many individual concepts as you can through free thinking and sketch them so they are available for further consideration. Sometimes called brainstorming, this step is fun and can be done individually or in a group. It is not recommended

Table 7.1 Concept Development Milestones

Concept Development Milestones	Necessary Steps Within the Milestone						
1. Documenting the Unmet Need	Idea	Requirements documentation	Concept development plan	–	–	–	–
2. Generating concepts and preliminary pro/con analysis	Pencil, pen, and paper sketching	Multiple concepts—brainstorming	Multiple concepts detailed sketches	List of pros and cons	–	–	–
3. Concept specification and down selection	Quantitative specifications (numbers)	Review pros and cons against specifications	Down select to 2-3 concepts	–	–	–	–
4. Feasibility and "concepting to scale"	Computer-aided design and engineering analysis to meet specifications	Key features breadboards built, tested, and results documented	Key features breadboard(s) design iteration, retest, and document	Design iterations to meet user and marketing requirements	Design iterations to meet manufacturing and cost requirements	Preliminary risk analysis	Design review

Continued

Table 7.1 Concept Development Milestones—Cont'd

Concept Development Milestones	Necessary Steps Within the Milestone						
5. Proof of concept	Fabricate device according to drawings and specifications	Preliminary product testing	Design iterations to pass preliminary product testing	Small number of final proof of concept devices built	Detailed engineering qualification testing	Design review	–
6. Product development under design controls	Design and development under design controls	Manufacture clinical quantities under design controls	Design verification testing under design controls	Design validation testing under design controls	Design history file completed for FDA submittal	–	–

that one starts designing in computer-aided design (CAD) software. It is costly and often the time invested in the CAD work becomes a driver of the design as opposed to the primary direction set in the product requirements document.

After the quick sketching from the brainstorming sessions, each idea must be further refined. In the end, you may come up with 5 or 6 viable concepts that sufficiently meet requirements. The documentation may come in the form of sketches, drawings, flowcharts, and anything else you can think of to better understand how to solve your problem.

Lastly in this milestone, the ideas that are just plain, not going to work, need to be eliminated. This is often done through a pro/con technique where you list the positives and negatives for each idea and make a judgment call on which ones should move forward. Criteria for elimination can range from unobtainable technology requirements to high cost that your market cannot bear.

Deliverables

- Multiple concepts in the form of:
  - sketches
  - drawings
  - flowcharts
- Pro/con table with possible Pugh rating matrix
- Refined list of possible concepts (generally 5-6 is a good number)

CONCEPT SPECIFICATION AND DOWN SELECTION

Developing a specification is our next step in refining, eliminating, and coalescing to a final viable concept(s). This is where you add concrete numbers to your sketches. Things such as design details, material selections, user needs, human factors, etc. are considered. Identifying specific details to the design often causes some concepts to be eliminated.

Specifications are directly related to requirements. Often, the requirements document developed in Chapter 4 serves as the outline for specifications. For example, a requirement stating, "The device must hold a surgical instrument" might have specifications as shown in Table 7.2.

EXAMPLE REQUIREMENTS AND SPECIFICATIONS

Requirements are general statements of what the device must do, whereas specifications describe how to do it. This is a critical link to efficient concept development, resulting in lower development risk due to missing any crucial details.

Table 7.2 Example Requirements and Specifications	
Requirement	**Specification**
R1—The device must hold the instrument in place during surgery	R1S1—Device length 205 mm +/− 10 mm R1S2—Device placement accuracy <0.5 mm at 205 mm length R1S3—Device should be able to sustain a force of 20 lbs R1S4—The moving parts must survive 15,000 cycles before failure
R2—The device must not interfere with the surgeons activities	R2S1—Device footprint <21″ square R2S2—Device height <42″

Now we go back and look at the pro/con table of each concept to determine if the addition of hard specifications caused some concepts to get stronger or weaker. We use this data to narrow down concept choices to the top 2-3 concepts if possible. Interestingly, we do not entirely discard the concepts that have fallen out. There may be some details in those designs that help to solve problems in the ones that have survived.

Clearly, this process is iterative, yet very important as it lays out the development path ahead.

Deliverables

- Refined pro/con list
- Table of requirements with preliminary specifications
- Refined concepts with preliminary specifications (2 or 3 documented concepts)

DESIGN FORMALIZATION AND "CONCEPTING TO SCALE"

This is a critical milestone in concept development because the product you are developing now meets the reality of physical design. The phrase "concepting to scale" specifically refers to designs that incorporate physical dimensions, tolerances, materials, manufacturing processes, and a wide variety of other design constraints driven by real-world limitations. If the product incorporates electronics and software, "concepting to scale" means developing the hardware, firmware, and software to a point that can be tested to an appropriate level. Electronic product development is different from mechanical development because different tools are used, but the process is the same.

Computer-Aided Design

Design formalization means moving beyond sketches, pro/con list, etc. to an actual device design, usually in CAD. Designing in CAD requires specifications because actual measurements are required to build the CAD models. If electronics and software are required, development kits with their specific electronic hardware are often employed to create a risk-reduced breadboard for analysis. These development tools further add scale to the concepts and are vital to developing useful prototypes that can be verified and tested.

CAD three-dimensional design tools allow for aspects of the design to be analyzed for optimal mechanical configuration and performance against specifications without actually building the device. The natural process would be iteration through give and take, balancing the requirements with design features and mechanics. CAD 3-D design tools allow for making changes and evolving the design as more information becomes available.

Computer-Aided Engineering Analysis

CAD engineering analysis is a useful tool to weed out unlikely solutions in an iterative fashion relatively quickly while conserving resources. CAD engineering analysis or finite element analysis can predict performance in many areas including:

- Strength and material analysis that predict mechanical performance such as device stiffness and the device's ability to handle force loads. Nonlinear versions of this type of analysis are effective in understanding the performance of rubbers and high-deformation materials
- Fluid analysis that predicts static and dynamic fluid effects such as how a vessel will maintain integrity under various pressures or how a nozzle might respond to changes in pressure or flow rate
- Thermal analysis that predicts the effects on heating and cooling with respect to temperature extremes and material expansion and contraction under thermal stress
- Vibration analysis that predicts the device's response to internal and external cyclical forces
- Electromagnetic interference analysis can predict the device's effect in creating and absorbing electromagnetic waves on the surrounding area during use

Software and Hardware Development Kits

Software and hardware development kits are another form of "concepting to scale." An example is developing a device that requires imaging. A wide variety of imaging (camera) development kits are available to various specifications. This type of kit often contains the imager, control printed circuit board (PCB), cables, and software and can be run with a laptop or desktop computer. Purchasing and experimenting with various development kits can prove out performance features required for your product prior to any custom development, saving money, time, and reducing development risk.

SW/HW development kits and mechanical design and analysis tools are not always employed during the concept development phase. In some cases, analysis tools will not be employed until the more rigorous product development phase under design controls because the development risk is very low.

Key Features Breadboard(s) Built, Tested, and Results Documented

In some cases, simplified breadboards consisting of development kits, fast prototyped parts, and purchased parts can greatly help early concept development. Breadboards are rough approximations of your product that give the team a fairly good idea of the concept and allow for some level of evaluation. Key details may incorporate very small components or technology-leading electronics or a new procedure that requires the clinician to do something differently. Any of these and more may lead you to developing breadboards to prove out the basics of your design.

Analysis Against User Requirements

User needs are of primary importance. Every product ends with the user accepting it or not. As you move through this milestone, your team may provide you with drawings, sketches, and/or renderings of what the product could look like. Physical models can be created with rapid prototyping to put shapes and geometries into clinician's hands. This is often done before a proof of concept (PoC) is built. In addition, when possible, it may be wise to build a simulator, allowing prospective clinicians to even better understand your technology or invention. The learnings from initial clinician reviews are critical to the process because follow-on user interviews are shaped by the initial results. For example, the user interview guide might be modified to reflect new learnings about a procedure developed from a breadboard.

The objective is to have a clear understanding of what the clinician wants before fabricating a prototype device.

Analysis Against Cost and Marketing Requirements

Some additional factors that we must also cover at this point are product cost and meeting marketing needs. With a preliminary concept design in CAD form, we can make some rough estimates on product cost. In addition to component cost or bill of materials, one must consider processing/manufacturing cost and assembly cost. In many cases, a new product can require process development effort. As an example, your device may have a component that requires special handling in the assembly. How that special component integrates with the overall product in a cost-effective way may take some additional investment beyond the actual product. All these costs need to be understood.

Revisiting marketing requirements is a good idea at this time. Assuming the concept design can achieve the desired clinical goals and meet technical specifications and user needs, one must measure against the marketing goals. An analysis of expected quantity that can be sold and meeting the target manufacturing cost and retail price become good indicators if it is worth continuing to move forward with development. If a design concept is going to cost 10 times more than the product it replaces, there needs to be an assessment of whether the added benefit justifies the added cost or hospitals will not purchase it. If it is a completely new product, the assessment is harder as it may not have a reimbursement code. The value of the product may lie in decreasing hospital stay, preventing disease reoccurrence, or fixing something that was previously not fixable. However, a path other than cost reduction is sometimes a hard way to justify a new product to purchasing organizations.

Risk—User, Patient, Project, Technical, and Regulatory

Risk is largely covered during the product development under design controls, but now is a good time to begin documenting any risks you may recognize. Although not a requirement of the concept development phase, sooner or later the project will need to meet the FDA regulatory requirements for product development. Ultimately, you will have to create a design history file (DHF), documenting most of your development efforts. The concept development stage is a gray area when it comes to required documentation, but any effort at collecting this information in safe electronic storage location will greatly assist you in assembling the DHF. The DHF is a requirement for product development under design controls.

Design Review

Design reviews can be held at any time during the development process; however, prior to passing on to the fabrication step, it is very wise to hold a design review and document the findings. Design reviews help to demarcate the transition from paper to device and focuses the entire team's attention on the specifics of the project. An accurate understanding of the likelihood of success can be determined in a good design review.

Deliverables

- Design documentation—mechanical and electronic
- Software documentation
- Engineering analysis documentation
- Fabrication documentation for suppliers
- Pro/con analysis revision
- Analysis against key user, marketing, and cost requirements
- Breadboards and testing results
- Preliminary risk list
- Design review(s) and approval to fabricate

PROOF OF CONCEPT

Lots of work and probably a fair amount of money have been expended by this time in the concept development phase. However, if all is aligned and the decision is to continue development, it is time to build the first PoC. Note we use the phrase "first proof of concept" as it is unlikely that the first device you build will be the one that goes into product development under design controls. It is the first real device that will enter some form of engineering qualification and testing we will cover in the next section.

Fabricating the Parts

There are a variety of resources available to build the first PoC. Assuming you have assembled an engineer or a team of engineers to help design, build, and test the device, they can also lead its fabrication. Some of the types of fabrication resources you may need include:

- Machining of plastic and metal components
- Molding of plastic components
- 3-D printing of various components, plastic, metal, and elastomers
- PCB fabrication
- Foam, rubber, or other elastomer components fabrication
- Purchased component (bill of material) management
- Others for various specialized fabrication requirements

Component Qualification Prior to Assembly

After going through many concept development phases in a wide range of products, one realizes how much has to come together for success. This comes from good planning and maintaining best design and engineering practices. For best results, each part must be checked against the drawings or other associated documentation for its adherence to the specifications prior to assembly.

Individual component qualification, some so simple as just taking measurements and making sure they are correct, can save many frustrating hours trying to debug why the first PoC is not performing as expected. Once all the components are acquired and checked for adherence to design intent, assembly can begin.

During assembly, it is a good idea to document the steps you go through. Often this is done by taking pictures, some well-staged, to capture assembly detail. Adding text to describe what is being done completes the process. This is a great way to begin the assembly documentation.

Preliminary Device Testing and Design Iterations

Initial assembly and product testing will likely manifest any number of changes to be made prior to engineering qualification testing. As engineering qualification can be quite extensive, especially if there is software involved, one can prepare by making any required small changes in tandem with some preliminary device testing, saving time and money.

The old adage "test early and often" is very true. Getting feedback in any way you can to improve the expected performance prior to full engineering qualification testing is critical. It provides for a better device and continues to inform the inventor on what the proper solution needs to be to meet all requirements.

Detailed Engineering Qualification Testing

Presuming the PoC has been successfully built, detailed engineering testing can begin. Testing can come in all forms, but it is smart to keep the testing directly related to expected performance. Concept specifications created earlier in this process can form the foundation of engineering qualification testing. However, there may be certain requirements created in the Forming a Solution phase that need to be tested as well. An example might be a laparoscopic device designed to improve suturing techniques. Although this requirement might not be an actual specification, the PoC will be less than useful if the surgeon fails to satisfy the requirement. A simple way to test the requirement would be to actually have a surgeon try the PoC device in a simulator.

The object here is to get through concept development with a very low risk of failure prior to entering the formal product development phase.

Deliverables

- Mechanical design and documentation
- Electronic design and documentation
- Software development and documentation
- Material selection research and documentation

- Quality records by checking each and every component against appropriate specifications. This includes fabricated and electronic components. Software has a specific set of requirements for quality records. It is highly recommended that someone in the organization become familiar with quality standards
- Assembly documentation
- Preliminary assembly of subcomponents with engineering testing of individual components (as necessary)
- Final assembly of integrated product with documentation, number to-be-determined based on need
- Engineering qualification testing of the integrated PoC device and documentation of performance against specifications and select requirements

All this work helps to avoid serial PoC failure, which can be very deflating to the overall product development process. The documentation detail allows the engineer to work efficiently to overcome performance deficiencies.

Resource Options to Assist Proof of Concept Development Efforts

There are a number of resource options to help create your first PoC including:

- You working in your lab designing, building, and testing the device
- Individual design and engineering contractors that provide a specific service to move development along
- Original equipment manufacturers that would gain by manufacturing the devices for you by amortizing the development cost in the future unit cost
- Universities and academic groups that will work through development through their intellectual property groups for a significant chunk of equity
- Multidisciplined design and engineering product development companies with a wide range of experience that work on a contract for hire basis

Each of these resources has pros and cons and must be considered as you move though the journey of creating a solid PoC.

PRODUCT DEVELOPMENT UNDER DESIGN CONTROLS

This chapter has walked you through the steps to get to a working device. However, the concept development and feasibility process has been completed with typical design and development skills, not under design controls required for FDA submittal.

The FDA adopted Section 820.70 product development and manufacturing standard in 1996. This product development methodology is documented in the ISO standard ISO 13485 and is often referred to as product design and development under design controls. The core tenet of the medical device development methodology is to design medical devices that are consistent with quality systems requirements worldwide. This is a broad mandate, but specifically the inventor must follow a heavily documented approach to defining, developing, testing, and validating user, safety, reliability, and a myriad of other requirements. This is a daunting task and is generally done by experienced medical device development professionals.

TRANSITION FROM CONCEPT DEVELOPMENT AND FEASIBILITY TO PRODUCT DEVELOPMENT

During the Concept Development and Feasibility phase, we laid out list of documents and deliverables. The purpose of these documents is to provide a foundation for transition to development under design controls. Some of the core deliverables are:

- Requirements document
- Preliminary risk analysis
- Engineering and analysis documentation
- Engineering qualification results

Basically, any documentation that tells the development story and provides traceability of the development process will ease design and development under design controls.

KEY TAKEAWAY POINTS

A successful Concept Development, Selection, and Testing phase is a very important threshold to attain. It provides you with the first prototypes to confirm the original intended use claims by enabling the user to see it, try it, and test it. It provides:

- ▶ confidence prior to moving to the very expensive formal product development phase

- ▶ a significant milestone in obtaining follow-on funding

- ▶ a foundation for the DHF that you will submit to the FDA after product development under design controls

- ▶ reduced risk of failure of the product in the eyes of the clinician, patient, marketing and sales groups, and regulatory bodies

- ▶ intense satisfaction seeing your PoC in your hands and those of your future customers

BIBLIOGRAPHY

1. Original Work by Paul DiCesare, Start, LLC, Co-author for This Chapter.
2. Stanford Researchers Publish Comprehensive Model for Medical Device Development. https://www.dotmed.com/news/story/9524.

CHAPTER 8

Engineering Resources: First Steps to Making a Tangible Prototype

JESSE RUSK, DAVID JACOBS

ABOUT THE AUTHORS

Jesse Rusk has worked within medical device product development for close to 15 years, with engineering leadership roles within product development consulting firms and medical device start-ups. He is a project manager for Boston Engineering, an ISO 13485–certified product development firm with a dedicated medical devices practice.

Dave Jacobs oversees Boston Engineering's Medical Devices practice. Previously, Dave served as chief operating officer at Scion Medical Technologies, a medical device developer and manufacturer with locations in the United States and China. Prior to Scion Medical, he was the vice president of operations at Interlace Medical, a medical device start-up acquired by Hologic in 2011.

Introduction

At this point, you have identified a market need, refined the product concept to capitalize on the business opportunity, and have justified moving forward with development. The next logical step is to generate a product prototype.

The definition of a "product prototype" varies significantly, and the scope of the product prototype will depend on your overarching business strategy. Early-stage prototype categories include:

- **Proof of principle/functional prototypes** that demonstrate an early operation of a product or component. Because these "breadboards" only focus on technical operation, they do not address size or other form factor requirements (see Figure 8.1, phase 2).

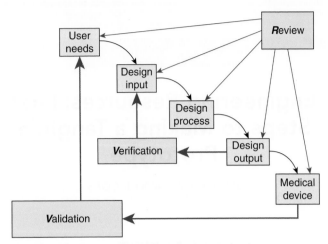

Figure 8.1 The Boston engineering phase-gate development process.

- **Aesthetic design prototypes** are nonfunctional units with external product packaging to get user feedback regarding ergonomics and other industrial design considerations.
- **Engineering prototypes** are full-production equivalent units that are intended to be used for formal design verification and validation activities.

This chapter focuses on the engineering prototype, typically separated into Alpha and Beta prototype development, which includes the product engineering, refining, and testing that lead to a final, commercial-ready product (See Figure 8.1, phases 4-6).

Defining Objectives for Alpha-Beta Prototypes

The typical goal for Alpha-Beta prototyping is to generate the test data and documentation required for regulatory clearance, although this can be a slow and costly process. It may be more appropriate in some instances to shed the burden of a formal medical device design control process if the acquisition parties do not require the level of precise, auditable data required for FDA submission. This may be the case if an acquirer plans to make design modifications or to follow their own development process. However, the decision not to lay the groundwork to support an FDA submission can be costly if a hopeful acquisition falls through and other potential buyers require more robust design traceability.

KEY CONSIDERATIONS TO SHAPE YOUR PROTOTYPE STRATEGY

Before cutting the first of many checks for product development, think through the following questions:

- Is the primary intention to bring the product to market or to create the best position for acquisition?
- If acquisition is the primary intention, what is the major milestone within the product lifecycle that will maximize return on investment (ROI)?
- What is the ultimate intention of the prototype?
- What is your timeline?

The Quality Management System

Assuming that the goal is to bring the product to market, the FDA requires a systematic approach to product development and associated design control. As such, entrepreneurs and other medical device developers are responsible for establishing internal processes that meet the Quality System Regulations and that document product development activities. These requirements are captured within the Code of Federal Regulations, Title 21, Part 820.

Some product development consultants have their own established design control processes that their clients can leverage to establish their quality management system (QMS). The value of this should not be underestimated for entrepreneurs. Implementation of a full QMS can typically cost $50-$100k, assuming there is minimal change required from the templates that a QA consultant would provide. A limited QMS, which references a partner's established development process, can be a fraction of the cost.

Project Phase Structure

Although there are many ways to structure the development process, the most widely used is the Waterfall model, a sequential process as shown in Figure 8.2 below.

A Waterfall model uses review gates after each significant development phase. It blocks subsequent activities until current phase tasks and deliverables are complete. This has the benefit of a controlled process with intrinsic review, at the detriment of the pace of development in some cases. Alternative methods such as Agile and Spiral models are not as prevalent within medical device designs.

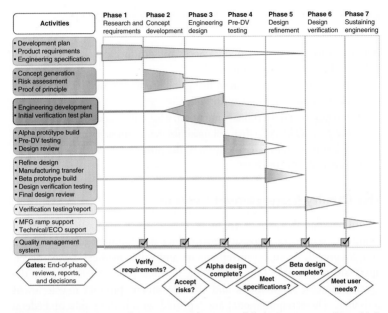

Figure 8.2 Application of design controls to waterfall design process. (From U. S. Food and Drug Administration. *Design Control Guidance for Medical Device Manufacturers.* 1997.)

THE PHASE-GATE DEVELOPMENT PROCESS

Translating the development activities into design phases typically results in four-to-seven distinct phases; an example phase structure is shown in the figure below. Some activities may overlap with work performed during prior concept generation. This may apply if the previous work was not performed and documented under formal design control.

The phase-gate process is designed to optimize product development via a consistent business process that often includes company development models and standard operating procedures. This process is designed to:

- Provide key check points along the development roadmap with defined goals and deliverables.
- Ensure that each phase supports all product goals—from features to manufacturability requirements.
- Identify and eliminate potential risks before they become costly, time-consuming problems.

In addition to the activities in each phase, Figure 8.2 also illustrates resource loading throughout the product development process.

Design Control Requirements for FDA Clearance

The FDA's Quality System Regulation, 21 CFR Part 820.30, details the design process requirements for most medical devices. The main regulatory areas for prototyping include:

Design Control Requirement	Description and Deliverable
Design and development planning	Plans that describe the activities, roles, and responsibilities throughout the development process.
Design input	Outlines design requirements that typically include: • high-level user and patient needs, and • low-level product requirements.
Design output	Provides documentation to evaluate if the product design conforms to the design inputs. This is typically accomplished by means of a traceability matrix, which links design inputs to supporting documents.
Design review	Provides a formal, documented review of design results, typically performed at the end of the each design phase.
Design verification	Provides testing (or related processes) to confirm that the design output meets the design input. Design verification should be quantifiable, with clear acceptance criteria.
Design validation	Conduct simulated or actual device use to confirm that the designed product meets the defined user and patient needs, and its intended uses.

Product Verification and Validation

Verification and validation both begin in the Alpha-Beta prototype phase, whereas other design control areas are initiated earlier in the process.

VERIFICATION FOR MEDICAL PRODUCTS

Verification activities confirm by objective evidence that the design output (i.e., the product design) fulfills all design input requirements and may be performed using either final prototypes or specialized builds that are designed for a subset of testing. Product developers must show how verification activities capture the expected output of the full variation allowed for the product (e.g., tolerances). This is typically performed either by testing "worst case" test builds or creating a statistical sampling plan with sufficient build quantities. Verification testing strives to be quantifiable and usually employs a range of fixtures and measurement equipment to isolate the particular product characteristic being tested.

VALIDATION FOR MEDICAL PRODUCTS

Validation activities—the process of confirming that the product meets the patient and user needs—can be more challenging. The validation process varies considerably depending on the medical product category. The FDA permits the use of "initial production units, lots, or batches, or their equivalents," which allows for use of prototype parts. This model assumes a justification can be made that they are both equivalent to production product and acceptable for use, given the validation activities proposed. The ability to perform validation activities before incurring the cost and time of generating production parts can be of significant benefit to entrepreneurs.

Capturing an Accurate Project Development Estimate

Most entrepreneurs partner with an external development firm and will use the cost estimates from firms as an input for funding goals. Many engineering firms typically do not have the context or visibility to propose a prototyping strategy to support both verification and validation activities.

The result is an underestimation of costs and time. By working through a preliminary strategy in concert with identifying a development partner, entrepreneurs can better position themselves for both adequate funding and more efficient use of those funds.

Selecting the Best Fit Among the Four Product Development Models

The following table lists benefits and drawbacks to each of the four models for product development and engineering:

Product Development Resource Type	Benefits	Drawbacks
Direct hires	• Known fixed costs, easier to estimate necessary funding • Retain learnings in-house for future projects • Potential to offset short-term cost through equity • Higher motivation due to design "ownership"	• Difficult to identify and retain good candidates • Costly if not fully utilizing resources • May have knowledge gaps • Need to handle employee overhead and logistics • Need to acquire product development software such as computer-aided design (CAD) tools • Need to implement, manage the QMS internally

Product Development Resource Type	Benefits	Drawbacks
Independent contractors	• Can "spin up" resources as needed; more cost-effective if full utilization is not necessary • Not responsible for employee overhead and logistics	• Difficult to find and retain good candidates • Contractors are typically experts, which may not be necessary for some tasks • May have knowledge gaps outside of their area of expertise • Availability not guaranteed (contractor may pursue more reliable work if your project experiences stops and starts)
Development firm	• Only pay for work performed • Typically has broad skill set and experience range, uses appropriate resource for a given task • Established design process and QMS • Manufacturing agnostic; can design product using optimal manufacturing techniques	• Hourly rate is typically higher than other options for similar level of experience • May have more issues during transfer to manufacturing because of separation of roles
Integrated development and contract manufacturing firm	• May be able to subsidize cost of development in later product production costs • Smoother transfer to manufacturing as it is handled by a single organization • Established design process and QMS	• Design capabilities may be limited, as it is not the company's main revenue stream • Typically designed to ensure compatibility with in-house manufacturing, which may result in a suboptimal product

For entrepreneurs, the risk of utilizing either direct hires or individual contractors as the main development resource is usually too high. Only in specific scenarios is it justified; examples include development of a novel technology that requires in-house expertise or having prior experience with a potential hire.

Keys to Evaluating Your Product Engineering Partners

The process of identifying and selecting an engineering partner is the same for both development firms and integrated contract manufacturers. After providing project background information, each firm should provide a detailed breakdown of anticipated development tasks, deliverables, resources necessary, estimated project timeline, budget range, and relevant capabilities.

CHECKLIST TO EVALUATE POTENTIAL PRODUCT DEVELOPMENT CONSULTING RESOURCES

The following are useful questions to raise during the selection process:

QUALITY-RELATED QUESTIONS

1. Is the firm ISO 13485–certified?
2. If the firm performs in-house manufacturing, are they FDA-registered?
3. Is the firm fluent in FDA, MDD, and product testing standards (ISO-14971, IEC-62304, IEC-60601, etc.)?
4. How often does the firm use its internal QMS versus a client's design control process?
5. Has the firm been audited by the FDA pertaining to a client's product? If so, what was the output of the audit(s)?
6. Has the firm established QMS for previous clients? Have those clients used the QMS to submit and receive product clearance by the FDA?
7. What is the firm's process for maintaining project quality/identifying and mitigating risk? (e.g., is there a dedicated director of quality position?; in addition to the project team, would senior management also be regularly involved in the project?)
8. What's the process for client communication?

RELEVANT EXPERIENCE

9. What was the firm's specific role for a relevant project/case study provided?
10. What was the firm's specific role in the relevant project(s), and which project team members are still with the organization?
11. Is the firm experienced in projects with a similar size and scope?
12. What portions of the proposed project will be outsourced, and who are the expected third parties?

13. How many other projects are the intended resources assigned to? Are there known resource conflicts in the future? If so, what mitigations are planned?

14. How does the firm handle costs that stem from development errors?

15. Can the firm provide client references, ideally for a project of similar scope/complexity?

16. How does the firm develop, manage, and share project data such as product CAD files?

17. How does the firm package and transfer product files to its clients and contract manufacturers?

18. Does the firm perform in-house verification testing? If so, what type of equipment is available for use?

WEIGHING THE EVALUATION CRITERIA

The recommendation is to focus more on the firm's capabilities and alignment of a firm's past projects than on the firm's bill rate. The cost of inefficiency, heightened risk, and time delays due to inexperience usually far outweigh variations in rates. There can be noticeable exceptions to this, and so ask for the bill rate structure of each firm. At minimum, limit the vendor search to firms that are ISO 13485–certified, with contract manufacturers that are FDA registered.

KEY TAKEAWAY POINTS

• ► The FDA requires medical devices companies to establish a formal, documented design process as part of a larger QMS.

• ► As the medical device manufacturer, it is your responsibility to generate this formal design process.

• ► There are multiple types of engineering resources available, although external development firms are typically the most appropriate for entrepreneurs, given their broad technical expertise and the ability for entrepreneurs to leverage their QMS.

• ► It is typically more important to find a firm that has prior experience developing similar products than their cost structure or advertised skill sets.

• ► Having a preliminary strategy on how to utilize prototypes for verification and validation activities will significantly increase the project estimates provided by development firms.

CHAPTER 9

Patent Strategy: How Do You Protect Your Intellectual Property?

DAVID J. DYKEMAN, ROBERT A. RABINER

ABOUT THE AUTHORS

David J. Dykeman is a registered patent attorney with over 20 years of experience in patent and intellectual property law and cochair of Greenberg Traurig's global Life Sciences & Medical Technology Group and intellectual property group in Boston. David's practice focuses on securing worldwide intellectual property protection and related business strategy for high-tech clients, with particular experience in orthopedics, medical devices, life sciences, and information technology. David has been named one of the top 250 Patent and Technology Licensing Practitioners in the world by *Intellectual Asset Management* magazine and is the founding chair of the ABA's Medical Devices Committee. David can be reached at dykemand@gtlaw.com or (617) 310-6009.

Robert A. Rabiner is a medical device entrepreneur and the Founder & Chief Technical Officer of IlluminOss Medical, Inc. located in East Providence, RI. Bob has led successful product and corporate enterprise launches, acquired and integrated new technologies, and directed external partnerships at a number of medical device companies. Prior to founding IlluminOss, he was the president of Selva Medical (sold to W.L. Gore in 2006) and was founder, president, and CEO of OmniSonics Medical Technologies. He has also held executive-level positions at American Cyanamid, United States Healthcare and Hospital Products Ltd., Australia. Bob has been a member of the World Economic Forum's Technology Pioneers Program since 2003 and is one of Fast Company's "Fast 50 Champions of Innovation" for his medical technologies. He is the named inventor on over 60 US-issued patents and over 125 issued patents worldwide and has many additional patent applications pending.

The authors wish to acknowledge and thank Brittany Schoenick for her contributions to this chapter.

Introduction

Protecting intellectual property related to orthopedic technologies presents a number of issues that deserve careful consideration. This chapter discusses strategies for orthopedic companies to build a strategic patent portfolio to protect their innovations and get a head start on competition.

Strategic Patent Portfolios

The orthopedic market is growing, and protecting innovations is more important than ever. Revenue in the orthopedic industry reached $48.1 billion worldwide in 2016 and grew at 3.2%, about $1.5 billion over 2015, according to estimates published in the Orthopedic Industry Annual Report.

Patents are extremely important for orthopedic companies in all stages. For early-stage companies, patents are often the only way for investors to place a value on a company's technology, as sales often cannot begin until after FDA approval. In this way, patents make up a significantly greater portion of enterprise value for early-stage medical device companies than other start-ups.

As an orthopedic company grows, patents become the currency to secure financing through venture capital or private equity investment. Patents can also lead to joint ventures, collaborations, and licenses with strategic partners.

For early-stage companies, the key is to develop a strategic patent portfolio, having comprehensive patent coverage around the company's innovations. The core technology must have adequate patent protection to provide technical flexibility and room to operate in a desirable market. To obtain broad patent protection, orthopedic companies should file an initial patent application covering the core technology, followed by additional patent applications covering key improvements. An orthopedic company should consider both current and future business objectives and analyze ways that competitors may attempt to design around its patents. By filing patent applications covering incremental improvements, orthopedic companies can expand their presence in the market and grow both varied and resilient patent portfolio.

Patents are likewise important for later-stage orthopedic companies that are generating revenue. Experts estimate that the average medical device and drug patent can have a net present value of almost US$200,000. Simply put, patents are a source of enterprise value that medical device companies cannot afford to ignore.

In addition to their monetary value, orthopedic patents also hold great strategic value. A strategic patent portfolio can be used both offensively as a sword, to strike out competitors, and defensively as a shield, to avoid competitor attacks. Offensively, the sword prevents competitors from making, using, selling, or importing the patented invention. Defensively, the shield can serve as a bargaining chip against a competitor that threatens to sue for patent infringement.

Patent law is currently in the midst of the biggest reform in the last 60 years with Congress, the executive branch, and the courts all changing the US patent system. The America Invents Act (AIA), passed by Congress and signed into law by President Obama on September 16, 2011, is now fully phased in. With the switch from a "first-to-invent" system to a "first-inventor-to-file" system, the patent, and the rewards, will now truly go to the early bird. This major switch adds a further incentive for companies to speed their development cycle to beat competitors in the race to both the patent office and the market.

In addition to the changes brought about by AIA patent reform, the US Supreme Court is refining the definition of patent eligible subject matter. The US Supreme Court has issued far-reaching opinions, impacting patents in cases such as the following:

- *Bilski v. Kappos,* June 2010: Patentability of a process
- *Mayo Collaborative Services v. Prometheus Laboratories,* March 2012: Patentability of method and diagnostic claims
- *Association for Molecular Pathology v. Myriad Genetics, Inc.,* June 2013: Patentability of genes
- *Alice Corp. v. CLS Bank International,* June 2014: Nonpatentability of abstract ideas and use of a computer

Each of the above US Supreme Court decisions has redefined what subject matter is eligible for patent protection.

Create Strategic Patents: A Timeline

In the light of changing patent environment, companies should get to know the patent "landscape" to determine the best return on their patent investment. Orthopedic companies should work with a patent attorney with a biomedical background who understands their technology and conduct a patent audit to assess the strengths and weaknesses of their current patent portfolio and also determine what competitor patents might pose threats to the company's business plans. Early-stage companies should direct their patent filing strategy to areas of open white space in the patent landscape to receive more valuable patents.

The patent audit should also make sure the company's patent strategy is complete to capture as much open white space in the patent landscape as possible and also plug holes that competitors can design around the company's patents. The patent audit should include a freedom-to-operate analysis of third-party patents to assess potential threats. By ensuring that the patent portfolio is strategic, complete, and up-to-date, the orthopedic company enhances its strength and value in the medical technology marketplace.

Start-ups should file patent applications as early and often as their budget permits. To ensure both US and international patent coverage, a patent application should be filed before any public disclosure.

Figure 9.1 outlines the process of building a patent portfolio, including filing a US provisional application, then filing a US utility application (left side) and a Patent Cooperation Treaty (PCT) international application (right side), and prosecuting the patent applications in the patent office resulting in issued patents.

Filing Patent Applications in the US and Other Countries

A patent portfolio can be an orthopedic company's most valuable asset, but there is a cost to build a strategic patent portfolio. A cost-saving strategy for early-stage companies is to file provisional applications, which provide 1 year of protection, followed by the fully developed US and PCT international patent applications. By filing a provisional patent application, early-stage companies can defer larger costs for up to 1 year and file follow-on provisionals to cover incremental improvements as they build their picket fence of patent protection.

Foreign patent costs can be delayed for an additional 18 months by filing a PCT international patent application. This gives companies time to further develop their product and potentially enter the market to help defray some of the patent costs.

PROVISIONAL PATENT APPLICATIONS

As of June 8, 1995, US law provides for "provisional" applications for patent, as well as regular or "nonprovisional" applications for patent. A provisional application has a life of 1 year and must be followed by a regular application for a patent to issue.

A provisional application establishes a priority date for later-filed regular applications that are based on the provisional. The priority date determines what references qualify as prior art in determining the patentability of the regular application, but does not determine the term of any issued

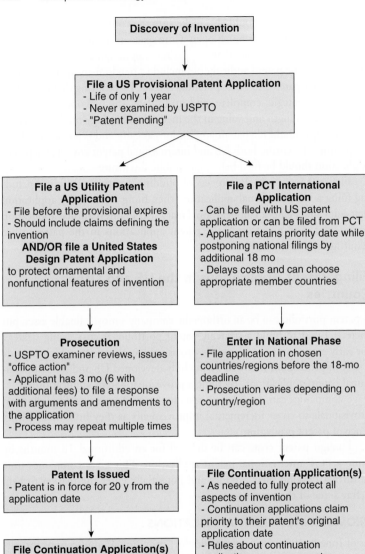

Figure 9.1 The Patent Application Process.

patent. The term of a US patent is 20 years from the actual filing date of the regular application, assuming all patent maintenance fees are paid. When a patent is issued, the provisional application filing date also establishes the date when the patent will be viewed as prior art against other applications.

For a regular application to gain the benefit of a provisional's filing date, certain requirements must be met. First, the regular application must be filed within 12 months of the provisional application. After 12 months, the provisional application is automatically abandoned. Second, each invention claimed in the regular application must be described in the provisional application in sufficient detail to comply with the description requirements of 35 U.S.C. § 112, as well as the drawing requirements of 35 U.S.C. § 113. Third, at least one inventor listed in the regular application must appear in the provisional application. The list of inventors in each application does not need to be identical; each may include inventors not found in the other application.

Other than these three requirements, there is no set form for provisional applications. Provisionals do not have to include claims or an oath or declaration. Provisionals can be of any size or page length, be cumulative of earlier provisional applications, and include multiple inventions.

Because multiple inventions can be placed in the same provisional application, periodic provisional applications may be filed, which include the results of an assortment of current research projects. If it later becomes apparent that some of these results should be patented, regular applications based on the provisional can be filed. This reduces the cost of securing a filing date for inventions of unknown importance.

US UTILITY PATENT APPLICATIONS

Utility applications include at least one claim and are examined by a patent examiner at the United States Patent and Trademark Office (USPTO). Patent examiners are generally well-versed in the basic technology of the patent applications that are assigned to them. A basic requirement for granting a US patent is that the inventor must sufficiently disclose the invention in the patent document so that a person skilled in the applicable art can build and use (or "practice") the invention. To fulfill this "enablement" obligation, the patent application must disclose details of how to make and use the invention. Drawings are also required if they are necessary to understand the subject matter of the invention.

The patent application must conclude with one or more "claims." The claims define the scope of patent protection. Claims must particularly point out and distinctly claim the subject matter of the invention. Generally speaking, the claims can be considered "word pictures" that define the contribution the inventor believes have been made, which will advance the progress of the useful arts. Just as there can be pictures that encompass a broad landscape or pictures that focus on detailed features, patent claims likewise can be broad (to provide wide coverage) or detailed (to focus on narrow improvements).

The patent claims will later determine whether infringement occurs by third parties, and thus the claims define and limit the exclusionary right that is granted to the inventor. In the United States, each and every element (or feature) of the claim, or its equivalent, must be found in the accused structure in order to establish patent infringement. Because of this, it is recommended that an experienced patent attorney drafts claims that allow the company the broadest range of protection.

For example, US Patent No. 9,265,549, entitled "Apparatus for delivery of reinforcing materials to bone," issued on February 23, 2016 with 38 claims including four independent claims covering systems for delivering a bone reinforcing mixture to a fractured bone or a weakened bone and methods for reinforcing a bone. The first page of US Patent No. 9,265,549 is shown on the following page. The patent application was filed in January of 2014 and received two office actions before it was allowed. As an example of the language required for a patent claim, independent claim 1 of the patent is reproduced below:

1. A system for delivering a bone reinforcing mixture to a fractured bone or a weakened bone comprising:

   a catheter having a proximal end, a distal end, and a longitudinal axis therebetween, wherein the catheter has at least one inner lumen for passing a bone reinforcing mixture therethrough;

   a balloon engaging the distal end of the catheter;

   a bone reinforcing mixture contained in the balloon when the balloon is in a cavity of the bone;

   at least one light guide extending through the catheter into the balloon to guide a light into the balloon to illuminate and cure the bone reinforcing mixture contained in the balloon; and

   a device engaging the balloon containing the cured bone reinforcing mixture.

US law requires that the true inventor or inventors be named in the application, and except for circumstances where the inventor refuses to sign or cannot be located, the inventor must personally sign the application and provide a declaration that the invention meets the statutory requirements of 35 U.S.C. § 102.

Prosecution of a US Patent Application

Patent applications, once filed, are assigned a serial number and sent to a particular examining group within the USPTO based on the technology. The patents are eventually assigned to an individual patent examiner who will review the application for the statutory requirements of sufficiency of disclosure and other formal requirements.

The patent examiner will conduct a search of prior patents and technical references (prior art) available at the USPTO to determine whether or not the claims of the patent application define an inventive advance, or "inventive step" over the prior art sufficient to merit the grant of a patent. Any previously disclosed, public inventions by an inventor may be construed as prior art against any subsequent inventions. After conducting a search and evaluating the application and prior art, the patent examiner will issue a written "office action," which points out any and all deficiencies of the patent application. The applicant is then entitled 3 months (or 6 with the payment of additional government fees) to respond to the office action with written amendments and/or arguments as to why the application meets the requirements for patentability and to request reconsideration of the application. The examiner may agree with or deny the applicant's arguments and may allow the application or issue a new office action.

The average amount of time from filing a patent application to issuing the patent (if a patent issues at all) can be 2 to 5 years. To address the large patent application backlog and demand for quicker patent issuance, the USPTO began offering Track One accelerated examination in 2012, which promises a final decision on patentability within 12 months for those applications paying a higher government fee.

Figure 9.2 is the first page of earlier referenced US Patent No. 9,265,549 owned by IlluminOss Medical, Inc., a clinical-stage medical device company revolutionizing orthopedic surgery. In addition to the US patent, foreign patents in the patent family have also been granted in 14 foreign countries including Europe (validated in 9 countries), Australia, Canada, China, Hong Kong, and Japan.

INTERNATIONAL PATENT FILINGS

Filing international patent applications further strengthens a patent portfolio and expands a company's presence in the global marketplace. Although foreign patent applications can be expensive, filing in strategic countries can be crucial to the commercial success of a medical product. North America currently dominates the global orthopedic device market. Although bioabsorbable implants, a growing elderly population, and increasing obesity in

US009265549B2

(12) **United States Patent**
Rabiner

(10) **Patent No.:** **US 9,265,549 B2**
(45) **Date of Patent:** **Feb. 23, 2016**

(54) **APPARATUS FOR DELIVERY OF REINFORCING MATERIALS TO BONE**

(71) Applicant: **IlluminOss Medical, Inc.**, East Providence, RI (US)

(72) Inventor: **Robert A. Rabiner**, Tiverton, RI (US)

(73) Assignee: **IlluminOss Medical, Inc.**, East Providence, RI (US)

(*) Notice: Subject to any disclaimer, the term of this patent is extended or adjusted under 35 U.S.C. 154(b) by 69 days.

(21) Appl. No.: **14/164,846**

(22) Filed: **Jan. 27, 2014**

(65) **Prior Publication Data**

US 2014/0142581 A1   May 22, 2014

Related U.S. Application Data

(63) Continuation of application No. 13/561,249, filed on Jul. 30, 2012, now Pat. No. 8,668,701, which is a continuation of application No. 12/875,460, filed on Sep. 3, 2010, now Pat. No. 8,246,628, which is a

(Continued)

(51) **Int. Cl.**
A61B 17/88 (2006.01)
A61B 17/72 (2006.01)
(Continued)

(52) **U.S. Cl.**
CPC *A61B 17/8822* (2013.01); *A61B 17/7275* (2013.01); *A61B 17/7291* (2013.01); *A61B 17/8816* (2013.01); *A61B 17/8836* (2013.01);
(Continued)

(58) **Field of Classification Search**
CPC A61B 17/7275; A61B 17/7291; A61B 17/8822; A61B 17/8836; A61B 17/8816; A61B 17/7097; A61B 17/8897; A61B 19/5202

USPC 606/62, 63, 13, 92 95, 108. 192; 600/101, 116. 178
See application file for complete search history.

(56) **References Cited**

U.S. PATENT DOCUMENTS

4,271,839 A   6/1981 Fogarty et al.
4,280,233 A   7/1981 Raab
(Continued)

FOREIGN PATENT DOCUMENTS

DE   40 28 466   3/1992
EP   0 709 698   5/1996
(Continued)

OTHER PUBLICATIONS

USPTO Office Action in U.S. Appl. No. 13/335,110 mailed Jul. 31, 2014.
(Continued)

Primary Examiner — Pedro Philogene
(74) *Attorney, Agent, or Firm* — Greenberg Traurig, LLP; David J. Dykeman; Roman Fayerberg

(57) **ABSTRACT**

An apparatus and methods for delivery of reinforcing materials to a weakened or fractured bone is disclosed. An apparatus for delivering a reinforcing mixture to a bone including a tube having a proximal end, a distal end, and a longitudinal axis therebetween. wherein the tube has at least one inner lumen capable of allowing a bone reinforcing mixture to pass therethrough; a balloon engaging the tube wherein the balloon expands from a substantially deflated state to a substantially inflated state upon the bone reinforcing mixture entering the balloon; and at least one light guide extending through the tube into the balloon to guide a light into the balloon.

38 Claims, 18 Drawing Sheets

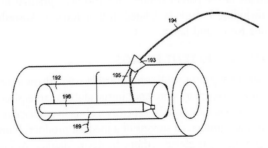

Figure 9.2 Initial page of US Patent No. 9,265,549 owned by IlluminOss Medical, Inc.

the United States will contribute to North America's continued leadership in the market, Europe is the second largest regional market for orthopedic devices, with increasing demand for drug-eluting stents and infusion pumps. Additionally, industry analysts predict that the Asia-Pacific market will be the fastest growing region in the world for orthopedic devices and is expected to reach $7 billion by 2022. Thus, orthopedic companies should consider patenting in the United States, Europe, Asia, and other countries of interest.

The United States is a member of two treaties: the Paris Convention of 1883 and the Patent Cooperation Treaty, both of which ease the application of international patents. The Paris Convention allows member countries from around the world to accept patent applications from citizens of 200 other member countries. The PCT is a central processing system used as an intermediate-stage patent application process. A single filing in the PCT system reserves an applicant's right to file the same application in any of the 152 PCT member nations.

The PCT can be entered upon filing of the original patent application or just before the end of the priority year. If a PCT is filed before the end of the priority year, the PCT will claim the benefit of the first-priority filing date. The applicant then has 30 months from the earliest priority date to exit the PCT system and file patent applications in the desired foreign countries.

The PCT international application acts as an effective temporary placeholder, allowing the applicant to delay foreign filing for 18 months while still retaining a priority date from the initial PCT application, allowing the applicant to keep the rights to the patent application while delaying cost expenditures as long as possible. During this time, an applicant may gain more knowledge about foreign markets and their own technology, allowing the applicant to submit a better application in only the countries that are the best fit for the product. This may be where the applicant expects to sell the product, in countries where there may be a prospect of licensing the patent rights or in countries where infringement is common.

Patent applications must be filed in each jurisdiction (country or region) where protection is needed. Costs increase with each application filed, so it is important to know where to allocate capital ahead of time. A company should consider filing in specific countries with a large target market for the product, countries where competitors' manufacturing facilities are located, and countries that export medical products to other regions through distribution channels. It is also important to consider the future: while a patent is in force for its 20-year term, a country's economy and markets may dramatically change.

It is also important to keep in mind that although some countries or jurisdictions such as Europe have an arguably quicker and less-expensive patent system, patent law and practice vary widely per country. For example, significant differences exist in the permitted number and structure of claims. These differences need to be navigated carefully to secure patent rights. Other jurisdictions, such as China, Korea, and Japan, have similar local differences and also require translations, which can add to the cost of applying for and prosecuting patents in these countries.

Although local differences may appear to be a deterrent to file patents internationally, it is still an important step to take to expand an orthopedic company's patent portfolio. The easiest way to navigate the international patent waters is to engage a strong patent attorney who has the ability to find and coordinate local patent attorneys in each country or jurisdiction of filing.

Additional Strategic Options

DESIGN PATENTS: DIFFERENCES BETWEEN DESIGN PATENT AND UTILITY PATENTS

When developing patent portfolios, design patents are often overlooked in favor of utility patents. Design patents may supplement a utility patent portfolio by providing additional protection covering the appearance of a medical device. For example, design patents can cover the appearance of femoral hip prostheses, an intramedullary nail, and even medical device packaging. Although generally having a more limited scope of protection, design patents can still deter potential infringers in the United States and foreign countries. For example, in a recent case involving smart phones, a substantial portion of the plaintiff's billion-dollar verdict was based on the infringement of design patents. Design patents may play an important role in protecting the orthopedic company's innovations and creating competitive advantages.

Both utility and design patents grant the owner the right to exclude others from making, using, selling, offering for sale, or importing the patented invention in the United States. Both utility and design patents also conclude with at least one claim that provides a concise legal definition of the invention. However, in most aspects, design patents and utility patents are very different.

Design patents protect the ornamental or nonfunctional features of a product. Design patents have no written description and are limited to one claim. The claim of the design patent covers only the exact product shown in the drawings. Design patents expire 15 years from the issue date. Design patents also do not require any maintenance fees after issuance. Design patents typically provide a more limited coverage than utility patents but are quicker, easier, and less expensive to obtain than utility patents.

Owing to these differences between the two patent types, design patents may supplement protection provided by utility patents, creating comprehensive product coverage.

LICENSING PATENTS

Licensing a proven technology is a quick way to begin building a patent portfolio. Orthopedic companies can license technology that is already patented from academic institutions and research hospitals. Licensing such technology not only comes with an existing patent portfolio but also can minimize the risks associated with new technologies and shorten the time to market. The inventors may have already tested the technology, established the proof of concept, and will likely be available to perform further research to improve the technology or serve as scientific advisors to the company.

Large medical device companies are another potential source to obtain proven technologies with patent protection. Often, large orthopedic companies own patented technologies that they are no longer pursuing for business reasons or anything related to the technology itself. Many promising technologies are sitting on the shelves of large orthopedic companies. Licensing such technology can benefit the large medical device company as well as the early-stage orthopedic company. The large company can recoup expenses incurred in connection with research and development of the licensed technology and reduce risks associated with further development and testing by effectively outsourcing these functions to the licensee. If the technology is successful, the large company can acquire it back or receive a royalty. At the same time, the early-stage company acquires rights to a technology that has already been tested and patent protected to some extent.

Cross-licensing with competitors is another method to enhance a patent portfolio. Cross-licensing opportunities arise when companies have overlapping patents, and practicing one patent results in the infringement of another patent. With cross-licensing, companies can mutually agree to share patents without the exchange of license fees and with a promise not to sue.

Ideally, start-ups should try to obtain an exclusive license with no (or a low) up-front payment and reasonable royalties tied to actual product sales, which may not begin for a number of years. Hospitals and research institutions are usually willing to negotiate a patent license because their primary mission is treating patients and curing disease, not forming start-up medical companies.

COMBINATION PRODUCTS

A growing trend in orthopedic patient treatment is combination products that combine biologics, drugs, and medical devices to improve treatment. By combining technologies, combination products provide patients with more targeted and specialized treatments that can improve the efficacy, safety, and delivery of medicines while minimizing side effects.

Combination products, however, face several unique hurdles in entering the marketplace. A sophisticated patent and regulatory strategy that emphasizes the benefits of converging technologies is necessary to succeed in the growing combination products market.

In orthopedics, bone fracture fixation devices combine biologics and orthopedic implants to regenerate bone growth. Hip implants can also be coated with anti-infective compounds to prevent infections. Additionally, combination products may combine diagnostics and therapeutics to predict, regulate, and monitor pathological responses. As new device and biologic combinations are created, vast opportunities and benefits exist for companies willing to develop complex combination products.

Implementing comprehensive patent coverage for combination products requires sophisticated and effective patent counsel. Because patent attorneys generally specialize in either biologics or medical devices, two separate attorneys may be needed to handle combination products. Ideally, these patent attorneys should work together in the same firm to fully and effectively prosecute patents directed toward each aspect of the product. Finding sophisticated patent counsel for combination products may be challenging but is crucial for maximizing patent coverage. Conducting a freedom-to-operate search early in the development process may assist the company in determining whether and how a company can market its combination product.

Problems and Pitfalls

INFRINGEMENT

Utility Patent Infringement, Remedies, and Damages

When an orthopedic company believes a third-party competitor is infringing one of its patents, the company should compare the infringing product sold in the market to the company's issued patent claims. A prefiling analysis should be conducted before any claims of infringement are filed to ensure patent claims are valid. All elements of the claim must be found in each alleged infringing product, either literally, or through what is known as the doctrine of equivalents.

Anyone can be sued who makes, uses, manufactures, or sells an infringing device. Contributory infringement can also be found under 35 U.S.C. 271(c) by whoever knowingly offers to sell or sells a component of a patent that constitutes a material part of the invention. The plaintiff must be the owner(s) of the patent unless substantially all rights have been licensed to a nonowner.

A company will want to work with an experienced patent litigator to determine the best possible venue for a legal suit. Some jurisdictions move quickly or slowly with respect to patent suits. Some jurisdictions favor local tendencies on certain issues, such as finding subject matter invalidity for software inventions. Other jurisdictions are more plaintiff-friendly. An experienced patent attorney should have a strategy for the best jurisdiction to accomplish the desired outcomes.

There are many possible defenses to a patent infringement cause of action. These include showing the patent has failed to clear at lease one of the requirements for patentability, patent misuse, inequitable conduct, laches, intentional delay in prosecution, or any number of infringement exemptions. These exemptions may fall under permitted research uses, regulatory uses, government uses, sovereign immunity, or patent exhaustion. A party may request a variety of different remedies such as destruction of the infringing product, an injunction to stop the infringing action, monetary damages, and equitable remedies and attorney fees. As patent litigation is one of the most intensive types of litigation, it is best to consult with an experienced patent attorney if this is on the company's horizon.

PATENT TROLLS

Patent trolls have recently invaded the medical technology industry, including orthopedics. Also known as patent assertion entities or nonpracticing entities (NPEs), patent trolls are businesses that acquire patents for the purpose of collecting royalties from companies whose products or practices allegedly infringe patents owned by the NPE.

Recently, patent trolls have become a bigger problem in medtech. Expect more patent troll lawsuits to be filed accusing medtech companies of patent infringement. Prudent medtech companies that receive demand letters or know of competitors that have received demand letters will weigh their options with legal counsel experienced in both medtech and NPE litigation. Congress may come to the rescue, but with millions of dollars at stake, do not expect NPEs to cede the battle quickly. The medtech industry would be wise to prepare for the patent trolls to invade medtech.

Conclusion

In the dynamic orthopedic market, a strong patent portfolio is crucial for securing investment and gaining market share. By working with a strategic and business-minded patent attorney, orthopedic companies can take advantage of the changing patent landscape to stake bigger claims in the orthopedic patent gold rush.

KEY TAKEAWAY POINTS

- ▶ Orthopedic companies should consider both current and future business objectives and contemplate ways that competitors may attempt to design around its patents.

- ▶ Failure to file a patent application prior to public disclosure will result in the loss of potential international patent rights.

- ▶ By filing a provisional patent application, early-stage companies can defer larger costs for up to 1 year and file follow-on provisionals to cover incremental improvements as they build their patent portfolio.

- ▶ Using the PCT international application process to defer a patent application while maintaining the priority date allows an applicant to keep the rights alive and options open while delaying expenditures as much as possible.

- ▶ Prudent medical device makers will hire experienced patent counsel to both protect their innovations from being appropriated by others and to provide freedom-to-operate opinions that allow orthopedic companies to avoid existing prior art.

BIBLIOGRAPHY

1. Patent Process Overview." United States Patent and Trademark Office. https://www.uspto.gov/patents-getting-started/patent-process-overview#step1.
2. Protecting Intellectual Property Rights (IPR) Overseas." United States Patent and Trademark Office. https://www.uspto.gov/patents-getting-started/international-protection/protecting-intellectual-property-rights-ipr.
3. *Patenting Strategies for Medtech Startups.*" Medical Design & Outsourcing. April 27, 2017. https://www.medicaldesignandoutsourcing.com/qa-patenting-strategies-medtech-startups/.
4. *5 Tips to Protect Your Medtech Startup's Innovations.*" Mass Device. April 17, 2018. https://www.medicaldesignandoutsourcing.com/5-steps-protect-medtech-startup-innovations/.
5. *Design Patents Provide Additional Protection for Products.*" Medical Design & Outsourcing. February 6, 2016. https://www.medicaldesignandoutsourcing.com/design-patents-provide-additional-protection-for-products/.

6. *The 5 Biggest Issues in Patenting Combo Products.*" Medical Design & Outsourcing. January 25, 2018. https://www.medicaldesignandoutsourcing.com/5-biggest-issues-patenting-combo-products/.

7. *Building a Strategic Patent Portfolio.*" MD+DI. August 21, 2015. https://www.mddionline.com/building-strategic-patent-portfolio.

8. David J. Dykeman Greenberg Traurig Biography. https://www.gtlaw.com/en/professionals/d/dykeman-david-j.

CHAPTER 10

Regulatory Basics: What Does It Take to Start Selling Your Device?

BECKY DITTY, RAHUL RAM

ABOUT THE AUTHORS

Becky Ditty, MS, is a consultant with the Biologics Consulting Group in Alexandria, Virginia. Prior to consulting, Ms Ditty worked for over 14 years for a leading medical device manufacturer. During that time, she was in various regulatory positions and supported research and development teams focus in areas such as computer-assisted surgery, interventional spine, and general surgical devices.

Rahul Ram is a consultant with the Biologics Consulting Group in Alexandria, Virginia. Prior to consulting, Mr Ram spent approximately 8 years as a scientific reviewer in various divisions in the Office of Device Evaluation (ODE), Center for Devices and Radiological Health (CDRH), and Food and Drug Administration (FDA).

Introduction

The orthopedic medical device manufacturer must comply with federal rules prior to marketing their devices to potential customers.

The labyrinthine web of laws, regulations, guidance documents, legal precedents, and references to the Food and Drug Administration (FDA; the federal agency responsible for enforcing federal medical device rules) may be intimidating to the newly initiated.

The purpose of this chapter is to provide a high-level overview of these rules and demonstrate that there is a simple way to make sense of them.

The beginning of this chapter is organized into the following areas:

- "Do I even need to follow FDA medical device rules?"
- *Background*: FDA Organization & FDA Rules
- "Which FDA device rules should I follow?" (All Devices)
- *Background:* FDA Medical Device Classification

- "Which FDA device rules should I follow?" (Class I Devices)
- "Which FDA device rules should I follow?" (Class II Devices)
- "Which FDA device rules should I follow?" (Class III Devices)
- "How do I comply with the FDA device rules that apply to me?"

The middle of this chapter discusses how to comply with specific FDA device rules, and the end of this chapter contains industry resources and references.

Do I Even Need to Follow FDA Medical Device Rules?

By far, most of the federal rules that the manufacturer must follow are FDA medical device rules, *if the orthopedic product is a medical device.*

WHAT IS A MEDICAL DEVICE?

A "medical device," as defined by the Federal Food, Drug, and Cosmetic (FD&C) Act (the watershed medical device legislation), is the following:

…an instrument, apparatus, implement, machine, contrivance, implant, in vitro reagent, or other similar or related article, including a component part, or accessory which is: recognized in the official National Formulary, or the United States Pharmacopoeia, or any supplement to them, intended for use in the diagnosis of disease or other conditions, or in the cure, mitigation, treatment, or prevention of disease, in man or other animals, or intended to affect the structure or any function of the body of man or other animals, and which does not achieve any of it's primary intended purposes through chemical action within or on the body of man or other animals and which is not dependent upon being metabolized for the achievement of any of its primary intended purposes

In summary, a medical device is a product that is used for medical diagnosis and/or treatment, or is intended to otherwise affect the human body and is not a drug or biologic.

If the product is *not* used for medical diagnosis or treatment and is *not* intended to otherwise affect the human body, *the product is probably not an FDA-regulated product and FDA rules would not apply.* If the product is used for medical diagnosis but is either a drug or biologic, FDA medical device rules most likely *do not* apply, but FDA drug and/or biologic rules *will* apply (FDA drug and biologic rules are not discussed here).

The determination as to whether a product is a medical device (and thus FDA medical device rules apply) is not to be taken lightly. To help manufacturers make this decision, FDA's Division of Industry and Consumer

Education (DICE) is available for free consultation. DICE is most easily available via call:

- Toll-free: +1 (800) 638-2041
- Local: +1 (301) 796-7100
- Hours of Operation:
  - 9:00 to 12:30 PM ET
  - 1:00 to 4:30 PM ET

BACKGROUND: FDA ORGANIZATION AND FDA RULES

The orthopedic device manufacturer has determined, based upon the FD&C Act definition, perhaps in consultation with FDA's DICE, that their product is a medical device.

Before we go any further, it is important to know some background regarding FDA and FDA rules.

FDA is a federal executive branch agency charged with regulating foods, drugs, cosmetics, and medical devices in the United States. To do so, FDA promulgates and enforces wide-reaching rules applicable to medical product manufacturers.

The following is a list of the different forms that FDA rules may take:

- **FDA-related laws:** laws are binding but are not generally written in practical terms. Laws are operationalized when they are translated into "regulations."
- **FDA-related regulations:** once a law is passed, it is translated into a set of binding regulations, which are codified in the Code of Federal Regulations ("CFR"). The CFR is organized into "titles"; Title 21 contains all FDA-related regulations. Titles are organized into "parts"; Parts 800-1299 ("21 CFR 800-21 CFR 1299") contain most FDA regulations related to that cover medical devices. Regulations specific to orthopedic devices are in Part 888 ("21 CFR 888").
- **FDA guidance documents:** guidance documents are publicly available (via FDA's website) sets of "recommendations" that represent FDA's current thinking on a topic. Though the recommendations of guidance documents are not binding, it is most practical to follow them.

Figure 10.1 is a reproduction of the current FDA organizational chart from the FDA website (https://www.fda.gov/AboutFDA/CentersOffices/OrganizationCharts/ucm393155.htm):

As per the diagram above, FDA is organized into 14 offices. The relevant FDA office for the orthopedic medical device manufacturer is the Office of Medical Products and Tobacco (OMPT). OMPT is further

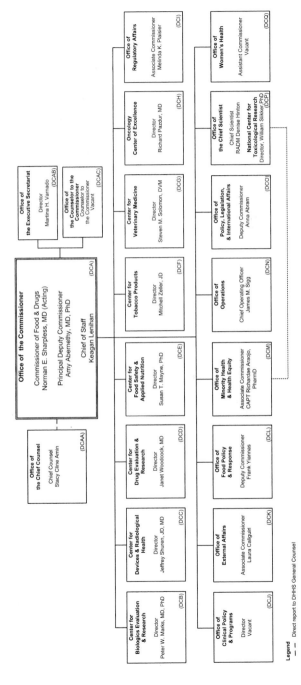

July 2019

Department Of Health And Human Services
Food And Drug Administration

Office of the Commissioner
Commissioner of Food & Drugs
Norman E. Sharpless, MD (Acting)

Principal Deputy Commissioner
Amy Abernethy, MD, PhD

Chief of Staff
Keagan Lenihan
(DCA)

Office of the Executive Secretariat
Director
Martina H. Varnado
(DCAB)

Office of the Counselor to the Commissioner
Counselor to the Commissioner
Vacant
(DCAC)

Office of the Chief Counsel
Chief Counsel
Stacy Cline Amin
(DCAA)

Center for Biologics Evaluation & Research
Director
Peter W. Marks, MD, PhD
(DCB)

Center for Devices & Radiological Health
Director
Jeffrey Shuren, JD, MD
(DCC)

Center for Drug Evaluation & Research
Director
Janet Woodcock, MD
(DCD)

Center for Food Safety & Applied Nutrition
Director
Susan T. Mayne, PhD
(DCE)

Center for Tobacco Products
Director
Mitchell Zeller, JD
(DCF)

Center for Veterinary Medicine
Director
Steven M. Solomon, DVM
(DCG)

Oncology Center of Excellence
Director
Richard Pazdur, MD
(DCH)

Office of Regulatory Affairs
Associate Commissioner
Melinda K. Plaisier
(DCI)

Office of Clinical Policy & Programs
Director
Vacant
(DCJ)

Office of External Affairs
Associate Commissioner
Laura Caliguiri
(DCK)

Office of Food Policy & Response
Deputy Commissioner
Frank Yiannas
(DCL)

Office of Minority Health & Health Equity
Associate Commissioner
CAPT Richardae Araojo, PharmD
(DCM)

Office of Operations
Chief Operating Officer
James M. Sigg
(DCN)

Office of Policy, Legislation, & International Affairs
Deputy Commissioner
Anna Abram
(DCO)

Office of the Chief Scientist
Chief Scientist
RADM Denise Hinton

National Center for Toxicological Research
Director: William Slikker PhD
(OCP)

Office of Women's Health
Assistant Commissioner
Vacant
(DCQ)

Legend
— —   Direct report to DHHS General Counsel
••••••   Formally reports to The Commissioner but day-to-day oversight is from Office of The Chief Scientist

Figure 10.1 FDA organizational chart.

organized into offices and centers; the relevant center for the orthopedic medical device manufacturer is the Center for Devices and Radiological Health (CDRH). CDRH enforces medical device regulations and writes medical device–related guidance documents.

WHAT FDA RULES SHOULD I FOLLOW? (RULES APPLICABLE TO ALL DEVICES)

Now that we know something about the organization of FDA and what forms FDA rules may take, what now?

The next task is to take stock of all FDA medical device rules that may apply.

The following set of FDA medical device rules apply to *all* medical devices (each of these types of rules is described in more detail at the end of the chapter):

- FDA "general controls":
  - Quality System Regulation (QSR): ensuring that the device manufacturer adheres to the principles of "quality"
  - UDI (unique device identifier): ensuring that medical devices (or their packaging) are labeled with an FDA-formatted identifier for tracking
  - Establishment registration and listing: updating FDA with current device manufacturing site(s) and updating FDA with a current list of marketed devices
  - Reporting, recalls, corrections, and removals: ensuring that FDA is kept current with events related to the medical device after being placed on the market

In addition to the set of rules above, there are four more sets of rules to consider (listed below):

- FDA device rules applicable to "class I" devices
- FDA device rules applicable to "class II" devices
- FDA device rules applicable to "class III" devices

To determine which rules sets apply to the orthopedic medical device, it is important to know something regarding device classification.

Background: FDA Medical Device Classification

FDA classifies medical devices into three classes:

- Class I (lowest risk)
- Class II (medium risk)
- Class III (highest risk)

Depending on the device class, different FDA device rules apply. Therefore, the device manufacturer must determine whether the device is class I, II, or III. The process of determining this is provided in more detail in Chapter 14.

The next three sections list FDA device rules that apply to a certain device class.

WHAT FDA RULES SHOULD I FOLLOW? (CLASS I DEVICES)

If the orthopedic medical device is class I (see Chapter 14 for more how to determine classification), the manufacturer must comply with the following types of FDA rules:

- FDA "general controls" (mentioned above; described in detail at the end of this chapter)

WHAT FDA RULES SHOULD I FOLLOW? (CLASS II DEVICES)

If the orthopedic medical device is class II (see Chapter 14 for more how to determine classification), the manufacturer must comply with the following types of FDA rules:

- FDA "general controls" (mentioned above; describe in detail at the end of this chapter)
- FDA "special controls" (described further below)
- FDA premarket notification ("510(k)") regulations (described further below)

WHAT FDA RULES SHOULD I FOLLOW? (CLASS III DEVICES)

If the orthopedic medical device is class III (see Chapter 14 for more how to determine classification), the manufacturer must comply with the following types of FDA rules:

- FDA "general controls" (mentioned above; describe in detail at the end of this chapter)
- FDA premarket approval ("PMA") regulations (described further below)

How Do I Comply With the FDA Device Rules That Apply to Me?

The remainder of this chapter is explanations of how to comply with FDA device rules. Some of the rules listed below depend upon the device class; it is important for the orthopedic medical device manufacturer to identify the class (i.e., I, II, or III) of their devices (please see Chapter 14 for more information on classification).

The next grouping of sections in this chapter discusses how to comply with the specific sets of FDA rules introduced above. These sections are the following:

- General Controls (for All Devices)—*Quality System Regulation*
- General Controls (for All Devices)—*UDI (Unique Device Identifier)*
- General Controls (for All Devices)—*Establishment Registration and Listing*
- General Controls (for All Devices)—*Medical Device Reporting*
- General Controls (for All Devices)—*Recalls, Corrections, and Removals*
- Special Controls (for Class II Devices Only)
- Premarket Notification ("510(k)") Regulations (for Class II Devices Only)
  - The De Novo Process
- Premarket Approval Regulations (for Class III Devices Only)

General Controls (for all Devices)—*Quality System Regulation*

Quality system regulations (QSRs), formerly good manufacturing practices (GMPs), provide a minimum framework of regulations that a manufacturer must comply with for the lifecycle of medical devices. The **QSR** is defined in 21 CFR 820 and includes 15 subparts, as identified below:

- General Provisions
- Quality System Requirements
- Design Controls
- Document Controls
- Purchasing Controls
- Identification and Traceability
- Production and Process Controls
- Acceptance Activities
- Nonconforming Product
- Corrective and Preventative Action
- Labeling and Packaging Control
- Handling, Storage, Distribution, and Installation
- Records
- Servicing, and
- Statistical Techniques

The specific subsections of the QSR that a manufacturer must implement are dependent on the activities the manufacturer performs and the types of medical devices manufactured. Some class I devices, such as tracheal tube cleaning brush (product code EPE) and nonsterile toothbrushes (product code EFW), are exempt from a majority of the QSRs. To determine if a class I device is exempt from the quality system requirements, either wholly or in part, search for the device's specific product code in the FDA's classification database (https://www.accessdata.fda.gov/scripts/cdrh/cfdocs/cfpcd/classification.cfm). The results identify if the product is GMP exempt. The results also identify if, even though the device is GMP exempt, the device must still comply with portions of the GMP, such as the records (820.180) and complaint file (820.198) requirements.

General Controls (for all Devices)—UDI (Unique Device Identifier)

In September 2013, the final rule for unique device identification requirements was established. The rule requires devices to be marked and labeled with a **unique device identifier** (UDI). The UDI requirements are being phased in over multiple years (Table 10.1). By 2022, the system will be fully implemented. UDI requirements are detailed in 21 CFR 830 Unique Device Identification and 21 CFR 801 Labeling.

Unique device identification requires that a devices package label includes the UDI in human-readable (plain text) and machine-readable (AIDC) format. For certain device classifications,e.g., implantable, life-supporting, life-sustaining, and reusable class III devices, the device itself must be marked with the UDI. The UDI is composed of two parts:

- Device Identifier—a mandatory, fixed portion of a UDI that identifies the labeler and the specific version or model of a device
- Production Identifier—a conditional, variable portion of a UDI that identifies one or more of the following when included on the label of the device:
  - the lot or batch number within which a device was manufactured,
  - the serial number of a specific device,
  - the expiration date of a specific device,
  - the date a specific device was manufactured, and
  - the distinct identification code required by §1271.290(c) for a human cell, tissue, or cellular and tissue-based product (HCT/P) regulated as a device.[2]

Some devices are exempt from UDI requirements, such as devices used in research and custom devices within the meaning of 21 CFR 812.3(b), and class I devices exempt from GMP requirements. For a complete list, refer to 21 CFR 801.30, 801.128(f)(2), and 801.45. A labeler may also

Table 10.1 UDI Compliance Dates[1]

Compliance Date	Requirement
1 y after publication of the final rule (September 24, 2014)	The labels and packages of class III medical devices and devices licensed under the Public Health Service Act (PHS Act) must bear a UDI. § 801.20. Dates on the labels of these devices must be formatted as required by § 801.18. Data for these devices must be submitted to the GUDID database. § 830.300. A 1-y extension of this compliance date may be requested under § 801.55; such a request must be submitted no later than June 23, 2014. Class III stand-alone software must provide its UDI as required by § 801.50(b).
2 y after publication of the final rule (September 24, 2015)	The labels and packages of implantable, life-supporting, and life-sustaining devices must bear a UDI. § 801.20. Dates on the labels of these devices must be formatted as required by § 801.18. A life-supporting or life-sustaining device that is required to be labeled with a UDI must bear a UDI as a permanent marking on the device itself if the device is intended to be used more than once and intended to be reprocessed before each use. § 801.45. Stand-alone software that is a life-supporting or life-sustaining device must provide its UDI as required by § 801.50(b). Data for implantable, life-supporting, and life-sustaining devices that are required to be labeled with a UDI must be submitted to the GUDID database. § 830.300.
3 y after publication of the final rule (September 24, 2016)	Class III devices required to be labeled with a UDI must bear a UDI as a permanent marking on the device itself if the device is intended to be used more than once and intended to be reprocessed before each use. § 801.45. The labels and packages of class II medical devices must bear a UDI. § 801.20. Dates on the labels of these devices must be formatted as required by § 801.18. Class II stand-alone software must provide its UDI as required by § 801.50(b). Data for class II devices that are required to be labeled with a UDI must be submitted to the GUDID database. § 830.300.

Table 10.1 UDI Compliance Dates[1]—Cont'd	
Compliance Date	Requirement
5 y after publication of the final rule (September 24, 2018)	A class II device that is required to be labeled with a UDI must bear a UDI as a permanent marking on the device itself if the device is intended to be used more than once and intended to be reprocessed before each use. § 801.45.
	The labels and packages of class I medical devices and devices that have not been classified into class I, class II, or class III must bear a UDI. § 801.20. Dates on the labels of all devices, including devices that have been excepted from UDI labeling requirements, must be formatted as required by § 801.18.
	Data for class I devices and devices that have not been classified into class I, class II, or class III that are required to be labeled with a UDI must be submitted to the GUDID database. § 830.300. Class I stand-alone software must provide its UDI as required by § 801.50(b).
7 y after publication of the final rule (September 24, 2020)	Class I devices and devices that have not been classified into class I, class II, or class III that are required to be labeled with a UDI must bear a UDI as a permanent marking on the device itself if the device is intended to be used more than once and intended to be reprocessed before each use. § 801.45.

Compliance dates for all other provisions of the final rule. Except for the provisions listed above, FDA requires full compliance with the final rule as of the effective date that applies to the provision.

request an exemption from the UDI requirements, as described in 21 CFR 801.55. FDA provides many resources to assist with UDI. Refer to FDA's website: Unique Device Identification—UDI or UDI Resources.

The main benefit of the UDI system is to facilitate a more accurate postmarket surveillance system, including adverse event reports and device recalls.

General Controls (for all Devices)—*Establishment Registration and Listing*

Most establishment (facilities) involved in the production and **commercial distribution** of medical devices to or within the United States is required to annually register and list the establishment and the activities the establishment performs on medical devices with the FDA. The registration process is the method the FDA uses to understand which establishments are performing regulated activities and should be periodically audited. Listing medical devices is the method the FDA uses to understand the type of devices an establishment is performing regulated activities on and the risk classification of those devices. Establishments performing activities on higher classification device types are audited by the FDA on a more frequent basis.

21 CFR Part 807 defines registration and device listing and also identifies which activities require a company to register. For example, all manufacturers, contract manufactures, contract sterilizers, and repackagers and relabelers must register. For a full list, refer to 21 CFR 807.20 or FDA website "Who must register, list, and pay the fee."

Unless an establishment has been granted a waiver from the FDA, the registration process must be performed electronically. Registration is completed in two steps. A company must first pay the registration fee using the Device Facility User Fee website (https://userfees.fda.gov/OA_HTML/furls.jsp?legalsel=2&ref=). The registration establishment fee is dependent on the fiscal year. For example, the establishment registration fee for 2018 is $4,624.

Once the company has paid the registration fee, the company must register and list via the FDA's Unified Registration and Listing System (FURLS)/Device Registration and Listing Module (DRLM) at https://www.access.fda.gov/oaa/logonFlow.htm?execution=e1s1). Foreign establishments that are required to register with the FDA must also designate a US agent. The US agent must reside in the United States and if requested, is responsible for assisting the FDA by communicating with the registered company (also known as the establishment or facility).

General Controls (for all Devices)—*Medical Device Reporting*

Once a device is marketed in the United States, device-related adverse events (21 CFR 803) must be captured and reported to the FDA by **Manufactures**, **Importers** and **Device User Facilities**. These reports are referred to as Medical Device Reporting (MDR).

- Manufacturer are required to submit device malfunctions that caused, contributed, or if repeated could cause or contribute to a death or serious injury. If the adverse event requires immediate remedial action to prevent unreasonable risk of substantial harm to the public, the event must be reported within 5 working days. Otherwise, manufactures must report adverse events within 30 days. Manufacturers submit MDRs to the FDA electronically through the FDA eMDR system.

- Importers must report adverse events relating to death or serious injuries to the FDA and the device manufacturer within 30 days of becoming aware of the event. Malfunctions must be reported only to the manufacture within 30 days. Importers also submit MDRs via the FDA eMDR system.

- Device User Facilities must report device-related deaths and device-related serious injuries (if the manufacturer is known) to the FDA and manufacturer within 10 days of the event. Device user facilities must also provide an annual report of device-related deaths and serious injuries to the FDA.

General Controls (for all Devices)—*Recalls, Corrections, and Removals*

Recalls, corrections, and removals are methods used to correct misbranded or adulterated devices that have been distributed.

- **Recalls** (21 CFR 7): a firm's removal or correction of a marketed product that the FDA considers to be in violation of the laws it administers and against which the agency would initiate legal action,e.g., seizure. Recall does not include a market withdrawal or a stock recovery. Typically, a recall is voluntarily initialed by a firm, however, in rare instances, FDA can mandate that a firm recall devices, per 21 CFR 810.10

- **Corrections** (21 CFR 807): the repair, modification, adjustment, relabeling, destruction, or inspection (including patient monitoring) of a product without its physical removal to some other location

- **Market Withdrawal**: a firm's removal or correction of a distributed product that involves a minor violation that would not be subject to legal action by the Food and Drug Administration or that involves no violation,e.g., normal stock rotation practices, routine equipment adjustments and repairs, etc.

- **Stock Recovery:** a firm's removal or correction of a product that has not been marketed or that has not left the direct control of the firm, i.e., the product is located on premises owned by, or under the control of, the firm and no portion of the lot has been released for sale or use

Market withdrawals and stock recoveries do not reduce a risk to health or remedy a violation of the act caused by the device and therefore do not have to be reported to the FDA. In contrast, recalls are initiated to reduce a risk to health or remedy a violation of the act caused by the device and must be reported to the FDA within 10 working days from the time the firm initiates the recall.

Premarket Notification ("510(k)") Regulations (for Class II Devices Only)

If the device is class II, then *clearance* via a premarket notification submission (also known as a "510(k)") is necessary.

A 510(k) submission is a set of documents, which demonstrate that the device is "substantially equivalent" to another class II device that is already being legally marketed. The device manufacturer must submit the 510(k) submission to FDA, and FDA will review the contents of the submission. If FDA agrees with the determination of substantial equivalence, they will issue a decision letter indicating that the device has been "cleared" for marketing in the United States.

The device manufacturer may not market the device until clearance has been obtained from FDA.

For more details on this process, please refer to Chapter 14.

DE NOVO PROCESS

If the device is class II but there is no similar class II device on the market, the orthopedic device manufacturer must avail themselves of the *De Novo* process.

For more details on this process, please refer to Chapter 14.

Premarket Approval Regulations (for Class III Devices Only)

If the device is class II, then *approval* via a premarket approval submission (also known as a "PMA") is necessary.

A PMA submission is a set of documents, which demonstrate that the device is "safe" and "effective" for its intended use. Unlike 510(k) submissions, PMA submissions are not centered around a comparison to a legally marketed device. Instead, a PMA submission will generally include a description of the device, testing (bench and clinical) to characterize performance of the device, and analyses/conclusions regarding how the device is safe and effective. Notably, the PMA submission also includes manufacturing information to demonstrate that the device can be consistently produced.

Unlike 510(k) submissions, "substantial equivalence" is not a relevant consideration for a PMA.

The device manufacturer must submit the PMA submission to FDA, and FDA will review the contents of the submission. If FDA agrees with the determination of safety and effectiveness, they will issue a decision letter indicating that the device has been "approved" for marketing in the United States.

Please note the difference in terminology between the 510(k) and PMA processes ("clearance" for 510(k) submissions, "approval" for PMA submissions).

The device manufacturer may not market the device until approval has been obtained from FDA.

For more details on this process, please refer to Chapter 14.

Industry Groups/Resources

Popular industry groups and publications that support medical device manufacturers include:

- Orthopedic Surgical Manufacturers Association (OSMA)—OSMA represents the manufacture of medical devices used in orthopedic surgical procedures. OSMA holds semiannual meetings to discuss the latest news in the orthopedic medical device industry (http://www.osma.net/resources.html).
- Regulatory Affairs Professional Society (RAPS)—is a global organization for those involved with the regulation of health care and related products, including medical devices. RAPS also provides a certification program for regulatory professionals (http://www.raps.org/Default.aspx).
- Advanced Medical Technology Association (AdvaMed)—the medical industry in the United States. Also offers training on common medical device topics, such as premarket notification, investigational device exemptions, and combination products (https://www.advamed.org/about-advamed).
- European Confederation of Medical Suppliers Association (Eucomed)—represents the medical industry in Europe (http://archive.eucomed.org/).
- Medical Device and Diagnostic Industry (MD&DI)—assists manufactures of medical devices and in vitro diagnostic products (https://www.mddionline.com/).
- Medtech Insight—reports on developments in the medical device, diagnostic, and biotech sectors (https://medtech.pharmaintelligence.informa.com/).

REFERENCES AND RESOURCES

1. Food and Drug Administration (FDA). *UDI Compliance Dates*. 2017. https://www.fda.gov/MedicalDevices/DeviceRegulationandGuidance/UniqueDeviceIdentification/CompliancedatesforUDIRequirements/default.htm.
2. Food and Drug Administration (FDA). *UDI Basics*. 2015. https://www.fda.gov/MedicalDevices/DeviceRegulationandGuidance/UniqueDeviceIdentification/UDIBasics/default.htm.

CHAPTER 11

Research and Development and the Importance of Testing

HANI HAIDER

ABOUT THE AUTHOR

Hani Haider is a Professor and Director of the University of Nebraska Medical Center Orthopaedics Biomechanics and Advanced Surgical Technologies Laboratory. He has led over 90 research grants/contracts in Nebraska, totaling over $10M, from 32 different orthopedic companies from the United States, Europe, and Japan. He has received 16 academic and international awards, four invention patents, and presented more than 300 scientific papers in journals and international conferences. He is the Chair of the US Technical Advisory Group and delegation to the ISO/TC 150 Committee on Medical Devices, member of the ASTM Executive Committee on Medical Devices, First Vice President and Director of IT and Scientific Review for the International Society for Technology in Arthroplasty, and Reviews Editor for the *Journal of Engineering in Medicine*.

Introduction

Technology for orthopedics devices and especially joint replacement surgery is now a mature industry, very different from its pioneering days of the second half of the last century. This was less than 60 years ago, later than transistors were commercially developed and the digital age had already by then started. Innovating orthopedic surgeons and engineers working together could literally "cut and try" new materials and devices quickly and experimentally iterate designs, sometimes with rudimentary testing if any at all.

The cart has been put before the horse; the artificial joint has been made and used, and now we are trying to find out how and why it fails

This was what Sir John Charnley noted[1] in 1955, the inventor and pioneer of the first total hip replacement (THR). His first choice of bearing was polytetrafluoroethylene (PTFE) or what we know as Teflon, the most commonly used self-lubricating bearing and bushing material in industry. PTFE failed miserably however for Charnley because of its low wear resistance and the extreme adverse tissue reaction caused by its wear debris particles. Charnley was sure of that, as he had injected PTFE particles into his own body's tibial bone to confirm the effect! It took boldness from one of Charnley's technicians to secretly try a new material introduced casually to him, previously used for impact bearings in mechanical machines. That was ultrahigh-molecular-weight polyethylene (UHMWPE) which succeeded. It is still used today as the gold standard bearing material in joint replacements, with a variety of modern processing techniques.

How different we are with today's medical device regulation and litigation climate. It is ironic, however, that despite the many years of learning and the seemingly harsher regulatory requirements, are we really that proud of the status today? It appears so many failures in implants still occur, with frequent large-scale recalls and legal retributions. Among many reasons are the higher "expectations," including those of patients. A patient of the 1950s had little choice on how to prevent the pain of arthritis, so any implant would be a blessing to reduce pain. In contrast, we now have patients almost expecting a totally pain-free joint with an almost normal level of activity after a joint replacement.

What was needed then and what is still needed now is more research and development (R&D), and much more testing. Yet, continuing consolidation of the orthopedics manufacturers through mergers and acquisitions, various extra taxes on medical devices, and added regulatory scrutiny and enforcement have possibly led to a decline, sometimes reaching neglect, of the importance of R&D and especially of in vitro testing.

This is the subject here but such a wide scope can never be given sufficient justice in the space of one chapter. Device testing and especially R&D or testing for the purpose of R&D are suffering from ever-decreasing budgets in relative terms especially compared with marketing costs and remain below single digits in percentage of overall costs of implant development.

We will first elaborate on why we need more R&D and more preclinical testing of orthopedic devices. We describe the new technologies, faster design and production cycles, and litigious "blame" atmosphere, which renders more R&D and testing as even more crucial. We then describe the types of testing required and how they vary with device classification and possible risks to the patients, emphasizing the important role and limitations of the regulation agencies. A brief description follows of some types of human, animal, in vitro and in silico (computational simulation) preclinical testing and the standards associated with some of them.

Research and Development Verification and Validation Testing

R&D, verification and validation (V&V) are integral tasks of any implant or medical device development process. In the medical industry, R&D refers to the process of innovation and conception of new devices or understanding in more depth aspects of their work. However, for most small innovative medical device companies, the R&D and product development functions can be so lightly staffed by few key personnel that they become indistinguishable. In this context, R&D for them literally encompasses V&V.

Verification is required at multiple stages of the design and development process to provide objective proof that the design requirements (specifications) are met. It is mostly done by testing, inspections, and in some cases computational simulation (see later section in this chapter). Such testing, whether done in house or outside the company premises, can be considered "internal" testing.

Validation is the process of objective evidence that the device or implant can deliver the user needs in terms of expected functional performance, expected longevity, and of course the safety requirements related to both. Typically, a whole implant system or individual components of it, as produced for clinical use, are assessed according to self-predetermined or externally recommended requirements such as official regulatory and testing standards.

Why We Need More not Less Research and Development and Device Testing

When there were no alternatives in the past and arthritic hip and knee patients could not really walk, any device design, even with suboptimal materials that could return patients to some mobility and less pain might have been tolerated. Today there are already plenty of good-working, tried, and tested joint replacement systems available, so bringing a new device to market has to be proven to improve rather than introduce unwanted problems. The same could be said and more so in trauma instruments such as plates, screws, intramedullary nails, etc. Therefore, one subtle reason why more R&D and testing of orthopedic devices is needed before a new device is clinically used is that orthopedics clinical problems such as lower and upper limb osteoarthritis or trauma are not life-threatening, and some alternatives are available. Therefore, first and foremost, implants must "do no harm" in terms of side effects.

New implant designs are always being introduced however, and they bring with them the need for more R&D and of course regulatory scrutiny.

There is an ever-increasing number of small manufacturing companies, typically founded by orthopedic surgeons who, for compliance or other reasons, no longer find it easy to consult with the large companies to have their ideas implemented. The competition from the rising number of small companies is currently unmatched by the rate of consolidation through mergers and acquisitions and is exasperated by more international competitions. Companies from Brazil, Korea, and lately in big numbers from China are fast emerging and introducing new products for their local markets, naturally aiming to expand outside them.

Strong impetus for more serious R&D and preclinical testing stems also from the stream of new emerging materials and technologies that are applicable to the field. Polyether ether ketone (PEEK) has been introduced for specific spine applications and in strengthened variations by additives such as carbon fiber. Innovations with shape memory alloys and superelasticity materials such as nitinol are being utilized. Additive manufacturing (popularly termed 3-D printing), especially now with metallic alloy material capability, opens new avenues for new orthopedic implant and instrument designs, which could not be practically manufactured before.[2,3] They may be light weight or customized to fit a patient-specific anatomy or have varying gradients of fused or interfaced materials for different functions, among many other emerging innovations.

Advances in coating technologies intended to reduce wear or provide metal ion diffusion barriers especially for metal-sensitive patients pose extra testing burdens for ever more complex regulatory claims, perhaps with mixed and unknown side effects or risk factors.[4] Many other types of coatings continue to emerge; those that encourage bone growth, are antibacterial and resist infection, elute drugs, and various other nanotube and other nanotechnology applications.[5] Implants made with hybrid materials and biodegradable materials[6] add their special requirements for function testing. So do smart orthopedic devices and instruments and implants that include sophisticated software and communications capabilities including wireless which brings in electromagnetic and other signal interference. Complicating all the above are resorbable material implants and the inevitable emergence of medical devices that combine a biologic agent or drug with an implant such as antibiotic-eluting hip and knee polyethylene bearings.[7] Finally, the increasing innovations in tissue engineering and regenerative medicine will bring their own challenges in preclinical testing. Except for animal studies perhaps, how can an implantable system, which relies on host human tissue for biological integration, be preclinically tested with confidence?

When all the above are combined with modern computer-aided design (CAD)/computer-aided manufacturing (CAM) and 3-D printing tools, which allow for much faster design and production cycles, it can easily be seen that testing, standardization for testing, and regulation, which depend on testing, would all lag behind. Ironically therefore, it can be argued that unless the speed of these modern advances is matched by an expansion and acceleration of testing methods and standards, the risks to the patients from some new technology solutions may rise instead of fall. Exceedingly rampant legal liabilities and a litigation atmosphere in the United States add to all the above. Increasing numbers of seemingly dedicated lawyers await any systematic implant failure in patients to seek retribution, which can go into the billions of dollars. This in itself would add to the burden and possible turmoil in optimizing how much and what type of R&D and preclinical testing are needed.

Therefore, very clear pressures point to the need for more and more R&D-based preclinical testing of orthopedic implants, yet the trends show less and not more investment in them. Therefore, the strategies and choices of what to test are even more critical.

General Approach for Research and Development of Medical Devices

FOOD AND DRUG ADMINISTRATION CLASSIFICATION OF ORTHOPEDIC DEVICES BASED ON RISKS TO THE PATIENT

What we test and how much testing is needed depends on the type of orthopedic device involved and the risks it poses to the patient if used.

Most new orthopedic devices are introduced because they bring "new claims" or promises of improvement to what is already available. This could be either in design or materials to improve function or longevity, more safety through easier surgical technique, faster surgery and more efficiency, or significant cost reduction. So, any claim of improved function or longevity needs to be technically tested in vitro, or it could be unannounced as a claim, leaving only the usually required tests to be done.

Generally, claims for superiority of a new implant design in any way are preclinically tested to verify that superiority is attainable with confidence and to screen for any new risks that the new design feature may introduce. All these issues to screen against are called risks and are sometimes called "risk controls." The appropriate testing for any orthopedic device may be available from the general scientific literature, international standards, and the published requirement by regulatory bodies, which screen such devices for clearance to be commercially sold and clinically used on patients. The principal relevant regulatory organization in the United States is the Federal

Food and Drug Administration (FDA). It has various published guidelines and requirements, and upon satisfaction of those including much data and testing by the device manufacturer, can issue "FDA clearance" for the device. In other countries, it could be the Chinese FDA, the Japanese FDA, the Conformité Européene (CE), and so on.

The FDA categorizes medical devices in the United States into one of three classes—class I, II, or III—based on the risks they present when used and the regulatory clearance controls necessary to have confidence in their safety and effectiveness. Class I devices generally pose the lowest risk to the patient, and class III devices pose the highest risk:

- Class I devices are deemed to be low risk and are therefore subject to the least regulatory controls. For example, dental floss is classified as a class I device.
- Class II devices are higher-risk devices than class I and require greater regulatory controls to provide reasonable assurance of the device's safety and effectiveness. For example, THR and total knee replacement (TKR) systems, and even condoms are classified as class II devices.
- Class III devices are generally the highest risk devices and are therefore subject to the highest level of regulatory control. For example, replacement heart valves are classified as class III devices.

Many wonder what minimal R&D testing must be done for an innovative orthopedic device. It depends on the FDA in the United States or regulatory classification in other countries in which the device is to be used. However, should it really be the minimal testing specified in the requirements one should aim for?

ON WHOSE SIDE IS THE REGULATOR?

The above device classifications were provided here, and are available with detailed guidelines in multiple other forms, especially by large regulatory bodies on their websites and through other publications and media. It is by nature of any such regulations that no matter how specific they promise to be, they remain relatively general. Some expertise is needed to plot the regulatory pathway for a particular device. As they become more advanced and complex in their materials and designs, the regulatory pathways also get complicated, inevitably requiring more data and testing. Various initiatives by the FDA attempt to speed up the clearing process, but understaffing, together with the growth in new technologies, materials, and devices mentioned above, makes this very difficult. Active participation by regulators in the standardization process in American Society for Testing and Materials (ASTM) International and International Organization for Standardization

(ISO) allows the responsibility and challenges of deciding "what to test, and how?" to be delegated to those organizations. This in itself poses a challenge and introduces a significant limitation as not all regulatory (e.g., FDA) implant reviewers can attend ASTM International or ISO meetings. A large gap and disparate levels of expertise can exist between individual regulatory reviewers. When they are also understaffed, the compounded problem of a hectically busy reviewer without the sufficient technical expertise can only imply failure somewhere in the process or dissatisfaction by someone along the way. Game-changing technologies, such as additive manufacturing and new composite and hybrid materials, add to that complexity and challenge.

With all the above, how should we see the regulator and individual reviewers, and whose side are they really on? The typical answer is they have a job to do, protecting the patient at large. However, when they are understaffed, overloaded, and potentially lacking in advanced technical expertise, would the manufacturer submitting for clearance of a new device somehow benefit from this i.e. would they be lucky? In the opinion of the author, it is precisely the opposite. The review of a submission is the last possible safety check to help implant manufacturers save their patients from possible adverse effects. Any feedback toward more safety and sparing the manufacturer from possible ramifications is very valuable. In recent years, medicolegal claims have meant losses of billions of dollars in settlement fines and compromised company reputation. In recent history, one technical oversight during manufacturing and quality testing, a (then) leading European manufacturing company of ceramic implants had to fold. Owing to almost similar reasons, the largest blue-chip European company lost its flare, changed its name, and then got absorbed for a fraction of its previous worth by another US company. Applying the same considerations to a new start-up company, innovating with a new implant, and seeking regulatory clearance, the risk to the company and the risk to the patient are intertwined. It would appear a harsh intricate FDA regulator with a critical eye for detail is the biggest ally of the manufacturer in the long term. What should really matter for the manufacturer in the end is that the implant successfully and safely works. The regulator and the manufacturer are on the same side.

Categories of Medical Device Testing

IN VIVO TESTING

In vivo means inside the body and that could be a human, animal, or any living organism. This contrasts with in vitro, which is sometimes termed bench testing and in turn contrasts with in silico, analytical and computational simulation testing. This section was divided to briefly describe some considerations for testing in animals and in humans, with some examples relevant to orthopedic implants.

Whether testing on humans or animals, the aim is to garner reasonable evidence for V&V (Figure 11.1) of safety and efficacy of the implant. This evidence aims to assure all stakeholders. In orthopaedics, these include the patients, the hospitals and surgeons who acquire and install the implants, regulatory bodies who guard for proper preclinical safety screening and finally, even payers such as medical insurance companies or government public health provision agencies such as Medicaid and Medicare in the United States.

In vivo testing should be designed to be as predictive as possible, with a predetermined selection of end points, observation of biomarkers, and a solid consideration of how they translate to risks in humans. These could range from predicting failure, or reaching or exceeding the performance or longevity of existing successful devices (predicates) of which some may be routinely clinically used as "gold standard."

In the field of orthopedic implants, examples of in vivo study end points include biocompatibility to avoid inflammatory response due to

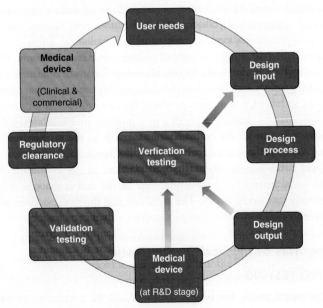

Figure 11.1 Research and Development verification and validation testing within the design cycle of a medical device.

debris or metal ion release. V&V testing should also demonstrate efficacy of function, e.g., noncemented fixation by demonstrating effective bone growth, implant stability, and so on. The selection of end points to assess should be based on what is new or being claimed by the tested device be it its material, a coating or processing, or by the new or modified design for improved function.

Testing on Animals

In drug safety generally, and in early medical device development, animal studies used to play a huge role and in some instances were the only possible preclinical tests done. In all cases, it is not only important to carefully select the animal species, but to determine the rest of the "model" as well in terms of conditions, detailed procedures, and evaluation of outcomes. A recent good summary of the merits and deficiencies of various species when evaluating a new material or device was provided by Wancket.[8] It describes the characteristics of the most commonly used species such as mice, rats, rabbits, guinea pigs, dogs, sheep, goats, and nonhuman primates and their suitability in studies of bone-implant materials. It usefully describes the relevance of a particular model to human bone physiology and pathology. In our earlier example of fixation of orthopedic implants to the bone, mice and rats provide good models. However, their limbs would be rather small for very detailed analysis and physical fixation-force measurements. On the other extreme, sheep and goats solve the latter size problem and offer bigger bone samples to perform slicing, clearer imaging, and force testing, but study costs would escalate with the required numbers of such large animals. Careful control of their habitat, diet, disease, and activities is required.

Generally, the model must as closely as possible match the human anatomy and clinical disease. The method of evaluation must be sensitive and repeatable enough to sufficiently discriminate between levels of observed outcome. It is also important when choosing a suitable animal model to select appropriate age, sex, and disease state, as well as species of the animal, to best match a human (say arthritic) bone. Taking the implant-bone fixation example again, if the implant is to fix to cortical or cancellous bone, it is important to identify those regions of the bones with minimum variations within each animal when testing at various sites (e.g., bone sections). When testing multiple animals, interanimal variations must be minimized for proper variable control. In any situation (single or multiple sites on single or multiple animals), the choice of appropriate "controls" is vital when comparing between implanted or nonimplanted cases or between (say) a coated implant and noncoated, and so on.

Failure mode analysis of an implant should be done first, defining what constitutes a failure and projects a risk to humans. A suitable animal model is then selected and justified through its biological relevance. Predetermined end points to assess are then carefully selected. The actual evaluation can utilize radiographic follow-up, imaging, and histology of implant and surrounding tissue explants, morphology, and of course infection, immunological, chemicals, and other pathology can be observed. Among the attributes that could be tested on animals are biofunctionality, which is the ability of an implant to desirably influence surrounding tissue. Chondrogenesis is another, which is the ability of an implant to induce or support regrowth of cartilage. Osteoinduction, osteoconductivity, and osteointegration[8] can be assessed as abilities to encourage bone formation or bone growth of tissue into a scaffold or implant surfaces as exemplified above.

In all studies on animals, animal welfare and related regulations have become exceedingly important, causing a shift toward smaller animal models, and shorter, better planned tests. Overall, it can be safely generalized that animal testing is a specialized and relatively costly activity, needing special resources and expertise. Like other things, much knowledge could be gained through a comprehensive literature survey. An alternative starting point is to refer to an international standard, ISO 10993 on Biological evaluation of medical devices, which has 20 parts. Its first part sets a general framework and guidelines for how to evaluate any device in vitro or in animal tests within a risk management process. Its second part provides a useful summary of animal welfare requirements, and the remaining parts delve into more detail about all the issues described above.

The author was involved in one study[9] to test the efficacy of an innovative nanostructured cubic zirconium surface coating by ion-beam–assisted deposition. It had potential in promoting osteointegration of noncemented titanium implants for arthroplasty in elderly patients. The animal model utilized 10 different 1-year-old rats in each of two groups (a and b), which were given a protein-deficient diet to simulate arthritic bone. One group received coated and the other uncoated (control) simplified titanium intramedullary nail implants inserted in their proximal femur bone. The third group (c) of 3-month-old rats received normal protein diet and the control implant. The question was whether the implant with the nanostructured zirconia surface would increase expression of markers of bone maturation within the remodeling of periimplant woven bone. The animals were euthanized 8 weeks after implantation. Transverse sections of femur-implant samples were used for histology, microcomputed tomography, and immunohistochemical evaluations. In group b, the expression of integrins, which were known to help osteointegration, was less than half of that in group c (the healthy young rats). The nanostructured zirconia surface used in group a prevented these deficiencies and prevented the impaired osseointegration in the elderly rats.

In the above study, simplified nail-like implants inserted in tiny femurs of small rats were assumed as surrogates of complex-shaped hip stems in humans. Also, the osseointegration evaluation using imaging and multiple other benchtop techniques on tiny slices of bone and nail sections in them was taken as indirect pointers to the efficacy of long-term fixation of hip stems in elderly arthritic humans. Such deviations between the rat model and the physiological anatomy and conditions of humans are not untypical. However, such a study with its relatively high speed, low cost, and small risk (using rats) contrasts very much with what it would have taken to test the same on humans. An equivalent human clinical study could neither be justified let alone (Institutional Review Board [IRB]) approved at such an early exploratory stage of implant technology innovation.

Clinical Testing in Human Patients

This topic is vast, covered by hundreds of textbooks, thousands of research articles, and official stringent regulations. It can be stated that all drugs, implants, and devices need to be clinically tested by observing the outcomes of their use in patients, even after regulatory clearance. "Clinical trials" are therefore part of the R&D development of an orthopedic device. The topic is wide and can be viewed from different perspectives such as that of an investigator (e.g., surgeon), a subject such as the patient or patient advocate (e.g., IRB) or that of a sponsor such as the R&D team of an implant manufacturer. Throughout the history of medicine, clinical trials were the norm and formed the ultimate testing of any new implant or medical device. The rich history of medicine is full of thousands of examples, but only in the last few decades has there been a substantial shift[10] toward more regulations, understandably requiring much more in vitro preclinical testing when possible.

Obviously, trials in humans are risky by nature, but when there are no "predicates" of similar devices, it becomes the only route if the evidence from prior R&D and all possible in vitro testing still points to significant potential benefit from the innovative device in humans. This by definition makes such trials appear very heavily regulated for technological devices that do not address fatal health conditions and for which there may be clinically available alternatives (c.f. contrast that to exploratory cancer drugs).

Outcomes Studies Through Implant Survival Analysis

For orthopedic devices, and joint replacement in particular, "outcomes" studies continue to dominate clinical studies. These studies typically log implant survival in vivo through some well understood and communicated metric. The most common is the Kaplan-Meier survival analysis,[11] logging the number of subjects or limbs treated in which the implant survived after installation surgery over a period of time. When performing or interpreting such analyses, a detailed understanding is necessary of how death of a subject is treated, e.g., implant survived till death, and how uncooperative subjects who refuse to continue to be in the study or are lost to follow-up for a myriad of other reasons are dealt with. Another factor is when an implant revision occurs not because of its failure but secondary to a different event such as limb fracture, infection, etc. When comparing Kaplan-Meier implant survival across different implants, surgeons, or hospitals, all these factors influence the results as well as inclusion and exclusion criteria of patients in the study (see below).

Outcome Studies Through Surgeon-Examined and Patient-Reported Functional Scores

Another big category of outcomes measures the surgery quality, patient satisfaction, and performance during follow-ups. The minimum of these are surgeon physical examinations and observations from radiological imaging, which tend to be mostly qualitative, e.g., evidence of implant migration, malalignment, instability and subluxation, infection, fractured cement mantle, periprosthetic fracture, etc. Some may involve minimal semiquantitative data, e.g., enumerated pain levels during activities, knee range of motion measured as the maximum flexion angle in degrees reached by the patient, location and area of radiolucency signifying osteolysis, and risk of compromised fixation and loosening.

Another category of R&D clinical evaluations are through quantitative metrics based on some objective surgeon measurements combined with patient-reported outcome measures (PROMs). They measure patient symptoms, pain, function, satisfaction, and expectations in fulfilling daily activities including walking, and stair ascent and descent. These metrics literally aim at the same thing, to be as objective and reasonably comprehensive and convenient as possible in capturing the patients' state at different stages prior to and post surgery. The metrics have historically emanated from different academic and clinical research centers, so they have differences in what they log and how data is processed. Therefore comparisons between implants, patients, and time are only possible by using the same metric. Examples for TKR are the Knee Society Score (KSS),[12] Knee injury and Osteoarthritis Outcome Score (KOOS), Western Ontario and McMaster Universities Osteoarthritis Index (WOMAC), and Oxford Knee Score. A single, validated, reliable, and responsive PROM addressing TKA patients' priorities has not yet been identified. Moreover, a clear definition of a successful procedure remains elusive.[13] Among the commonly used ones for the hips are the Harris Hip Score (HHS) and the Oxford Hip Score (OHS).

Gait Studies and 3-D Tracking of Motion of Patient Limbs

This category of clinical studies is traditional and fundamentally quantitative by using 3-D camera and computer tracking technology of patients, bodies or individual limbs. Several high-accuracy cameras take time-synchronized reflected infrared or normal photos or video streams of patients with multiple reflective markers distributed in clusters attached to various parts of the subject patient body. Postprocessing analysis of the recorded photos or video stream using segmentation, triangulation, and stereotactic algorithms helps determine pose of the patient limbs relative to each other or from the relative positions of markers within predetermined clusters. For example, through a point cluster technique,[13] reasonable accuracy of knee and hip kinematics could be determined during different activities including walking gait, stair climbing and descent, upper limb motions to track shoulder kinematics, etc. More benefits could be gained when combining and correlating gait data with time-synchronized force measurements using force plates located on the laboratory floor. The measurements could be further combined with electromyographical (EMG) force measurements, representing relevant dynamically contracting patient muscles.[14,15]

Kinetic and kinematic measurements of patients with implants during various activities have contributed substantially to our understanding of the in vivo performance of implants throughout the history of joint replacements. As with all other categories of clinical studies, awareness and care should be taken of the limitations inherent in such measurements. The most significant is that the markers are usually attached to the patient's skin external to the body. Naturally, this partly limits the accuracy of 3-D tracking of internal bones and smaller internal implant components whose positions and orientations can only be indirectly estimated because of the compliance of soft tissue and skin.

Fluoroscopic Measurements of Implant Kinematics

This technique has continuously boomed in the last 25 years and is now widely used. It utilizes single or biplanar fluoroscopic X-ray imaging to estimate the implant kinematics in vivo during dynamic patient postures and activities. Typically, the three-dimensional positions and orientations (pose) of implants are determined by registering at each instant/pose the 3-D CAD model of the implant to its corresponding image or pair of time-coincident orthogonal radiographs. The images are taken using flat-panel detectors and image intensifiers in custom setups. Some of the latest of these can be made to move in the lab to closely follow and continuously image the patient joint during motion (e.g., walking). Using proprietary software (although there are now open-source code versions available), the implant kinematics are tracked in 3-D post processing to an accuracy of approximately 1 mm for in-plane translations and about 1° in three rotations. In recent developments, CT-segmented and CT-reconstructed 3-D bone models of the patient could also be tracked using fluoroscopy and thus pose of bones and implants is determined. Multiple studies have led to useful comparisons of in vivo kinematics of various TKR designs[16,17] and some findings have inspired new TKR design concepts.[18]

Roentgen Stereophotogrammetric Analysis

Roentgen stereophotogrammetric analysis (RSA), sometimes also known as radiostereometric analysis, is a technique used to monitor the subsidence, migration, or wear of implant components in the bone of a patient. It relies on the basic concept of roentgen stereophotogrammetry, which is over a hundred years old. RSA in joint replacement however has been introduced and clinically and commercially boomed in the last 30 years.[19]

The 3-D pose of objects is localized in roentgenograms (radiographs) through small metallic markers used as fiducials for measurements on each object. In modern RSA, prior to and during surgery, special tantalum marker injectors are used to safely embed tiny tantalum beads (≤1 mm diameter) within bones (e.g., the proximal tibia) and in UHMWPE hip bearing components and on the surfaces of metallic implant components (e.g., a metallic acetabular shell). These beads can be seen in X-ray images and act as fiducial markers. Calibration cages, with measurement, analysis, and visualization software, are initially calibrated to scale and register images to distances and angles (see Figure 11.2 for an example of such setup in the author's lab). The same calibrated setup is then used at post surgery follow-up intervals to image the patient's surgical site. The bones and components are assumed perfectly rigid, and therefore if any of them move or rotate relative to another even within fractions of a millimeter or degree, the cluster of beads on them also shifts relative to others. Two simultaneous plane X-ray radiographic images are taken at each stage and analyzed using the same software to accurately measure such minor changes of relative position or orientation.

RSA is used routinely today to detect migration of implants in hip arthroplasties or other artificial joints and prosthetic UHMWPE wear. As with any other quantitative computer- and imaging-based system, it is vital to estimate and verify the accuracy and precision of RSA prior to clinical

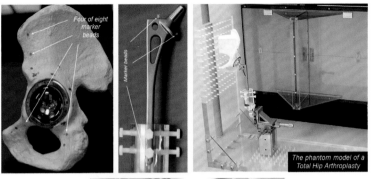

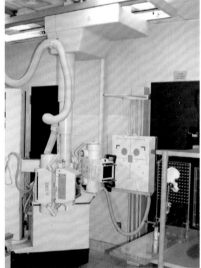

	Pelvis/Cup	Pelvis/Stem	Cup-Stem
Precision (mm)	0.013 – 0.071	0.023 – 0.182	0.029 – 0.230
Accuracy (mm)	±0.026 – ±0.139	±0.033 – ±0.536	

Figure 11.2 Roentgen stereophotogrammetric analysis (RSA) calibration and verification setup and results within the author's laboratory in Nebraska.[18]

use. Astounding accuracies have been reported, to <86 μm in some cases, from phantom studies with conservative simulated wear and migration distances of <0.2 mm in each direction.[20] In 2006, the current author's own RSA phantom study[21] (Figure 11.2) estimated accuracy and precision with larger simulated distances and verified precision to 0.23 mm and accuracy to ±0.5 mm (both of which were still very impressive), showing RSA to be the most precise method at that time. However, its results should always be viewed with these uncertainty figures in mind.

The general methodology of calibrating an RSA setup and the practice for determining femoral head penetration into acetabular components of THR using clinical radiographs have been standardized in ASTM F2385-15.[22] This standard therefore offers a good starting point for the novice user.

Martell Computational Radiographic Method

This method is more traditional and has been gradually improved by John Martell, MD of the University of Chicago into a widely used validated computer-assisted hip analysis software. X-ray radiographs are analyzed, either in two-dimensional or two oblique X-rays to improve accuracy.[23] Simpler and perhaps expectedly less precise, the Martell method is as routinely used today as RSA to measure UHMWPE wear of hip replacements in vivo. Some studies reported sensitivity of a few tens of microns.[24] The Martell method as essentially a bearing penetration hip wear measurement method is also (nominally) covered by ASTM F2385-15.[22]

In Vivo Telemetry Force Measurements

This type of testing has been so far limited to the field of academic R&D but has produced very useful results to help implant technologists for over 20 years. Special implants (see example of one of the earliest in Figure 11.3) are equipped with embedded strain gauges, wireless inductive electrical charging circuitry, signal conditioning, processing, and wireless communication, all safely sealed within. After surgical insertion, and in planned experiments, the implant is powered inductively from outside the body. It is able to measure the joint forces passing through the implant and transmit logged data externally to be received by proprietary mobile equipment carried by the patient.

This type of technology has enabled physical verification of compressive forces in the knee joint that had previously been estimated[25,26] by theoretical computational methods aided by empirical gait lab measurements (examples of these will be covered later; see pages 160-164). Expansion of the method has enabled the measurements of anterior-posterior (AP) forces and internal-external (IE) torques in TKRs in more than one patient undergoing a variety of daily activities.[27] The Julius Wolff Institute, of Charité—Universitätsmedizin Berlin, has produced a comprehensive set of telemetry measurements in a variety of human joints such as hips, knees, and shoulders in patients performing a wide variety of controlled and monitored

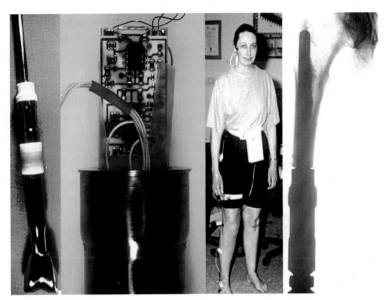

Figure 11.3 Telemetry of a distal femoral replacement from which compressive forces on the knee were measured in vivo.[22,23]

activities. Their study results have been widely published,[28,29] and even their actual detailed numerical results are publicly available in their well-known "OrthoLoad" database on their (similarly named, Orthoload) website.

Clinical Study Design and Ethical Considerations

In any and all clinical trials, there are serious challenges at all stages of the process. In the design of any clinical study, procedures have to be very clear. This includes patient selection and inclusion/exclusion criteria, enrollment, IRB, and patient consent involving multiple-party (company sponsor, hospital, surgeon, and patient) contracting. Subject selection and recruitment are critical, to make them suitable for a specific study or as historic or new controls. Surrogate and final end points for assessment must be defined beforehand. A statistical plan on selecting sample size acceptance criteria (e.g., superiority or equivalence) must all be prepared beforehand. Decisions on blinding/masking subjects or investigators, the roles, and communications of those conducting the study procedures and the disciplines for maintaining or modifying the plan during the study must all be clearly made beforehand and adhered to. Of course data measurements, recording, integrity, analysis, confidentiality, and reporting details free of inventor or consultant bias are also crucial.

All the above processes offer numerous ethical considerations, especially in the cases of high-risk implants.[30] Commercial factors can be involved too, such as new devices that could be marketed for a profit once proven in a clinical trial; these naturally bring legal liabilities into play. Even after clinical trials, these issues continue with the implementation of adverse event monitoring and reporting and feed into the larger implant registries, which are becoming more and more important.[31] Finally, clinical "outcome" studies are today the mainstay of the medical device surgeon academic and industrial R&D community. These range from the highly sophisticated random prospective trials in which the study is all planned properly in detail of patient inclusion/exclusion, and randomization of controls before any surgeries are done. More frequently published, however, are the retrospective smaller studies, usually conducted with the help of or exclusively by surgeon-resident trainees who examine outcomes of multiple patients, sometimes years after they are examined or treated. Variable control is much less robust in such retrospective studies, with modest sample numbers especially when they involve uncommonly used implants or surgical procedures. Even if such limitations were left aside, the observer or measurement (e.g., of radiographic records) can suffer from intraobserver and interobserver inconsistency. Adding to all that, the pressure to publish research naturally skews such studies to be naturally (statistically) underpowered. Some end up over-conclusive or report statistically significant but clinically insignificant results.

All these issues are further complicated with the international dimension. For example, harmonization with other regulatory bodies (e.g., CE marking) may encourage compromises and cutting corners. It is never easy to know how to absorb clinical data conducted in foreign settings, especially when it may have been done to circumvent stricter regulations and to save costs.

All in all, however daunting, complex, time-consuming, and costly, in vitro testing may sound at first, these difficulties pale in comparison to what are essentially much more complicated, longer term, more costly, properly planned clinical trials.

IN VITRO TESTING

In vitro testing of medical implants, sometimes called bench testing, refers to practical experiments performed outside a living body (i.e., not in vivo). These tests are generally carried out in a controlled laboratory environment, at various levels of complexity depending on the simulation. Such testing is by nature preliminary, aiming to verify, and predict, typically implying further clinical tests or observations should follow. The precursory and supposedly economical nature of in vitro testing makes it directly and frequently useful during design iterations of a product. It may comprise screening or assessment to guard against the toxic risk of an implant (e.g., biocompatibility), and to determine whether the implant can safely and effectively deliver the functionality intended, and to assess the longevity or durability of the implant and estimate if it can fulfill the required or expected duty in vivo.

Biocompatibility

In a previous section, we stressed the importance of the "do no harm" principle in medical device design and screening. Therefore, the first and most basic design criterion for orthopedic devices is to ensure that the materials are biocompatible and the least harmful to the body in the short and long terms. This is the central theme for biomaterials applications in medicine. Just as with whole devices, functionality is as important as longevity. So, here too, biocompatibility means not only absence of a cytotoxic effect but also positive effects in the sense of biofunctionality, i.e., the promotion of biological processes which are intended as the aim of the application of a biomaterial.

Prior to implanting a device in humans, it is vital to ensure that the device's materials will not cause unwanted biological reactions. As note earlier, the most extensive and widely recognized international standard for biocompatibility testing methods for medical devices is ISO 10993 in 20 parts. Due to the breadth of these standards, we will only address some of the more important considerations.

As with mechanical testing, it is preferred that compatibility testing be performed using the final, sterilized device materials. However, a company may be able to justify that testing of a device raw material is representative of the final device in sterilized form. FDA scientists do consider the biocompatibility of the bulk device material, but it is also important to investigate the specific processing and finishing steps used in a particular device and also to assess any by-products created by the device either chemically or mechanically. Chemical material extracts are used in many of the ISO 10993 tests, which allow for evaluation of any chemicals that may potentially leach from the device's materials inside the body.

Another common type of "by-product" of a device, especially in orthopedics and spine, is wear debris. Particulate wear debris is generated when two or more bearing surfaces within the device articulate against each other under a load in vivo. This articulation may be by design such as in total knee, hip, or disk replacements or other articulating devices or it could be unintentional when components are misaligned or become loose and wear against each other. Although there are materials that are more wear resistant than others, and although wear rate is affected by many variables such as load and lubrication regime, any two materials that articulate under a load will eventually experience wear through adhesive, abrasive, or fatigue mechanisms, or any combination of the aforementioned. The question is how much debris will be generated over the service life of the device, and what is the expected size and morphology of this debris. Wear debris poses a biological concern which may vary depending on the size, the material, and the body's ability to isolate and tolerate it. As with other orthopedic joints, the physiologic response to debris could lead to other unwanted biologic reactions such as osteolysis or degradation of the surrounding bone. It is important that developers evaluate how susceptible their device is to the generation of wear debris and to justify whether the debris will be tolerated by the human body without causing an unacceptable biological response. This evaluation is typically conducted through a combination of mechanical testing to generate wear debris, evaluate the wear rate, and characterize the debris by estimating the distribution of particle shape and size. In some untested cases, animal testing is performed to estimate the biological response of the wear debris.

The literature is abundant with multiple publications and there are some standardized methods for how to prepare, isolate, and characterize UHMWPE wear debris from joint simulator wear tests.[32,33] The challenge is that the debris particles are usually embedded in complex lubricant serum proteins, and these proteins need to be digested in order to isolate the particles without damage. Then, their size and shape distributions need to be characterized when they are billions in number with varying three-dimensional shapes and sizes. Sophisticated electronic imaging techniques and software processing are used, but they are essentially two-dimensional, and most elongated particles (e.g., fibril shaped ones) would not necessarily lie in the plane of the image.

The debris from wear of orthopedic joint replacement devices can also be smaller-size ceramic particles, but they are ceramics and less harmful physiologically. Debris can also be in the form of metallic wear particulates and also in ionic form from corrosion. Each of these on its own is a subject of study of their own. One very strong technique used by many labs recently is inductively coupled plasma mass spectroscopy (ICP-MS), which allows detection of parts in a billion of almost any metal element. This allows comparisons of the amounts of overall metal debris in any tiny representative sample specimen (of say simulator test lubricant) to great accuracy. However, the technique relies on turning the whole sample into a plasma, combining particulate and ionic forms of debris into one. The experience of the author has been that one little submicron metallic (e.g., cobalt-chrome alloy) particle present in the specimen may skew the results by adding so much more in comparison to another specimen that has no particle, but only metal ions. This very issue remains the subject of discussion in standards committees on how to reliably compare metallic ionic debris from orthopedic joint replacement devices.

Mechanical Testing

Mechanical testing is the most pertinent for orthopedic devices, and forms the core tools in their R&D. Both function and durability need to be verified and validated by testing, and each requires different types of tests. We will describe and give examples of each category separately.

Mechanical Function Testing of Implants

Function needs to be tested to verify that an implant can perform as intended clinically. Depending on the definition of "function," it is sometimes easy, sometimes difficult, and sometimes impossible to test and verify in vitro. The following are examples with an artificial knee or hip replacement.

The main clinical function of these joint replacements is to provide a new articular bearing surface to worn cartilage in osteoarthritic patients who suffer great pain due to (among other things) the bone rubbing against bone in the severely worn areas. If the function is defined as "reduce or eliminate pain," then this is literally impossible to test in vitro, as pain is only felt by a patient and could only be tested clinically after surgery. The same could almost be said if the functional end point to assess was "proper walking gait," etc.

Another aspect of function could be defined as the "ability to surgically insert an implant to properly and rigidly fit." The functional aim here is to verify that the implant can be inserted to replace worn cartilage surface areas on typical patients' bones and that it will fit rigidly. This is easily assessed either qualitatively or, better, quantitatively. A simple test can be a simulated surgery setup with synthetic (sawbone) models. The subject implant together with its appropriated instrumentation is tested by a surgeon or trainee, with or without supervision. The test could verify that the implant and instrumentation can be inserted successfully prior to clinical implementation. In this case, the end points are qualitative, e.g., whether the surgeon found it easy to do, the implant covered the bone appropriately, etc. Or the assessment could be quantitative such as measuring the time of the surgery or parts of it or measuring the accuracy of implant alignment after insertion, and so on.

More advanced benchtop testing would quantitatively assess the fixation of (say) an uncemented knee replacement baseplate. In the author's laboratory, a novel medium-size test project took few weeks to setup (Figure 11.4). In this test the linear and rotational multiaxial micromotions were measured, and the rigidity of initial uncemented fixation were compared between a new total knee replacement (TKR) baseplate versus a similar (predicate) tibial component.

Some implant function tests address aspects of the overall system (e.g., artificial joint) performance. Using TKR again as an example, the testing of its range of motion and constraint has been the subject of much R&D,[34]

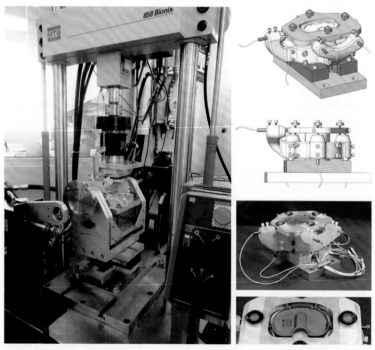

Figure 11.4 Four-axis MTS (MN, USA) test frame system in the author's laboratory used to conduct micromotion (or efficacy of uncemented fixation onto bone) testing of a total knee replacement baseplate. (Top right) 3-D CAD (computer-aided designs) of sophisticated fix- turing attached to a synthetic tibial bone model. The fixture holds seven different miniature displacement sensors (linear variable displacement transducers [LVDTs]) against a plate, which is also shown manufactured and assembled in photos below. The plate was rigidly fixed with set-screws to the outer edge of the tibial tray implant (bottom photo). The white cords are the cables from each of the seven LVDTs. The setup allowed accurate few-micron range measurements of relative linear and rotational motions in various directions between the tibial baseplate and the bone model to assess and compare early uncemented fixation.

and an ASTM standard (F1223) has been developed for the testing method. Constraint is the inverse of "laxity" of the knee joint, and the testing referred to here is of the constraint inherent in the implant system itself. It is known that the overall constraint/laxity of a replaced knee joint depends partly on the soft-tissue ligament structure, implant position, and its alignment after surgery. But, it also partly depends on the detailed design shape and conformity of the TKR implant articulating surfaces, which influence the resistance the implant shows against motion in the anterior-posterior (AP) plane and internal-external (IE) rotation. The resistance in each mode can be mechanically tested by applying a constant compressive (approximately one human body weight) force, applying a varying AP force to the tibial component, and plotting the relative AP motion versus AP force in both directions. This is also done in IE rotation, plotting imposed IE torque versus IE angle. Both result in a nonlinear laxity curve with some hysteresis due to frictional and viscoelastic effects.[34] The slope of the laxity curves and the limits of AP or IE motions can be estimated to compare different implants, articulating surface shapes and materials. The resulting characteristic curves, become like kinetic-kinematic signatures representative of how much each implant design would contribute to the overall constraint of a TKR in a patient.

The foregoing are a few examples of R&D testing methods for assessing the function of a TKR in vitro. More thorough descriptions of various approaches have been published,[35,36] including Oxford-rig–type simulators[37,38] and fully fledged knee simulators.[11] These are sophisticated custom-built physical simulator machines to help assess the factors that influence in vitro performance of artificial knee joint designs.

There are various functional tests on Total Hip Replacement systems too. Examples range from simple (CAD) geometry-based characterization of articular surface coverage, measurement of friction one-dimensionally in a pendulum-like setup,[39] or measuring hip friction three-dimensionally during hip simulator wear testing.[39-41] Some of these methods have been adopted as international standards or are on the way of being so with ongoing standards development. More methods are required and will inevitably slowly emerge for the shoulders, ankles, elbows, and spine.

There are other examples of widely used tests on other aspects of function. Take the efficacy of modular interlocks between a TKR UHMWPE bearing and its metallic baseplate. The function is for the interlock to work, and the strength of that is tested in various directions: anterior loading, posterior, medial and lateral, and lift-off modes. In each case, the UHMWPE bearing component interlock to the baseplate is characterized to verify it to be sufficiently rigidly fixed if its dislodging force or moment is found to exceed prescribed acceptance values.

Mechanical Testing of Implant Durability

The longevity of an implant in the human body is a critical safety factor to avoid surgical complications and revision surgery. Let us consider hip and knee joint replacements, which are among the most successful intervention surgeries in the history of medicine. They relieve patients of severe pain, providing them mobility, and help preserve other aspects of their overall health. Yet, even after 50 to 70 years of arthroplasty technological R&D, and with the current 1 million surgeries performed per year in the United States, projected to double in another decade,[16] revision rates are still occurring at 8% to 16%.[42,43] This amounts to tens of thousands of typically elderly patients who will have to endure a risky and expensive revision surgery a significant proportion of which are still related to implant failure causes. Naturally, some implant designs have been better than others, and only preclinical testing can help screen and discriminate between them.

In the majority of cases, mechanical failure of a knee or a hip system is due to materials or design. But faulty surgical installation or misuse, and/or unusual patient activities may also cause mechanical failure. Most implant designers attempt to make implants as forgiving as possible to pre-empt the latter surgical and patient factors.

The type of implant testing needed depends on the type of failure risk to be screened.

Some failures can be sudden and catastrophic to cause an immediate compromise of the function of the implant and possibly pain and damage to the patient, requiring urgent rectification or revision surgery. Examples of this are excessive deformation or fracture of an implant component caused by lack of strength, fatigue resistance, or other faulty design or material reasons. More specific examples are outright fracture of a TKR tibial baseplate, disassociation of the UHMWPE bearing component from the baseplate due to failure of the modular interlock features, or fatigue and fracture of a hip stem. The latter risk is the subject of the most commonly performed mechanical screening test covered by multiple international standards such as ISO 7206.

Other mechanical failure modes can be more gradual through accumulative damage, which can take years, but is as severe in overall final effect. The most common example is "wear" or corrosion of joint replacement bearing systems. Over years of clinical use, the principle risk to patients from wear is the UHMWPE wear debris, which can be in the form of billions of tiny micron-size particles released into the joint space. These particles can cause an inflammatory response in the bone adjacent to the implant, which can result in osteolysis (bone resorption), which can ultimately end in implant loosening and total failure. Most joint replacement systems (hips, knees, shoulder, ankles, and spine) use UHMWPE as the gold standard soft bearing component, articulated against CoCrMb metallic alloy components. Artificial knee implant wear has been described extensively in the literature.[44] In short, the ultimate risk to patients from joint replacement wear using UHMWPE bearings is generally termed as aseptic loosening due to osteolysis caused by UHMWPE particulate debris. Only a few hundreds of milligrams of UHMWPE material loss due to wear would cause enough osteolytic burden to risk implant loosening failure.

In hips, the threshold of osteolysis and eventual loosening failure may be caused by wear in excess of 0.1 mm bearing thickness reduction per year.[45] In TKR, bearing thickness reduction threshold rates are not easy to estimate as the articular surface conformity and bearing geometries generally vary. In either case, testing to screen for such small amounts of mass reduction of the bearing material makes in vitro wear testing of knee and hip testing much more complex and requires sophisticated wear joint simulators. The history and development of knee wear test methods in simulators, and the international standards that ensued are the subjects of multiple text book chapters,[46] R&D papers,[47,48] and international standards.[49,50] Multistation knee wear simulators typically have six degrees of freedom of motion, with at least four actuated in synchrony with dynamic multiaxial loads. The human walking gait cycle is simulated at a physiologically realistic frequency of one walking step per second (1 Hz), typically to 5 or even 10 million gait cycles in each test, which is equivalent to a patient walking for 5 to 10 years.

Comprehensive setup, including jig and fixture design and manufacture, implant alignment, and simulator tuning add to the multimillion cycle running time of each test, interrupted once a week or so for cleaning, gravimetric wear measurements, and lubricant replacement. Each test can therefore take 3 months at best and more likely 6 months. That is why these simulators usually have multistations (e.g., 3, 4, 6 or even 12) to allow some comparison in each test between different implant groupings. With multistations, 6 degrees of freedom motion on each, with multiactuators working 24 hours a day, these simulator machines are therefore very expensive and are typically considered major capital investment items beyond the capabilities of the average academic laboratory or test house. Also, the specialized "know-how" required to accurately perform testing drives most small companies and R&D centers to outsource testing to specialized labs (Figure 11.5) that have invested many years in such capital equipment and related specialized skills.

Sometimes the history of development of various test methods[46] results in the emergence of two or more different ways of simulating and testing the artificial joint to assess its wear in vitro. For example, the TKR wear testing

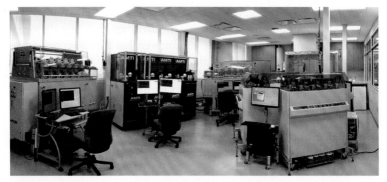

Figure 11.5 Knee, hip, and general orthopedic joint simulator room at the Orthopedic Biomechanics and Advanced Surgical Technologies Laboratory in Omaha, Nebraska (NE). It houses multiple simulators including four separate force-control knee simulators with full computer control and data logging (each simulator has four separate test stations). There are also two AMTI (Watertown, MA) hip wear simulators with 12 test stations and eight separate soak control stations on each. The lab also has four separate stations of the AMTI "Vivo" generalized joint test machine with virtual soft-tissue simulation and 3-D axis transformation capability on each. Finally, there is an AMTI Orthopod six-station pin-on-disk testing machine, and a variety of friction and other testing equipment.

example and international standard ISO 14243-1[49] referred to above are known as the "force control" test methodology. In force control, the TKR AP linear motion and IE rotation in the simulator (i.e. AP and IE kinematics) "result" from standardized AP force and IE torque dynamic waveforms input (actuated) by the machine in synchrony with flexion angle and compressive force waveforms. This allows the same AP and IE kinetics to be used to test different designs of TKRs, and the kinematics of those knees would vary and are measurable on the simulators to facilitate comparisons of different TKR designs or conditions.[36] A simpler alternative method with severe limitations[46] is the "displacement control" wear testing, which prescribes standardized AP and IE motions (kinematics) to be enforced (input) directly, regardless of TKR design variations. The latter method also has a published international standard (ISO 14243-3[51]) to cover the earlier design simulators, which employ only that method.

The foregoing section was intended to briefly provide the reader with awareness and examples about wear testing methods. The reader can access more specialized coverage of it elsewhere.[46] Note also that THR wear tests are also available in two versions, also covered by two standards (ISO 14242-1 and ISO 14242-3), with wear measurement procedures in ISO 14242-2.

All the wear testing methods above are of whole joint systems, simulating in vitro their loading and motions during gait activities to screen for implant design as well as materials. In many circumstances, a new bearing material needs to be evaluated, or different variations of a material processing need to be tested and compared, e.g., techniques of cross-linking of UHMWPE, coatings on bearing materials to enhance wear resistance, etc. Naturally, these ultimately need to be tested when used in an implant system on a knee or similar wear joint simulator.[4,52,53] However, it is wise and more economical to precede these tests with simpler material wear testing, which can compare the materials without having the implant design considerations involved. Pin-on-disk (POD) tribological wear testing is the most appropriate and widely used for orthopedic bearing materials.[54] It is important in POD testing to use appropriate and physiologically realistic loads, stresses, and articular motions to make the tests relevant and to make them useful in predicting longevity of bearing materials in vivo. For example, for wear of UHMWPE bearing materials, it is vital to incorporate cross-shear by having repeated cross-paths and not simple reciprocating motions. Again, like simulator wear testing, much R&D has been published and can be reviewed[54] about this subject, but the most relevant international standard on the topic (ASTM F732[55]) is rather too general. It currently lacks coherently prescriptive methodology and therefore needs a major revision to make it more useful.

In summing up this section, mechanical testing of durability and longevity, preclinical in vitro evaluation of orthopedic implants, and especially joint replacement systems are at the heart of R&D. Such testing can range from the simple fast tests for strength, fatigue, and fracture as described above, to testing of single components or testing interlock strengths of modular components. There are also advanced tests of materials and systems on POD testers reaching all the way up to full joint simulator wear testing.

Computational Simulation Modeling for Research and Development and In Silico Testing

In R&D about an implant or device, it is sometimes necessary to hypothesize or ask questions that have not been answered before. Such R&D process is traditional and essential, and inherently carries risk of unreliability as it inevitably delves in unchartered "what if?" types of questions and scenarios. It is frequently too costly and time-prohibitive if such questions are all to be addressed by practical laboratory experiments. Even a physical prototype specimen of an implant is difficult and expensive to make in small quantities for testing. It would also require setting up the laboratory apparatus, progressing through the learning curve, building jigs and fixtures, and conducting testing that could, by nature, take time (e.g., testing which involves prolonged fatigue loading). This becomes more critical when it is not certain that a new speculative implant concept, design, or detailed implementation will work as intended, or when a hypothesis or question would result in the desired answer. An alternative to practical experimentation, which is becoming increasingly useful as well as popular, is the use of predictive theoretical models and numerical simulation using computational methods. These have advanced in the last 30 years to provide economical solutions for many problems. It is sometimes termed "in silico" testing and is used as an analogy to in vivo and in vitro testing, considering that the core of the simulation processing occurs in silicon chips in computers. In silico testing today means performed on a computer or by computational modeling and simulation.

Some functional attributes of implant design or aspects of design and materials are analytically predictable or are at least determinant for comparison purposes. Using basic theory manually performed or implemented using commercially available computational simulation software tools can provide economical and valuable quick answers to screen out designs, that would turn out to be dysfunctional and wind up wasting valuable design time and testing resources.

In what remains of this section, we will generally and very briefly describe or remind the reader of the principles behind two main computational simulation approaches that can help reduce cost and accelerate development early in the design process of orthopedic implants.

Theoretical, Lumped Parameter Simulation Computational Modeling

A system comprising an orthopedic implant interacting with soft tissues such as muscles or ligaments can be modeled as discrete bodies interacting using simple physics rules. For example, their 3-D translational positions and orientations (sometimes termed "pose") and movements can be determined by Newton's laws of motion, using lumped parameters. Each component is characterized by its mass, simplified shape, positions, and velocities and/or acceleration. The stresses and strains (and thus risk of deformation or fracture) can be determined using linear elastic (Hook's law) or nonlinear elastic and plastic deformation rules using suitable parametric descriptors such as Young's modulus and Poison ratio, applied to a model of their simplified geometrical shape and with the loading applied to it externally or from a connected component. The friction between components can also be modeled using parametric descriptors such as coefficient of friction, or friction can sometimes be assumed zero in simplistic models. Even advanced surface characterizations such as surface energy, contact angle (for wettability and lubricity), and so on can be conducted today using modern modelling techniques.

On the extreme of simplicity, an elementary model of a bone (say tibia) can be solved using beam theory, assuming the bone to be cylindrical, of certain diameter, length, and Young's modulus. The bone could be positioned in a pose relative to the ground, with a certain ground-to-foot reaction force emanating from the gravitational forces (human body weight) at a certain phase of a walking gait cycle or other static or pseudosteady state posture. The forces and moments in the middle section of the tibia can be estimated with reasonable accuracy using linear and rotational equilibrium with a free body diagram. This simple model can be advanced/complicated further more by adding a knee joint (in the form of a "black box") on top and modeling the action of the quadriceps muscle pulling in one direction at one point (hence the "lumped" parameter terminology) to provide the extensor mechanism, and balancing moment necessary for the leg's rotational equilibrium. Such solutions that can be seen in almost all traditional biomechanics textbooks would then show the compressive force on the knee to reach multiples of the assumed human body weight. If there was an implant (e.g., tibial component of a TKR) inserted on the bone, this simple model can estimate the compressive and shear forces on the metallic baseplate and with similar simplifying assumptions, the overall forces and average stresses on a polyethylene bearing insert on top.

The computational aspect adds much power and ease to systematically help the user define the simplified geometry and lumped parameter model characteristics of the individual components, the simplifying assumptions for the solution method (e.g., neglect friction in some connections, and/or neglect inertia/acceleration forces in some, etc.). The software data structure combined with user choices organizes the model equations to be solved, and which are the given known variables versus the desired unknown ones. The computational power becomes essential when many, e.g., tens of components can be combined into a big model, resulting in hundreds of equations and sometimes not enough knowns to directly solve them, so iterative solutions become the only way forward.

It is common for such computational model solvers to treat all objects (e.g., human musculoskeletal system segments as in Figure 11.6) as rigid bodies, joined together kinematically simulating human joints and influenced by external forces such as gravity/human body weight and other internal forces from simulated muscle action. Linear or nonlinear spring-like elements can be added to simulate ligaments or any other soft-tissue constraint elements.

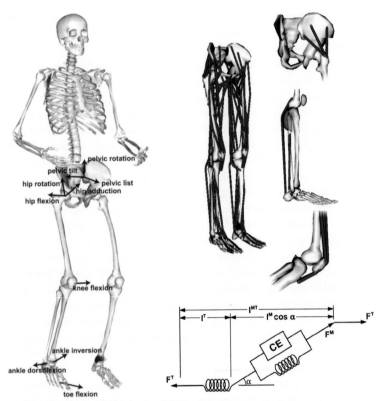

Figure 11.6 Model by Rajagopal et al[38] depicting a whole human musculoskeletal system (left), the muscles modeled and their attachment points (top right), and the theoretical model parameters of a muscle acting through its tendon. (Walker PS, Heller Y, Cleary DJ, Yildirim G. Preclinical evaluation method for total knees designed to restore normal knee mechanics. *J Arthroplasty*. 2011;26(1):152-160. doi:10.1016/j.arth.2009.11.017.)

The initial or input boundary conditions for such a model can either be assumed, e.g., initial joint angles and bone segment velocities, or can be based on gait lab data measured by a motion capture system. The computation utilizes any external force and motion inputs and the theoretical rules such as described earlier to determine the other segment motions. The solution can be used to estimate, for example, what muscles (if modeled) contributed how much to make the whole system motion consistent. When known motions (kinematics) are used to compute forces and moments for a lumped parameter modeled system, it is called an *Inverse Dynamics* solver.

A pioneering example of a lumped parameter computational model using mainframe computers during the 1970s was developed by the late Professor John Paul. Paul and Morrison[25] modeled the forces on the human knee. They used multiple muscles with assumed attachment points, and assumed zero friction at the knee joint, and fed the model with kinematics from gait studies, which measured force-plate data of ground-foot reaction forces synchronized in time with kinematics or posture. They successfully computed the internal forces on the knee during different phases of the walking cycle. The forces computed reached multiple body weights during the stance (load-bearing) phase. The compressive force plotted versus the phase of a walking gait cycle is now the widely-known "Paul Curve," a good estimate still used today in ASTM and ISO standards[9,49,51] for knee wear testing.

On the other extreme, examples of modern computational models[56] used in the academic field are those from Dr Scott Delp's team of the University of Stanford, which originated and resulted from a very comprehensive research program over many years, and it was partially commercialized. The *Anybody* suite of software (by AnyBody Technology/Denmark) is another modern system, which is more aggressively commercialized. As expected, such tools are very flexible in the user interface and can handle large numbers of musculoskeletal body segments, and input force or kinematic data, and incorporate implants for simulation. Some models can handle more physiologically realistic bone shapes with anatomical articulating surfaces, which can roll or slide against each other and predict the detailed joint motions based on "collision detection." They utilize the valid assumption that the shapes of virtual 3-D models of rigid or semirigid surfaces cannot in physical reality penetrate into each other. So, when the motions determined computationally are constrained by that condition, the simulation becomes more physiologically realistic for relative motion at joints and can account for how implant component bearing surfaces articulate against each other.

Caution is always necessary not to extrapolate too much from such models, due to the many simplifying assumptions made. Obviously any stress analysis for trusses, beams, and other simple structures applied to biomechanics of bone and implants can be dramatic simplification. In the example above, if the articular bearing is that of a knee replacement, the contact and friction of the relatively soft UHMWPE bearings is complicated by some compliance, viscoelastic deformation, creep, and even shape memory effects. This type of modeling also usually implies mass to be concentrated at the center of gravity of an object with the complex shape of (say) a bone simplified as a line segment or cylindrical bar. Most importantly, in traditional mechanical and structural engineering applications, the ultimate goal is to estimate theoretically predicted maximum stresses to verify them to be below the material's yield strength to prevent fracture or fatigue. Such structures are also given a large safety factor of say 2-3. This is frequently not possible in many orthopedic implant applications such as trauma plates, knee and hip replacement metallic components, and UHMWPE bearing components, which can seldom be over engineered due to space limitations and to maintain bone conservation and less invasion of other anatomic structures.

One example to illustrate the above is the contact of a metal femoral knee component implant on an UHMWPE bearing. It undergoes high-enough stresses to produce at least viscoelastic deformation and sometimes even plastic deformation in the UHMWPE. So, when models such as the above assume purely rigid articulating surfaces, regardless of how little friction they assume, they are neither equipped with the theory nor any empirically based rules to model the complex contact with, and viscoelastic deformation of UHMWPE.

Finite Element Analysis Computational Modeling and Simulation

Finite element analysis (FEA) is a big subject described in multiple textbooks, hundreds of case studies, and published research papers.[57] Armed with the solution concepts highlighted in the previous section, we will only here describe the essential principles and what differentiates the FEA computational approach from above. The earlier modeling depicted objects (e.g., bones, or implant components) as whole rigid body segments of different shapes. In FEA, each object is divided into many much smaller and more manageable block elements with simple shapes (e.g., tetrahedral or hexahedral). These elements are characterized at points and nodes, representing their material properties, and their state including position and orientation, and stress and strain in all dimensions. The elements are meshed such that their corner points or vertices are common and shared. They are made small enough in size and large enough in number to be able to represent any complex geometry of the whole component, including curved edges, contoured surfaces, or spatially changing mechanical properties within one object. Elements are made smaller still (finer mesh) in regions of fast-changing geometry or expected stress concentration, to represent high gradients of change in these properties and thus higher accuracy and more spatial resolution of the results. All elements in the mesh are ascribed mechanical and other properties, which can vary with region or objects or even on an individual element basis (see example later in this section, and Figure 11.7), and so would the given boundary conditions such as contact or external loading prescribed for them.

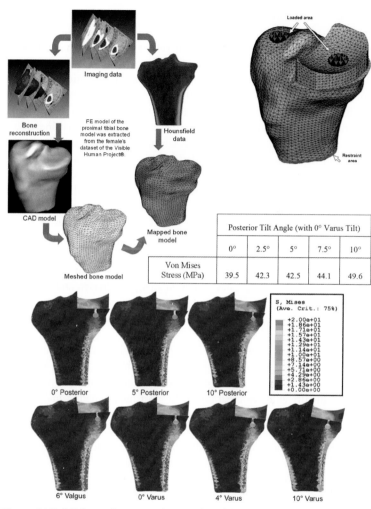

	Posterior Tilt Angle (with 0° Varus Tilt)				
	0°	2.5°	5°	7.5°	10°
Von Mises Stress (MPa)	39.5	42.3	42.5	44.1	49.6

Figure 11.7 3-D finite element analysis study[58] of the bone stress distribution of aligned and misaligned novel designs of tibial components for unicondylar knee arthroplasty performed by the author's laboratory between 2000-2005. Top left shows the Finite element analysis (FEA) mesh generation from CT data with totally distributed bone material properties. Top right shows the implant incorporated within the solution domain and the loading boundary conditions. Bottom shows a sectional view of the resulting von Mises stress distribution. CAD, computer-aided design.

The computational solver data structure can end up with thousands or millions of elements and even higher numbers of equations to solve expressing the same type of theoretical rules as described in the modeling of the previous section. For example, mechanically, the strain of an element is proportional to its stress during elastic deformation, linked by Young's Modulus. This is one, and the most common, rule among many possible others, which also incorporate 3-D nonuniformity (anisotropy) considerations. In FEA however, the rules are applied to each individual (simple) element at a time, where the solution for the element is simple, and thus provide high fidelity (for the element). When combined, for the whole mesh of all elements that closely models the complex shape object or assembly, the overall accuracy becomes only subject to rounding errors that are negligible in modern computers and of course subject to how closely the theory applies (e.g., in rigid elastic model solvers, the stresses anywhere must not be in excess of elastic deformation or large errors would emerge, and so on). Iterations are required until the resulting strains and small changes of element shapes are consistent to continue to mesh with adjacent elements, which might have different strength, stresses, and strains. In this manner, the solution converges with an estimate of the internal spatial stress distribution within each modeled segment. This is typically termed an "implicit solution".

When the inertia and acceleration considerations are also taken into account, the model becomes an explicit FEA solution, allowing the positions and motions of the segments to be determined at different time steps, dynamically driven by external forces. In most such dynamic analyses, the computational solution time step must be slow enough in propagation compared with the acoustic wave speed through the object's materials so that the mechanical effects from all elements have time to propagate and affect all other elements in representing the transient state of the system.

An example of a (then-pioneering) study[58] from the author's own laboratory was performed in 2002-2005 and presented in 2006. The stress distributions (Figure 11.7) in a novel uncemented unicondylar knee replacement design and in the tibial bone underneath it were estimated by FEA using Abaqus software (Dassault Systèmes/France). We attributed fully distributed Young's Modulus material properties to the bone model, which were different for each FEA mesh element. These were input automatically into Abaqus from a data file, mapping each mesh element to a property value. We generated the data file ourselves using simple code we wrote in the Fortran programming language. For input and to represent the shape of the bone model, we used data we produced from processing CT imaging of the knee bones from a dataset of the Visible Human Project[59] using Mimics software (Materialise/Belgium). The latter helped us segment and reconstruct the CT imaging (DICOM format) into surface models, and then these were converted to volumetric models. The 3-D models of the bone were meshed using software tools into a suitable mesh file to be input into Abaqus for FEA. Mimics software was also used to extract and download data tables, mapping each bone CT imaging pixel in 3-D coordinates to its corresponding Hounsfield Unit (HU). These HU values represented the X-ray radiodensity at each pixel from the CT data. This was in a way similar to a DICOM file but only for the bone of interest.

Our Fortran program, using this data as input, mapped the radiodensity values of each imaging pixel into an actual bone density and then Young's Modulus value in SI Units using known (published) relations between HU, bone density, and Young's Modulus. At that stage, the two data sets from the two different systems (imaging pixels from CT and the FEA mesh for Abaqus) were obviously different data structures. The former contained 3-D coordinates of imaging points with related material properties. The latter represented 3-D–shaped FEA mesh elements.

The main and final task of the Fortran program was to ascribe for each bone model mesh element for the FEA analysis from Abaqus, a Young's modulus value. The value in each case was computed by spacial interpolation and averaging of the properties of all the geometrically neighboring imaging pixel elements, from the imaging data table originating from Mimics. As can be seen, this looks rather complicated and was novel in 2002. The good news for the reader is that all this is now much easier to do and almost fully automated with modern versions of the same software tools.

Like any other modeling, FEA suffers various weaknesses, especially if the theoretical model (rules) governing how each element behaves is too simplistic. Rigid elastic modeling was the earlier example, especially when viscoelastic and plastic deformations were involved. Contact mechanics and the effects of friction and lubrication are also often too simplified. Of course the effects of creep and shape memory of some polymers such as UHMWPE add much more complexity. Very often, scientific publications would present predictions of UHMWPE wear in TKR using FEA solvers, neglecting even the wear-amplifying effects of cross-shear in the modeling of material removal. Cross shear is known to multiply the wear rates multifold and needs special modeling, which has not been fully successful as yet.

We mentioned earlier that FEA solutions are useful for producing estimates to answer "what if" type of questions. The results cannot be fully relied on, however, for final design or V&V purposes without comprehensive validation by physical mechanical testing. Experimental validation tests need to have the important variables of geometry and conditions such as loading varied across a suitable range before enough confidence is attained in the FEA solution, and before generalization and extrapolation are justified. The ASTM had recently put many years of effort to establish FEA modeling method practice guides, coupled with validation and a round-robin set of tests by multiple labs. This started with predicting strength and stress distribution of THR femoral stems. This culminated in 2013 with the publication of one standard, ASTM F2996-13 "Standard Practice for Finite Element Analysis (FEA) of Non-Modular Metallic Orthopedic Hip Femoral Stems." There is currently ongoing work on another to predict failure of TKR tibial baseplates. Notice the suitable choices in both cases, easily fitting the rigid body elastic modeling assumptions, with no temperature effects and no complex contact or frictional conditions, which could risk complicating the solutions. Even with that, validation is still required by regulatory bodies to minimize human errors, which could occur in FEA meshing, boundary and other input conditions, and in the final converged solutions.

Medical Device Testing Standards

In the previous sections, the emphasis was on R&D data for V&V as part of the implant design process. It is paramount for any R&D effort to capitalize from the previous work of others. This usually starts with a literature survey and continues with learning, training, and collaborations with experts. When previous R&D had involved testing, which is expected to have been commonly done by others, it is very sensible to check if there are any standards on how testing should be done. International standards represent the distilled understanding and consensus of most stakeholders who have dealt with a given test method or procedure before. This becomes crucial if the R&D team is not familiar or lacks expertise in the subject, and vital if the R&D work and its results are in preparation of a regulatory clearance submission. Standards help specification of materials and components that are used in the manufacture and assembly of medical devices. They can be used as they are to assess or demonstrate conformity with existing specifications, and for V&V of device performance or longevity. They can also provide reference or comparison with self-developed custom test methods. Some standards provide guidance on how to start compiling data for clearance or approval of marketing applications. Finally, standards are essential for quality management purposes.

In their most basic form, standard test methods aid the R&D team to demonstrate conformity with relevant regulatory requirements. This speeds up the regulatory review because it gives a better and partially predetermined understanding and expectation of the data to evaluate the safety and/or effectiveness of a device. When standards are international, they also represent agreed and clearly documented technical requirements for global harmonization.

There are two international Standards Development Organizations (SDOs), which are most relevant for orthopedic devices, and they are ASTM International and the ISO. Each covers standards, guides, and technical reports for a very wide range of products and services, well beyond medical devices. ISO/TC 150 standards and ASTM International are used by many manufacturers and regulatory bodies. Therefore, each has an appropriate specialist committee structure, which will be briefly described next.

AMERICAN SOCIETY FOR TESTING AND MATERIALS INTERNATIONAL STANDARDS

In ASTM International, committee F04 on Medical and Surgical Materials and Devices is the main committee covering orthopedic implants. Formed in 1962, ASTM Committee F04 fosters the development of standardized test methods, specifications, guides, performance standards, nomenclature, and definitions of terms for medical and surgical materials and devices. The committee also encourages research and sponsors symposia, workshops, and publications to facilitate the development of such standards.

There are over 140 other technical committees (TCs) in ASTM International, and some may overlap or relate to the work of F04 regarding orthopedic technology. For example, committee F42 is recent and formed in 2009 on Additive Manufacturing Technologies. It combines expertise from a much wider field than medical devices but takes into consideration and benefits from experts within the medical field including the orthopedic industry. F42 has a current membership of approximately 400 people and meets twice a year, usually in January and July, with about 100 members attending 2 days of standards work preeminently on all aspects of Additive Manufacturing Technologies. It has six technical subcommittees only (contrast that with the more mature F04 described below).

Committee F04 has approximately 900 individual members (who could be thought of as experts). F04 has developed hundreds of standards, 300 standards of which are currently active, and are published in the Annual Book of ASTM Standards, Volumes 13.01 and 13.02. The committee members physically meet twice annually, in May and November, with about 190 members attending over 3 or so days of technical meetings. This is sometimes preceded by a symposium or workshop on relevant topics in the field of medical/surgical materials and devices. For example, the last workshop that was held at the time of writing of this book chapter was on medical implant coatings and standards on how to tests them. The author was among the organizing committee for this workshop, which was attended by about 100 people. On the day, the author gave a technical presentation of research findings from the testing of ceramic coatings on hip and knee replacement systems.[60]

F04 has a hierarchical structure of four major divisions, Division II of which is on orthopedic devices (chaired by the author). F04 has 34 technical subcommittees spanning a variety of topics on materials, orthopedic devices, testing, tissue engineering, and medical/surgical instruments. Worthy of note is SC F04.22 "Arthroplasty." For the last many years, this has been chaired by Mr. John Goode, who is a most accomplished leader from the FDA's device review team and who has also been for many years the chair of ISO/TC 150 committee on implantable devices (described in the next section). For example, F04.22 is separate from F04.25 on "Spinal Devices". Very different examples of other subcommittees (SCs) within ASTM F04, which relate to topics covered in this chapter are F04.16 "Biocompatibility Test Methods" and F04.39 "Human Clinical Trials."

The documents produced by ASTM International are principally "standards documents," whose name/number (e.g., F1223-14) usually starts with a letter, in this case "F" stands for the committee (F04), which developed it and thus major area/topic, then a number signifying the document/standard unique subject, followed by a dash, and then a number signifying the year (in this case 2014) version of that standard. The current applicable standard is the one that has the relevant document number and latest year. Previous versions are uniquely preserved and can be referred to differentiate them from later versions for comparison, historic compliance, and other such reasons.

ASTM International standard documents can be "Test Methods," the most relevant type like most of the ones mentioned so far in this chapter, such as "ASTM F1223-14 Standard Test Method for Determination of Total Knee Replacement Constraint." There are also ASTM International "Specification" documents (described next) and various other less-known category types, including Classifications, Practices, Guides, Terminology or Definitions, Reference Radiographs, Reference Photographs, Tables, and Charts. Some of these category names are self-explanatory, but none are as important for our topic as Test methods and Specifications. Test methods prescribe methods of testing, from the description of the scope and rationale, term definitions, citations of other standards, to the experimental setup, test sample selection, materials, testing procedure, and all the way to what should be reported from the testing.

The title of the category of "Specification" standards does not make it clear how important its standards are for new implant development and the direct relevance to this book. In short, an ASTM International specification standard describes what type of implants a system comprises, what standardized materials they can be made of, what is required to formally and fully describe the implant system in terms materials and their processing, design shape, dimensions, and variations, and what standardized and nonstandard preclinical tests should be conducted to ensure patient safety. It is clear from the latter point at least how useful a specification standard is for any R&D team embarking on development of a new implant. It is important to remind the reader that the actual regulatory clearance requirements for any implant depend on the regulatory body, and in the case of the FDA in the United States, it is available through their relevant guidelines published on their official websites. However, since the FDA is represented on the ASTM International and ISO standards development committees among others, the FDA regulatory requirements stated in their guidelines usually cite and echo appropriate ASTM specification standards if they exist and can go beyond.

An example of a widely used ASTM specification standard is "ASTM F2083-12 Standard Specification for Knee Replacement Prosthesis." It defines what can be classed as a TKR, distinguishing between primary and revision prostheses, the minimum allowable flexion range, fixed versus mobile bearing knee designs, and generic categories based on three levels of constraint (e.g., how a hinged knee is categorized as "highly constrained" vs. the other extreme of laxity of say a "nonconstrained" cruciate-retaining TKR). It also covers components of modular designs and distinguishes between cemented versus uncemented components. Basic descriptions of appropriate materials and prosthesis geometry are also provided. Additionally, the characteristics determined to be important to in vivo performance of the prosthesis are also defined.

F2083-12 makes it clear that the choice of standardized materials is understood to be a necessary but not sufficient assurance of function or longevity of the device. It also prescribes an array of in vitro tests, which need to be performed on a TKR. Among them is range of motion and constraint (through ASTM F1223), fatigue testing of baseplates (F1800), contact area and stress, and modular interlock mechanism strength (not standardized yet), and of course wear testing (ISO 14243-1, -2 and -3). In some cases, when a standardized test only describes a methodology without specifying performance acceptance criteria (e.g., F1800 and F1223), the specification standard (F2083) would state the required fatigue test loading level, and number of cycles and specimens to be tested (performance requirements). In the F1800 case as an example, the minimum is to test five specimens, to successfully reach runout at 10 million cycles, at 900 N sinusoidal loading with R = 0.1. The F2083-12 specification standard also states at what conditions a test should be performed, e.g., at various flexion angles and other conditions for constraint testing based on F1223. The above is by no means an exhaustive list or description of what ASTM 1223 contains, but it gives an idea and examples of the type of content and requirements in it.

The same exists for hips with similar content (viz. ASTM F2033-12 Standard Specification for Total Hip Joint Prosthesis and Hip Endoprosthesis Bearing Surfaces Made of Metallic, Ceramic, and Polymeric Materials). Shoulders and ankles have them too (viz. ASTM F1378-17, and ASTM F2665-09 (2014) respectively, although they both currently lack specific wear test methods, which currently are work-in progress for standardization. The author confesses to have drafted the first version of the latter (Ankle Specification) standard based on similar content in the knee, and omitting to address (or prescribe) at that time any wear test methods as they were lacking.

Finally, the ASTM F04 committee also facilitates liaison with other ASTM committees and other organizations with mutual interests. Among the most important is ASTM SC F04.93 "US TAG ISO/TC 150—Implants for Surgery," which will be described in the next section. TAG stands for "Technical Advisory Group"; so through this ASTM SC (with short name "US Tag"), the United States as a country handles balloting and voting on ISO standard development matters. The author of this chapter has recently been elected as Chair of the US TAG. Three task forces have been setup to reform and upgrade how the United States disseminates ISO standard ballots, facilitates discussion, solicits feedback from a wide variety of stakeholders, collates comments, synthesizes, and distills them into coherent votes and how comments are to be explained and defended in actual ISO meetings. As mentioned in an early section of this chapter, the stakeholders include all the country's implant manufacturers, regulatory bodies (e.g., FDA), surgeons, hospitals, payers, and of course patients. So this is a mammoth task, which should and can be done much better in the future.

It must be mentioned that ASTM International is truly so, international. Only the venues of its two meetings a year circulate in various North American locations. ASTM has over 30,000 members from more than 140 countries. Anyone, from any country, can join to be a member and actively participate in ASTM F04 or join an SC. The author has attended literally all the ASTM F04 Medical Device meetings in the last 18 years. These forums have become a haven to all those wishing to learn and influence orthopedic device standards, regulatory requirements, and how testing is done. The annual subscription fee per person is only nominal, allowing literally free attendance to the relevant physical and online ASTM meetings. Each member's organization, whether a >10,000 employee multinational blue-chip company, or a small one- to two-person start-up company, or an academic R&D lab or a one-person consultant or scientist, or any other, has only one single official vote that counts for that organization/entity. However, every individual member alone, or from any organization, has an equal opportunity to discuss, to be heard, and a chance to comment on and improve standards. Thus lies a huge strength of the ASTM International method as it is really inclusive of all expertise wherever it comes from, and this is therefore reflected in the good quality of most of its standards.

INTERNATIONAL ORGANIZATION FOR STANDARDIZATION

ISO is the world's largest developer of international standards. Founded in 1947, it is an independent, nongovernmental organization whose members are the national standards bodies of 162 countries. It has fostered the development and publication of more than 22 thousand international standards, covering almost all aspects of technology and business. ISO's Central Secretariat is in Geneva, Switzerland, with about 135 people working full-time to coordinate its activities.

There are nearly 250 different ISO Technical Committees (TCs) that develop standards. The TC that deals with our topic is ISO/TC 150 titled "Implants for Surgery," which has >150 standards, and >50 under development. TC 150 has an internal structure of 15 working groups (WGs), and 7 SCs. An SC has long time span, covering a particular area, and can expand in standards. A WG of TC 150 has a specific task, e.g., establishes one or a series of standards on a topic and then disband. The WG topic can span the scope of multiple SCs. The following are the current ISO/TC 150 WGs and SCs:

- SC 1 Materials
- SC 2 Cardiovascular implants and extracorporeal systems
- SC 4 Bone and joint replacement
- SC 5 Osteosynthesis and spinal devices
- SC 6 Active implants
- SC 7 Tissue-engineered medical products (TEMPs)

The active ISO/TC 150 WGs include:

- WG 7 Fundamental standards
- WG 10 Use and retrieval of surgical implants
- WG 12 Implant coatings
- WG 13 Absorbable metal implants
- WG 14 Models of tissues for mechanical testing of implants
- WG 15 Neurosurgical implants

It can be easily seen how some of these WGs can directly relate to orthopedic technology but equally so to cardiovascular and other implants.

Each TC 150 SC has within it semipermanent or temporary WGs. For example SC 1 "Materials," has under it SC 1/WG 1 "Ceramics," SC 1/WG 2 "Metals," and SC 1/WG 3 "Plastics." And similarly, so does SC 4 and also SC 5, which is broad and has in it SC 5/WG 1 on "Osteosynthesis devices" (i.e. orthopedic trauma plates and screws, etc.) and SC 5/WG 2 on "Spinal Devices."

For some countries other than the United States, and especially those which are new to standardization activity, the ISO is the SDO they see as the most relevant. The main players in the ISO operative procedures are the "member bodies," such that there is one member per country. This is inherited from the formation of the ISO under its charter; each country is represented and helps in the discussions and development of standards through the (country's) "experts." When it comes to ballots and voting on standards, and commenting on work-in-progress standardization documents, each member body (i.e. country) has one vote. The author was a member of the task force, which drafted the latest revision of the ISO/TC 150 strategic business plan. The ISO general regulations and that plan assert the right and responsibility of each member body to vote, representing their stakeholder's interests and objectives. TC 150 and its SCs encourage all members to actively engage in the work of the committee and provide constructive input through nominated experts.

This general principle is good, in that it is inclusive of all, including developing countries, to participate and to be influential. After all, the acronym of the name ISO reminds us of the Greek "isos," meaning "equal."

Olle Sturen, the Secretary General of ISO in 1969, profoundly commented.

Political nationalism will most probably prevail for as long as we live. Economic nationalism is about to disappear. And technical nationalism has disappeared!

This becomes truly so if each country's delegation would include actual "experts" in the ISO/TC 150 meeting to contribute to the technical discussions for better standards. This however becomes difficult unless each country's delegation was to include tens of specialist experts to attend and discuss the different standards, which may occur simultaneously in different meeting rooms. The United States regularly does so, such that in the recent years, the US delegation has been more or less consistently the largest, typically exceeding >80 delegates, out of the whole world's total of around 200-220 in each annual meeting.

A good proportion of member bodies (or other countries) naturally send smaller delegations. Many of them send as little as 1-2 people even, and some attend irregularly and therefore frequently send none. When standards ballots are cast, many countries seem to vote "approval" on draft standards most of the time. It is not known how many specialist experts actively participate in meetings or discussions within those countries to establish these votes. A negative vote requires comments to justify them, or as constructive input on work items. It seems natural and easy for any member body to vote "approval" on ballot items for which they have little to no expertise. Therefore, the ISO process has tended to be inadvertently biased to favor new proposals or push working documents along with relatively little critique. Sometimes well-considered "disapproval" votes from countries which happen to have experts may not carry sufficient weight in committee discussions. Such member body "disapproval" votes that include constructive criticisms and suggestions for improvements, when faced with a significant number of seemingly routine "approval" votes, may struggle or find it too late to persuade the majority to slow down the progress of a document before their comments are adequately addressed. It is theoretically possible, and this has happened in some extreme cases, that tens of experts and comments from a very large country which such experts would lose in ballots through their single (country) vote, versus a multitude of approval votes coming from other countries. This author calls this phenomenon as a "democracy of science," which is a complicated notion if not hazardous to say the least.

The new ISO/TC 150 strategy planning document now recommends that rather than voting "approval" in such a situation, when lacking stakeholder specialist or local experts participation, a vote of "abstain" is encouraged by default, according to the ISO directives. This is appropriate even if it means that on multiple ballots on a particular topic, member bodies would end up repeatedly voting "abstain." If applied, this would solve the problem of naturally allowing new standards to be started and to continue without adequate technical scrutiny and especially in the cases of potentially duplicating a standard from another SDO, a subject covered next.

DUPLICATION OF STANDARDS

For coherence of international standards, any duplication of work which may result in similar standards on the same subject between SDOs must be avoided. Duplication can lead to confusion if standards written on the same topic contain different or conflicting information or instructions. Such standards, over time, would inevitably "grow apart" as each may be revised independently. Duplication also wastes valuable resources including those needed to develop standards in areas of unmet need. This has been a severe problem between ISO/TC 150 and ASTM International's F04 committee, especially in joint replacement and other orthopedic technology. In one or two cases, when the author was responsible for the area of joint replacement wear, this was fundamentally addressed between 2003 and 2009. The equivalent ASTM standards, which were at the time work-in-progress guidance documents in knee replacement wear testing for example, were withdrawn in favor of the (then) more mature ISO 14243-1, -2, and -3 standards for knee wear testing. To bring all the US-based stakeholders on-board (tens of manufacturing companies, test labs, FDA, and other stakeholders), these two ISO standards were drastically revised after much technical discussion in the ASTM International meetings. The revisions were formally carried out within the ISO/TC 150 process, and still do, but the technical discussions about what to revise were carried out within the ASTM International meetings, which were typically attended by more experts and facilitated for longer and richer technical discussions. So, in wear testing of hip and knee replacements, only ISO 14242-1, -2, and -3 and ISO 14243-1, -2, and -3 (respectively) are the standards being currently followed all over the world and discussed for revision.

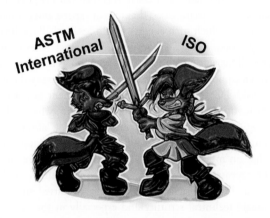

Much duplication with many (national) standards organizations has been previously avoided by transferring into the ISO/TC 150 the national (say, British BSI or German DIN) standards and making them ISO documents by agreement. Unfortunately, the same has not happened with ASTM International. It is estimated that >70 or so ISO standards and ASTM International duplicate standards have occurred over the years in orthopedic materials and technology. A good example is ISO 14897 on fatigue testing of knee replacement tibial component baseplates. When this ISO standard was first written (around 1997-2000), it had exactly mirrored the content of the then ASTM F1800 standard. But, since then, the ASTM F1800 has had multiple revisions, but the ISO standard had very little revision and they have thus unintendedly diverged. In these situations, what is needed is either for one SDO to withdraw its duplicating standard or the two get harmonized to be exactly the same. The latter route is not easy and is now an ongoing effort with the ISO 14879 and F1800 example.

In general principle, ISO/TC 150 has categorically discouraged duplication in its own directives (Part 1, Annex C) where it is required for any new standard proposal to first provide "… a listing of all relevant documents at the international, regional, and national levels," to be examined for overlap or duplication. The new standard proposal should include a plan on how to avoid or minimize this by widening the scope of the original standard. In practice however, these directives have not been strictly enforced by the individual ISO/TC 150 SC and WG chairs and secretaries, thus unintentionally leaving the duplication problem to grow to what it is today. ISO/TC 150 has recently setup a duplication prevention task force (which includes the author of this chapter), which worked for >2 years and produced a guidance document for additional steps to minimize and avoid duplication of work. Among its plans is to identify the exact standards, which duplicate, and prepare a plan of either withdrawal or harmonization on a one-by-one basis. The ASTM International F04 committee has since started a similar parallel effort to avoid future duplication. Despite the inevitable bureaucracy and some natural competition between ASTM International and the ISO organizations, there are many grass-root volunteer leaders who help in both. They diligently perform the technical work on standards and have dedicated much effort to make the two SDOs collaborate rather than compete to fulfill the unmet standardization needs and to help implant manufacturers plot a clearer and safer V&V route for the benefits of patients.

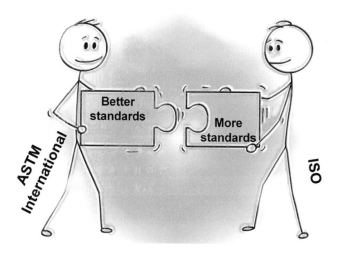

Concluding Remarks

We started this chapter highlighting how the number of orthopedic implant and device manufacturing companies has grown in the United States, and in many other countries. We also highlighted the emergence of new materials and technologies (e.g., additive manufacturing, coatings, etc.) and how that has required more R&D, V&V, and preclinical testing. R&D and testing are clearly cost-center activities; they do not generate revenue but the opposite for most implant manufacturing companies. Therefore economical pressures have made it difficult for them to sufficiently expand investment in device R&D and preclinical evaluation to match the technological advances and growth in product variety.

We described the regulatory classifications of orthopedic implants based on levels of potential risk to patients. The reader can safely conclude from all the above that R&D for truly innovative implants can be complex, costly and takes time. Therefore most tend to incrementally improve existing implants and devices, which have already been granted regulatory clearance and have an extensive body of testing and supportive R&D data behind them. This was partly the basis of the 510K clearing process, which relies on comparisons to existing clinically successful implant predicates. In doing so, it is paramount to compromise to find a balance between the significance, incidence, and severity of the clinical problem addressed, with the advantages and risks of the proposed new or modified implant solution. The balance should fill the gap between in silico and in vitro R&D data, and the unknowns of efficacy and long-term safety in large-scale human usage over many years.[61]

The categories of preclinical V&V testing were described, starting from animal studies when suitable. The importance was emphasized of choosing the appropriate animal model, variable control, and what observations should be planned beforehand. As always, we briefly mentioned the deep ethical issues involved. We then delved in much more detail into in vivo clinical studies in humans, by logging outcomes through Kaplan-Meier survival analysis and commonly used patient-reported functional scores. We then described the principles of more technical quantitative clinical R&D methods on patients with implants, including biomechanic gait studies and fluoroscopy kinematic measurements. We described RSA and other more conventional (Martell) radiographic studies of implant subsidence, migration, and wear. We finally visited telemetry measurements of implant forces on some R&D patients within the larger scope of biomechanic gait studies.

R&D through in vitro testing of implants was described with much detail, differentiating between bench simulations to assess implant function from those assessing implant durability such as fatigue and wear. Some of these expensive tests could be preempted by cheaper and more flexible in silico testing, where FEA or lumped parameter analysis can provide very useful estimates in the early stages of a design process.

In all the above, we pointed to particular ASTM International and ISO testing standards when appropriate, and explained how specification standards, when they are available, are useful umbrella reference documents to find out what testing methods should be done for a given implant type. The standardization process through ASTM International and ISO and their committee structures were explained in some detail to encourage the reader to participate. After all, one very good way to understand what and how testing standards are used is to actually participate in the discussions when they are created or revised. It is surprising to many how easy and open these standards forums are, and how educational it is to listen to those who derive standard test methods from the years of experience of testing themselves.

Overall, there is a tendency for large and small companies to be too conservative with their R&D approach. There is an inherent fear of "failing" in a test and what that may entail in the design process. Owing to economical pressures and technological advances (e.g., CAD/CAM, rapid prototyping, and additive manufacturing), design iterations can run faster today but are frustrated by much slower in vitro testing, especially if the results from such testing would suggest design changes. However, engineers, scientists, and surgeons who undertake R&D for innovative orthopedic implants need to be willing to subject their innovations, to and sometimes fail in, preclinical implant testing. Otherwise, they will be blind-hooded in false perceptions and veneration of their particular design and that can generally cause them to be left behind in the innovation race. Implant R&D and testing should be so integral to the design process and not for regulatory clearance purposes alone. Failure in preclinical testing should only mean "have not succeeded yet." All in all, R&D and implant V&V are the surest way for patient safety, market share, potential profits, retaining employee talent with good morale, and building a reputable brand. We conclude this R&D chapter by emphasizing three things: testing, testing, and testing!

REFERENCES AND RESOURCES

1. Charnley J. Arthroplasty of the hip, discussion. South African Orthopaedic Association (1955). *J Bone Joint Surg.* 1956;38:592.
2. Haider H, Ponnusamy KE, Giori NJ, Anderson PA, Nassr A. One Layer at a time; rapid prototyping in orthopaedics. What is the state of the art in orthopaedic 3D printing? *AAOS Now.* 2015.
3. Ponnusamy KE, Haider H, Anderson PA, Nasser A, Giori J. Customizing patient care with rapid prototyping. instruments, implants and more from 3D printing. *AAOS Now.* 2015.
4. Haider H, Weisenburger JN, Namavar F, Garvin KL. Why coating technologies for hip replacement systems, and the importance of testing them in vitro. *Operat Tech Orthop.* 2017;27(3):152-160. doi:10.1053/j.oto.2017.05.003.

5. Su EP, Justin DF, Pratt CR, et al. Effects of titanium nanotubes on the osseointegration, cell differentiation, mineralisation and antibacterial properties of orthopaedic implant surfaces. *Bone JointJ.* 2018;100-B(1 suppl A):9-16.

6. Wong HM, Yeung KW, Lam KO, et al. A biodegradable polymer-based coating to control the performance of magnesium alloy orthopaedic implants. *Biomaterials.* 2010;31(8):2084-2096.

7. Suhardi VJ, Bichara DA, Kwok S, et al. A fully functional drug-eluting joint implant. *Nat Biomed Eng.* 2017;1:0080. doi:10.1038/s41551-017-0080. Epub 2017 Jun 13.

8. Wancket LM. Animal models for evaluation of bone implants and devices: comparative bone structure and common model uses. *Vet Pathol.* 2015;52(5):842-850.

9. Dusad A, Chakkalakal DA, Namavar F, et al. Titanium implant with nanostructured zirconia surface promotes maturation of peri-implant bone in osseointegration. *Proc Inst Mech Eng H.* 2013;227(5):510-522.

10. Stengel D. The changing landscape of product development and randomized trials. *J Bone Joint Surg Am.* 2012;94(suppl 1):85-91.

11. Goel MK, Khanna P, Kishore J. Understanding survival analysis: Kaplan-Meier estimate. *Int J Ayurveda Res.* 2010;1(4):274-278.

12. Insall JN, Dorr LD, Scott RD, Scott WN. Rationale of the knee society clinical rating system. *Clin Orthop Relat Res.* 1989;(248):13-14.

13. Ramkumar PN, Harris JD, Noble PC. Patient-reported outcome measures after total knee arthroplasty: a systematic review. *Bone Joint Res.* 2015;4(7):120-127.

14. Andriacchi TP, Alexander EJ, Toney MK, Dyrby CO, Sum J. A point cluster method for in vivo motion analysis: applied to a study of knee kinematics. *J Biomech Eng.* 1998;120(6):743-749.

15. Andriacchi TP. Biomechanics and gait analysis in total knee replacement. *Orthop Rev.* 1988;17(5):470-473.

16. Banks SA, Hodge WA. 2003 Hap Paul Award Paper of the International Society for Technology in Arthroplasty. Design and activity dependence of kinematics in fixed and mobile-bearing knee arthroplasties. *J Arthroplasty.* 2004;19(7):809-816.

17. Dennis D, Komistek R, Scuderi G, et al. In vivo three-dimensional determination of kinematics for subjects with a normal knee or a unicompartmental or total knee replacement. *J Bone Joint Surg Am.* 2001;83-A(suppl 2 Pt 2):104-115.

18. Banks SA, Harman MK, Bellemans J, Hodge WA. *Making sense of knee arthroplasty kinematics: news you can use.* In: *70th Annual Meeting of the American Academy of Orthopaedic Surgeons.* New Orleans, LA: AAOS; 2003(Scientific Exhibit 302).

19. Selvik G. Roentgen stereophotogrammetry. A method for the study of the kinematics of the skeletal system. *Acta Orthop Scand Suppl.* 1989;232:1-51.

20. Bragdon CR, Malchau H, Yuan X, et al. Experimental assessment of precision and accuracy of radiostereometric analysis for the determination of polyethylene wear in a total hip replacement model. *J Orthop Res.* 2002;20(4):688-695.

21. Haider H, Mupparapu S, Lyden ER, Stoner JA, Garvin KL. *Our Estimate for Accuracy and Precision of Radiostereometric Analysis in a Total Hip Replacement Using a phantom model.* 2006.

22. *ASTM F2385-15 Standard Practice for Determining Femoral Head Penetration Into Acetabular Components of Total Hip replacement Using Clinical Radiographs.* 2015.

23. Bragdon CR, Martell JM, Estok DM II, Greene ME, Malchau H, Harris WH. A new approach for the martell 3-D method of measuring polyethylene wear without requiring the cross-table lateral films. *J Orthop Res.* 2005;23(4):720-725.

24. Garvin KL, White TC, Dusad A, Hartman CW, Martell J. Low wear rates seen in THAs with highly crosslinked polyethylene at 9 to 14 years in patients younger than age 50 years. *Clin Orthop Relat Res.* 2015;473(12):3829-3835.

25. Morrison JB. The mechanics of the knee joint in relation to normal walking. *J Biomech.* 1970;3(1):51-61.

26. Taylor SJG, Walker PS. Forces and moments telemetered from two distal femoral replacements during various activities. *J Biomech.* 2001;34(7):839-848.

27. D'Lima DD, Steklov N, Chien S, Colwell CW Jr. In vivo knee moments and shear after total knee arthroplasty. *J Biomech.* 2007;40(suppl 1):S11-S17.

28. Bergmann G, Bender A, Dymke J, Duda G, Damm P. Standardized loads acting in hip implants. *PLoS One.* 2016;11(5):e0155612.

29. Bergmann G, Bender A, Graichen F, et al. Standardized loads acting in knee implants. *PLoS One.* 2014;9(1):e86035.

30. Barker JP, Simon SD, Dubin J. The methodology of clinical studies used by the FDA for approval of high-risk orthopaedic devices. *J Bone Joint Surg Am.* 2017;99(9):711-719.

31. Maloney WJ. The role of orthopaedic device registries in improving patient outcomes. *J Bone Joint Surg Am.* 2011;93(24):2241.

32. Stratton-Powell AA, Tipper JL. 33-Characterization of UHMWPE wear particles. 2016:635-653. doi:10.1016/B978-0-323-35401-1.00033-8.

33. International Organization for Standardization. *ISO 17853 Wear of Implant Materials – Polymer and Metal Wear Particles – Isolation and Characterization.* 2011.

34. Haider H, Walker PS. Measurements of constraint of total knee replacement. *J Biomech.* 2005;38(2):341-348.

35. Walker PS, Haider H. Characterizing the motion of total knee replacements in laboratory tests. *Clin Orthop Relat Res.* 2003;(410):54-68.

36. Haider H, Walker PS, DesJardins J, Blunn G. Effects of patient and surgical alignment variables on kinematics in TKR simulation under force-control. *J ASTM Int.* 2006;3(10).

37. Maletsky LP, Hillberry BM. Simulating dynamic activities activities using a five-axis knee simulator. *J Biomech Eng.* 2005;127(1):123-133.

38. Walker PS, Heller Y, Cleary DJ, Yildirim G. Preclinical evaluation method for total knees designed to restore normal knee mechanics. *J Arthroplasty.* 2011;26(1):152-160. doi:10.1016/j.arth.2009.11.017.

39. Sonntag R, Braun S, Al-Salehi L, Reinders J, Mueller U, Kretzer JP. Three-dimensional friction measurement during hip simulation. *PLoS One.* 2017;12(9):1-20.

40. Haider H, Weisenburger JN, Garvin KL. Simultaneous measurement of friction and wear in hip simulators. *Proc Inst Mech Eng H.* 2016;230(5):373-388.

41. Haider H, Weisenburger JN, Naylor MG, Schroeder DW, White BF, Garvin KL. *Friction of various hip replacement materials and designs captured during testing on hip simulators.* In: *23rd Annual Congress of the International Society for Technology in Arthroplasty (ISTA).* 2010.

42. McGrory BJ, Etkin CD, Lewallen DG. Comparing contemporary revision burden among hip and knee joint replacement registries. *Arthroplasty Today.* 2016;2(2):83-86. doi https://doi.org/10.1016/j.artd.2016.04.003.

43. Kurtz S, Ong K, Lau E, Mowat F, Halpern M. Projections of primary and revision hip and knee arthroplasty in the United States from 2005 to 2030. *J Bone Joint Surg Am.* 2007;89(4):780-785.

44. Haider H. 7.10 wear: knee joint arthroplasty. In: Ducheyne P, ed. *Comprehensive Biomaterials II*. Oxford: Elsevier; 2017:152-174. doi:10.1016/B978-0-12-803581-8.09359-0.

45. Walker PS. Biomechanics of total knee replacement designs. In: Mow V, Huiskes R, eds. *Basic orthopaedic Biomechanics and mechano-Biology*. Chapter 15. 3rd ed. Philadelphia, PA: Lippincott Williams & Wilkins; 2004:657-702.

46. Haider H. *Tribological assessment of UHMWPE in the knee*. In: *UHMWPE Biomaterials Handbook – Ultra-High Molecular Weight Polyethylene in Total Joint Replacement and Medical Devices*. Elsevier, Inc; 2016:553-578.

47. Haider H, Walker PS, Blunn GW, Perry J, DesJardins J. *A four channel force control knee simulator: from concept to production*. In: *Proceedings of the 11th Annual Symposium, International Society for Technology in Arthroplasty [ISTA]*. 1998:213-214.

48. Walker PS, Blunn GW, Perry JP, et al. Methodology for long-term wear testing of total knee replacements. *Clin Orthop Relat Res*. 2000(372):290-301.

49. International Standards Organization (ISO). *ISO 14243-1 Implants for Surgery — Wear of Total Knee-Joint Prostheses —Part 1: Loading and Displacement Parameters for Wear-Testing Machines With Load Control and Corresponding Environmental Conditions for Test*. 2009.

50. International Standards Organization (ISO). *ISO 14243-2 Implants for Surgery — Wear of Total Knee-Joint Prostheses — Part 2: Methods of Measurement*. 2016.

51. International Organisation of Standards (ISO). *ISO 14243-3 Implants for Surgery– Wear of Total Knee-Joint Prostheses– Part 3: Loading and Displacement Parameters for Wear-Testing Machines With Displacement Control and Corresponding Environmental Conditions for Test*. 2014.

52. Haider H, Weisenburger JN, Kurtz SM, et al. Does vitamin E-stabilized ultrahigh-molecular-weight polyethylene address concerns of cross-linked polyethylene in total knee arthroplasty? *J Arthroplasty*. 2012;27(3):461-469.

53. Muratoglu OK, Bragdon CR, Jasty M, O'Connor DO, Von Knoch RS, Harris WH. Knee-simulator testing of conventional and cross-linked polyethylene tibial inserts. *J Arthroplasty*. 2004;19(7):887-897.

54. Haider H, Baykal D. Wear assessment of UHMWPE with pin-on-disc testing. In: Kurtz SM, ed. *UHMWPE Biomaterials Handbook – Ultra-High Molecular Weight Polyethylene in Total Joint Replacement and Medical Devices*. 3rd ed. Elsevier, Inc; 2016:553-578.

55. ASTM International. *ASTM F732-00 Standard Test Method for Wear Testing of Polymeric Materials Used in Total Joint Prostheses*. 2006.

56. Rajagopal A, Dembia CL, DeMers MS, Delp DD, Hicks JL, Delp SL. Full-body musculoskeletal model for muscle-driven simulation of human gait. *IEEE Trans Biomed Eng*. 2016;63(10):2068-2079.

57. Taylor M, Prendergast PJ. Four decades of finite element analysis of orthopaedic devices: where are we now and what are the opportunities? *J Biomech*. 2015;48(5):767-778.

58. Haider H, Mupparapu S, Barrera OA, Garvin KL. "*3D finite element analysis of the bone stress distribution of aligned and misaligned tibial components in unicondylar knee arthroplasty*." In: *Transactions of the 52nd Annual Meeting of the Orthopaedic Research Society*. Chicago. March, 2006.

59. Ackerman MJ, Spitzer VM, Scherzinger AL, Whitlock DG. The visible human data set: an image resource for anatomical visualization. *Medinfo*. 1995;8(Pt 2):1195-1198.

60. Haider H, Weisenburger JN, Namavar F, Garvin KL. *Why coating technologies for hip replacement systems, and the importance of testing them in vitro*. In: *ASTM International Workshop on Coatings for the Medical Device Industry*. 2018.

61. Malchau H, Bragdon CR, Muratoglu OK. The stepwise introduction of innovation into orthopedic surgery: the next level of dilemmas. *J Arthroplasty*. 2011;26(6):825-831. doi:10.1016/j.arth.2010.08.007.

CHAPTER 12

What Is Needed to Produce Medical Devices in Large Volumes?

KUSUMAL JOSEPH SILVA

ABOUT THE AUTHOR

Kusumal Joseph Silva—US Patent Holder (Patent#: 5193989—Allied Signal Inc.). Certified Manufacturing Engineer up to year 2000 (SME Certification Institute—Dearborn MI.). Director of Quality and Engineering at Ortho-Precision Products Inc.

Design for Manufacturability

Manufacturing engineering representation at the design level is crucial in order to:

a. Design features based on the capabilities of the equipment available.

b. Establish dimensioning and tolerancing based on the capability and repeatability of the equipment available.

c. Minimize the complexity of workholding methods for fabrication.

d. Minimize the use of special cutting tools and maximize use of standard cutting tools those are readily available that can reduce the cost and improve delivery.

e. Determine the types of inspection equipment necessary to control manufacturing processes through **SPC** (statistical process control) methods.

f. Concurrent engineering (design/manufacturing) can reduce lead time of the transition from design to production tremendously.

Manufacturing

g. Identification and traceability; documents of traceability must be on file from the end user, all the way up to the raw material foundry (who performed, who inspected and approved each task). Each production order and shipment must have a "Lot#" assigned and laser marked on the component for the purpose of traceability.

h. PFMEA (process failure mode and effects analysis) must be performed to access and rate the risk factors of each process and to mitigate corrective/preventive actions proactively.

i. Equipment: Most orthopedic fixation hardware are hardly straight nor flat. They are commonly either machined into curved shapes on multiaxis machines or machined flat and formed/bent into curves. In order to be on the competitive edge of the market, the equipment must be versatile and efficient with multiaxis capabilities in order to machine many features in a single holding (chucking). Optical comparators and coordinate measuring machines (CMMs) are commonly used to inspect curved surfaces, profiles, and dimensional relationship among features.

j. Installation Qualification (IQ), Operational Qualification (OQ), and Performance Qualification (PQ) must be performed to assure the equipment is in optimum working order. PQ must be repeated periodically in order to access and maintain the accuracy of the equipment.

k. All software must be validated initially and at revisions there on after.

l. Records of the following must be kept on file for traceability:
   i. Raw material certifications
   ii. Equipment produced on
   iii. Certificate of compliance (CoC) for special processes such as heat treatment, anodizing, and passivation
   iv. Personnel who performed operations and inspected the medical device including the inspection records, the quantity, the signature, and the date

Quality Control

m. 100% inspection at the end of the process is never 100% effective, considering the fatigue factor of inspectors, and if a defect is detected, it would be too late to recover the loss. Solution is to build the quality into the process through **SPC** by controlling the dimensions against established **control limits** rather than the **specification limits** (specification limits are established by the design engineer based on the fit, form, and function of the component). Control limits are established by the manufacturing/quality engineer based on the condition of the machine, environmental factors, and human factors if any of the processes are operator interactive. Control limits are much narrower than the specification limits.

n. A system and procedures must be established to control nonconformance material and prevent nonconformance material escaping to the end user.

o. Quality control (QC) equipment must be calibrated periodically, and immediately following a repair, and records must be kept on file.

Resources

p. Human resources must be trained to fully comply with the quality management system (QMS) standard operating procedures, forms, and work instructions. Training records must be kept on file.

q. Types of equipment: Bones are never flat or straight. They are curved, and there are no two bones exactly alike. Machining equipment widely used in orthopedic industry are computer numerical control (CNC) Swiss turning lathes, multiaxis CNC milling centers, bending and forming machines, and surface finishing equipment such as tumblers, buffers and polishers, and bead blasters. Most orthopedic components are cannulated. It requires a specialized process known as gun drilling.

r. Equipment must be on a preventive maintenance program to keep in optimum condition and to reduce unexpected downtime.

Facilities

s. Vast majority of implantable orthopedic trauma fixation components are made out of titanium (Ti 6AL4V-ELI). Titanium is flammable material. For safety of the personnel and the expensive equipment, appropriate fire extinguishers must be placed at the vicinity of all equipment that machine titanium with easy access.

t. Pest control plan and procedure must be established in order to avoid contamination. Food shall not be allowed in all product manufacturing, inspection, and storage areas.

u. Hazardous waste must be disposed of properly.

Quality Management System—ISO 13485:2016(E) (Available at https://webstore.ansi.org)

v. Following documents and a system to maintain the documents must be established:
  i. Quality manual
  ii. Medical device file
  iii. Control of documents
  iv. Control of records

w. Management responsibility:
  i. Management commitment
  ii. Customer focus
  iii. Quality policy
  iv. Planning:
    1. Quality objectives.
    2. QMS planning.
  v. Responsibility, authority, and communication:
    1. Each employee's responsibilities and level of authority shall be documented.
    2. A management representative shall be appointed to control the QMS requirements.
    3. An internal communication system to flow down the effectivity of the QMS to all employees.

    vi. Management review:
      1. A periodical meeting to discuss the effectivity of the QMS and actions required to maintain and improve the QMS.

x. Resource management:
    i. Human resources
    ii. Infrastructure
    iii. Work environment and contamination control

y. Product realization:
    i. Planning
    ii. Customer-related processes
    iii. Design and development
    iv. Purchasing
    v. Product and service
    vi. Control of monitoring and measuring equipment

z. Measurement, analysis, and improvement:
    i. Monitoring and measurement
    ii. Control of nonconforming product
    iii. Analysis of data
    iv. Improvement

Permits and Certifications

a. QMS must be certified by a qualified third party, and the certification must be maintained by internal/external audits or fully compliant to the ISO13485:2016 international standard.
b. Must be registered with Food and Drug Administration (FDA) as a medical device manufacturer (annually).
c. Must be licensed by the "Department of Public Health" of the locality as a medical device manufacturer.

Typical Process Flow

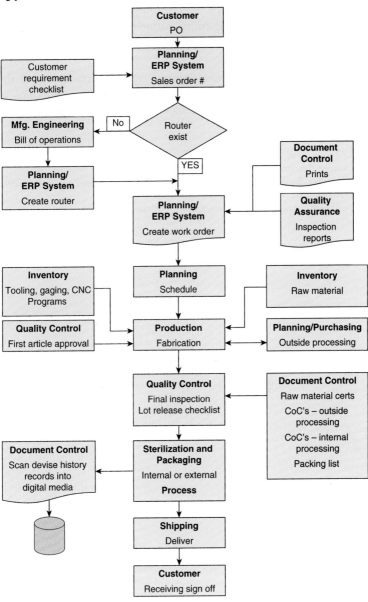

KEY TAKEAWAY POINTS

- ▶ In order to produce medical devices in large volumes, an organization must fully understand the critical nature of the product functioning as an implant in a human body such as fit, form, and function and cleanliness.

- ▶ Also, the organization must maintain records of traceability of the materials, processes, equipment, involved personnel, compliance to regulatory requirements, and licenses according to the local codes.

BIBLIOGRAPHY

1. ISO 13485: Regulatory Requirements. FDA. https://webstore.ansi.org.
2. Licenses: Department of Public Health of the Locality.
3. Machining Equipment: Ex: STAR CNC Machine Tool Corp., Tsugami CNC, Marubeni Citizen-Cincom, HAAS CNC, OKK Corp.
4. Inspection Equipment: Ex: Brown & Sharp, Mitutoyo, Starrett.

CHAPTER 13

FDA Marketing Authorization: How to Get Your Device on the US Market

JENNIFER A. DAUDELIN,
DEBORAH LAVOIE GRAYESKI,
TERRY SHERIDAN POWELL

ABOUT THE AUTHORS

Jennifer A. Daudelin, MSJ, is a consultant with M Squared Associates, Inc. in New York, NY. Ms Daudelin has over 20 years of experience in the medical device industry, with expertise in the regulation of orthopedic devices, diagnostic cardiology devices, peripheral vascular devices, donor organ transport systems, and craniomaxillofacial, ENT, and dental devices. Jennifer was part of the regulatory team that received the first Food and Drug Administration (FDA) 510(k) clearance for antibiotic bone cement.

Deborah Lavoie Grayeski, JD, RAC, is a consultant with M Squared Associates, Inc. in New York, NY. Ms Grayeski has over 15 years of experience in regulatory and clinical affairs for the medical device and biologics industry and serves as a member of an Institutional Review Board (IRB). Ms Grayeski spent 7 years with FDA, in the Center for Biologics Evaluation and Research, Office of Cellular, Tissue and Gene Therapies (now the Office of Tissues and Advanced Therapies).

Terry Sheridan Powell, MA, RAC, has over 20 years of regulatory affairs and clinical research experience in the medical device industry. Ms Powell has extensive experience in FDA submissions for device types including orthopedic joint reconstruction and trauma, spinal fusion, bone substitutes and bone growth stimulation, peripheral vascular, gastroenterology, urology, physical medicine, and general hospital.

Introduction

Medical devices marketed in the United States are regulated by the Food and Drug Administration (FDA) in accordance with the Federal Food, Drug, and Cosmetic Act (FD&C Act) and its amendments. As discussed in Chapter 11, General Controls apply to all classes of medical devices marketed in the United States. In addition to the General Controls, many medical devices require authorization from FDA before the devices can be legally marketed. The type of premarket application needed to obtain marketing authorization depends on the classification and classification regulation of the medical device. In general, the concepts in Table 13.1 will apply.

In addition, marketing applications that require inclusion of supportive clinical data (usually for class III devices) may require performance of a clinical study. Such studies are completed prior to submission of a marketing application and, if performed in the United States, require an investigational device exemption (IDE). This chapter will review how to determine device classification, describe the most common types of premarket applications, and explain how to get early FDA feedback on the likely regulatory pathway for a new device. The types of applications discussed here include:

- 513(g) Request for Information
- Pre-submission (Q-Sub)
- Premarket Notification (510(k))
- De novo (Evaluation of Automatic Class III Designation)
- Premarket Approval (PMA)
- Investigational Device Exemption (IDE)

Table 13.1 Type of Marketing Authorizations Required Before Placing the Device on the US Market

Class I Devices: Usually None[a]	Class II Devices: Usually 510(k)[a]	Class III Devices: Usually PMA[b]	Unclassified[c] Usually 510(k)

[a]FDA has exempted many (but not all) class I devices and some (but not most) class II devices from the 510(k) requirement. However, the exemptions are subject to specific limitations, and a 510(k) is still required if the new device exceeds the limits of the exemption. It is important to check the specific classification regulation applicable to a device, including the limitations on any exemption.
[b]Class III devices require a PMA unless they are preamendment devices (on the US market prior to the passage of the medical device amendments in 1976), and PMAs have not been called for, in which case, they require a 510(k).
[c]An unclassified device is a preamendment device (on the US market prior to the passage of the medical device amendments in 1976) for which a classification regulation has not been promulgated.

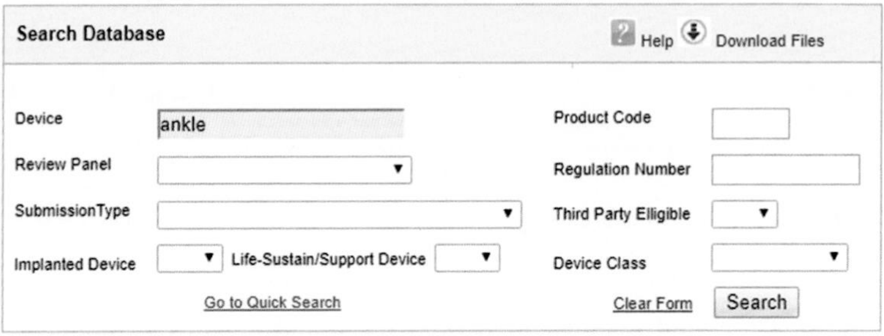

Figure 13.1 FDA Product Classification Database Search—ankle.

This chapter does not describe regulatory authorizations for special use circumstances, such as Humanitarian Use Devices,[a] expanded access (compassionate use),[b] or special circumstances for custom devices.[c]

How to Classify Your Device

The classification of a medical device determines its regulatory pathway and the type of premarket application required. Medical device classifications are found in the US Code of Federal Regulations (CFR). To find the classification of a device, check the FDA's product classification database (link provided in the reference).[d]

For example, typing the word "ankle" into the *Device* search field (Figure 13.1) will return existing product codes and associated regulations relating to ankle devices (Figure 13.2).

Click on any device result for further details, including the type of submission required. For example, if you click the entry for product code HSN, it describes a type of ankle prosthesis that is semiconstrained, intended for

---

[a]For more information on Humanitarian use Devices and Humanitarian Device Exemptions, see FDA website, "Humanitarian Device Exemption" at: https://www.fda.gov/medicaldevices/deviceregulationandguidance/howtomarketyourdevice/premarketsubmissions/humanitariandeviceexemption/default.htm.

[b]For more information on Expanded Access (Compassionate use), see FDA website, "Expanded Access: Information for Physicians" at: https://www.fda.gov/NewsEvents/PublicHealthFocus/ExpandedAccessCompassionateUse/ucm429624.htm.

[c]For information on custom device exemptions, see FDA Guidance Document, Custom Device Exemption Guidance for Industry and Food and Drug Administration Staff, issued September 24, 2014. https://www.fda.gov/downloads/medicaldevices/deviceregulationandguidance/guidancedocuments/ucm415799.pdf.

[d]US FDA: Product Classification Database at https://www.accessdata.fda.gov/scripts/cdrh/cfdocs/cfPCD/classification.cfm.

Product Code	Device		Regulation Number	Device Class
HSN	Prosthesis, Ankle, Semi-Constrained, Cemented, Met ...	Ankle Joint Metal/Polymer Semi-Constrain...	888.3110	2
ISH	Component, External, Limb, Ankle/Foot	External Limb Prosthetic Component	890.3420	1
ISW	Assembly, Knee/Shank/Ankle/Foot, External	External Assembled Lower Limb Prosthesis...	890.3500	2

Figure 13.2 FDA Product Classification Database Search—sample search results for "ankle."

cemented use, and manufactured from metal and polymer components. The submission type required is a 510(k) (Figure 13.3). Clicking the link to the regulation number (in this example, 888.3110) provides additional information about the characteristics and intended use of devices classified under this regulation. In cases where the submission type is 510(k) exempt, clicking the regulation number will also describe the limitations of the 510(k) exemption.

When researching the classification of a new device, it is important to consider how closely the new device, materials, technology, and intended use align with the regulation description and with other existing devices legally marketed under the same classification regulation, because differences in these characteristics can place the new device into a different classification with a different submission type.

Another way to determine the regulatory pathway for a new device is to check the marketing applications FDA has granted for other similar devices on the market. FDA maintains searchable databases for all cleared 510(k) s[e] and approved PMAs.[f] The databases can be searched by device name, manufacturer name ("applicant"), or product code.

For example, searching the 510(k) database for product code HSN will return existing 510(k)s for Prosthesis, Ankle, Semi-Constrained, Cemented, Metal/Polymer (Figure 13.4).

Click on the link to any 510(k) number to see the record for that 510(k). Each 510(k) record usually includes a link for "510(k) Summary," which provides the FDA clearance letter, the associated indications for use statement, and a summary of the information that supported the 510(k),[g]

---

[e] US FDA 510(k) Premarket Notification Database at https://www.accessdata.fda.gov/scripts/cdrh/cfdocs/cfpmn/pmn.cfm.

[f] US FDA Premarket Approval (PMA) database at: https://www.accessdata.fda.gov/scripts/cdrh/cfdocs/cfPMA/pma.cfm.

[g] The 510(k) Summary or clearance letter may not be available in some cases, for example, if the clearance is very old, or if the Sponsor instead provided a 510(k) Statement (a certification that the Sponsor will make available all information included in the 510(k) on safety and effectiveness within 30 days of request by any person).

New Search		Back To Search Results
Device	Prosthesis, Ankle, Semi-Constrained, Cemented, Metal/Polymer	
Regulation Description	Ankle joint metal/polymer semi-constrained cemented prosthesis.	
Regulation Medical Specialty	Orthopedic	
Review Panel	Orthopedic	
Product Code	HSN	
Premarket Review	Office of Device Evaluation (ODE) Division of Orthopedic Devices (DOD) Joint and Fixation Devices Branch One ¿ Knees/Shoulders/Elbows/Ankles/Toes (JFDB1)	
Submission Type	510(k)	
Regulation Number	888.3110	
Device Class	2	
Total Product Life Cycle (TPLC)	TPLC Product Code Report	

Figure 13.3 FDA Classification Database—description of product code HSN.

New Search		Export to Excel | Download Files | More About 510(k)	
Device Name	Applicant	510(K) Number	Decision Date
Hintermann Series H2 Total Ankle System	Dt Medtech Llc	K171004	11/07/2017
Invision Total Ankle Revision System	Wright Medical Technology, Inc.	K171067	09/11/2017
Prophecy Invision Pre-Operative Navigati	Wright Medical Technology, Inc.	K170968	08/16/2017

Figure 13.4 FDA 510(k) Database—select results for product code HSN.

typically including a high-level description of the performance testing that was done, and whether clinical data was needed. Similarly, when searching the PMA database, you can click on a PMA number[h] to see the PMA letter, approved device labeling, and a Summary of Safety and Effectiveness Data (SSED), which provides a detailed summary of the nonclinical and clinical testing that supported the approval decision. Checking the 510(k) Summaries or PMA SSEDs for similar devices provides insight into the type of information and testing that has previously been adequate to support a 510(k) or PMA marketing applications, and provides examples of the indication for use language (what the manufacturer can say the device should be used for) that FDA has accepted for those devices.

The FDA Product Classification Database and a review of the 510(k) clearances or PMAs for similar legally marketed devices can be helpful but do not always provide a clear answer. A new device may have characteristics that are different from or not specifically mentioned in the regulations, or the device may be sufficiently novel that no regulation seems to apply. Other methods for getting information about device classification and

---

[h]Filter the search of the PMA database for supplement type "Originals Only" to quickly locate the original approval letter with device labeling and SSED. Leave the supplement type field blank to see all PMA and PMA supplement records.

regulatory requirements include contacting the FDA's Division of Industry and Consumer Education (DICE) at 1(800) 638-2041 or (301) 796-7100 or DICE@fda.hhs.gov, contacting the FDA Office of Device Evaluation Branch Chief for the applicable product type,[i] or working with a medical device regulatory consultant. In cases where a formal documented response from FDA is needed, a 513(g) Request for Information can be submitted to FDA.

513(g) Requests for Information

A 513(g) Request for Information is a mechanism for getting FDA's opinion about the classification of a device and any applicable regulatory requirements. It is not a marketing authorization. This type of submission is optional. A 513(g) request is a relatively simple submission type that does not require extensive documentation or device testing. A 513(g) request should include:

- A cover letter.
- A device description in sufficient detail to provide a good understanding of the device concept, materials, technology, method of use, etc., and how it compares to any similar devices legally marketed in the United States.
- What the device will be used for.
- Proposed labeling or marketing material for the device (drafts are acceptable) and for similar devices legally marketed in the United States (if available).

FDA will respond in writing to a 513(g) request within 60 days of receipt. The FDA's response typically contains information outlining FDA's position on:

- The applicable device class and classification regulation.
- The type of FDA submission required prior to marketing the device (510(k), PMA, or neither).
- Other general or specific regulatory requirements that may apply.

Further information on the 513(g) process, contents, and format can be found in the FDA guidance document on 513(g) requests.[j]

---

[i] FDA's CDRH Management Directory by Organization at: https://www.fda.gov/AboutFDA/CentersOffices/OfficeofMedicalProductsandTobacco/CDRH/CDRHOffices/ucm127854.htm.
[j] FDA Guidance Document: FDA and Industry Procedures for Section 513(g) Requests for Information under the Federal Food, Drug, and Cosmetic Act: Guidance for Industry and Food and Drug Administration Staff https://www.fda.gov/downloads/medicaldevices/deviceregulationandguidance/guidancedocuments/ucm209851.pdf.

Although a 513(g) is optional, it can be useful when the classification is difficult to determine by other methods. It can also provide assurance for potential business partners or investors that the regulatory classification and likely regulatory pathway for the device are defined.

Pre-Submission Program: Getting Early Input From the Food and Drug Administration

A Pre-submission (known as a Q-sub) is a way to solicit FDA feedback before submitting a marketing application or IDE application. A Q-sub is useful when early FDA feedback, which is not otherwise available from FDA's website or device-/issue-specific FDA guidance documents, could help guide device development efforts and testing plans, or clinical study design. A Q-sub is an optional submission type and is not a marketing authorization. Some uses of the Q-sub are to seek FDA's input on specific questions related to:

- Proposed nonclinical testing intended to support a marketing application, particularly when the testing will use new, nonstandard, or otherwise unfamiliar test methods or will be lengthy/costly to conduct.
- Important clinical study design elements such as appropriateness of key safety and effectiveness measures, planned sample size, and statistical approach.
- Planned regulatory submission strategy if the approach is unusual for the device type, or the regulatory pathway is not well established for the device type.
- Whether a planned IDE study is significant risk (SR) or nonsignificant risk (NSR).

A Q-sub can be submitted early in the device or study development process. The content requirements for a Q-sub are less rigid than other types of FDA submissions, but it is important to provide sufficiently detailed information about the device, its intended use, and specific questions, so that FDA can provide meaningful feedback. It is not productive to simply ask FDA what they want or how to test a product. The Q-sub works best when the submitter first thoroughly reviews available regulatory information and issue- or device-specific FDA guidance documents and then lays out a proposal, with specific questions for FDA.

FDA generally responds within 75 days to a Q-sub request (sooner for a study risk SR/NSR determination). The Q-sub can request written feedback or a meeting. If a meeting is requested, it will typically be scheduled at around 75 days.

The Q-sub process is not subject to an FDA user fee, but there are specific content requirements for Q-sub eligibility and administrative completeness, and format requirements (eCopy) that must be met for the Q-sub to be accepted by FDA for review.

Information on the Pre-submission process and how to submit a Q-sub request is provided in the FDA guidance document on the Pre-submission program.[k]

The 510(k) Process

A premarket notification, also referred to as a 510(k), is generally required for class II devices. A 510(k) submission demonstrates "substantial equivalence" of a new device to a legally marketed predicate device.[l] A legally marketed predicate device is one that has been found substantially equivalent or "cleared" by FDA and is similar to the new device in terms of intended use and technological characteristics. Technological characteristics include design, materials, energy source, or other features of the device. The new device would fall under the same regulation number and product code as the predicate device. Depending upon the type of device or special features, an FDA guidance document may exist to cover additional testing or performance requirements to be addressed in the 510(k) submission.[m] Differences in intended use such as different patient populations and expanded or new indications, as well as, novel materials, novel design features, or significant differences in design features from the predicate warrant a presubmission meeting with the FDA. These changes do not necessarily signal a raise to a class III device but could require additional bench testing or possibly clinical data for the 510(k) submission.

The following testing is typically required for 510(k) submissions:

- Biomechanical testing: This testing is usually performed to a standard, i.e., the American Society for Testing and Materials (ASTM), International Organization for Standardization (ISO), etc. related specifically to the type of device or to test a specific design feature.

[k]Requests for Feedback on Medical Device Submissions: The Pre-Submission Program and Meetings with Food and Drug Administration Staff. Issued September 29, 2017. https://www.fda.gov/downloads/medicaldevices/deviceregulationandguidance/guidancedocuments/ucm311176.pdf.

[l]FDA Guidance Document. The 510(k) Program: Evaluating Substantial Equivalence in Premarket Notifications [510(k)]. https://www.fda.gov/ucm/groups/fdagov-public/@fdagov-meddev-gen/documents/document/ucm284443.pdf.

[m]Search for FDA Guidance Documents. https://www.fda.gov/RegulatoryInformation/Guidances/default.htm.

Some standards include performance criteria, and in other cases direct comparison to the performance of the predicate device is required to demonstrate substantial equivalence.

- Biocompatibility: Biological assessment (and typically testing), in accordance with ISO 10993, is required for all devices that have direct or indirect contact with the patient.[n] The level of testing required is dependent upon the type of the device, i.e., implant, invasive instrument, etc., and level and duration of contact. Reliance on the predicate device of the same materials with the same manufacturing processes can be used to show biocompatibility.

- Sterilization: For devices supplied as sterile, information on the sterilization method, sterility validation method, and sterility assurance level must be provided.[o] In addition, all implants and devices labeled as "nonpyrogenic" must include pyrogenicity testing to address bacterial endotoxin levels.

- End-user sterilization: Devices supplied nonsterile, but requiring sterilization prior to use, must include a set of validated sterilization instructions demonstrating that the device can be appropriately sterilized by the hospital, clinic, or other end user.

- Packaging: Packaging for the devices must be able to withstand transport of the device and in the case of sterile devices, maintain sterility for the labeled shelf life. Accelerated shelf-life testing is acceptable for the 510(k) submission.

In addition to performance testing, the 510(k) submission also requires a detailed description of the device; a statement regarding the intended use of the device; labeling such as labels, instructions for use, and surgical techniques; 510(k) Summary; and required FDA forms.[p] The 510(k) Summary becomes public information and must contain certain required elements but should not include any confidential or proprietary information. FDA forms include the CDRH Premarket Review Submission Cover Sheet and Medical Device User Fee Cover Sheet.

---

[n]FDA Guidance Document. Use of International Standard ISO 10993-1, "Biological evaluation of medical devices—part 1: evaluation and testing within a risk management process". https://www.fda.gov/ucm/groups/fdagov-public/@fdagov-meddev-gen/documents/document/ucm348890.pdf.

[o]FDA Guidance Document. Submission and Review of Sterility Information in Premarket Notification (510(k)) Submissions for Devices Labeled as Sterile. https://www.fda.gov/ucm/groups/fdagov-public/@fdagov-meddev-gen/documents/document/ucm109897.pdf.

[p]FDA Guidance Document. Format for Traditional and Abbreviated 510(k)s. https://www.fda.gov/MedicalDevices/DeviceRegulationandGuidance/GuidanceDocuments/ucm084365.htm.

The review time for a 510(k) is designated by the statute as 90 calendar days; however, that 90 days does not include times when the 510(k) is "on-hold."[q] The 510(k) process begins with an administrative review to determine if all the information submitted is adequate to allow the FDA to start a substantive review. This administrative review or Refuse to Accept (RTA) takes approximately 15 days. If any items are missing, the FDA will notify the submitter/sponsor and request those items. This "on-hold" time is not part of the 90-day review cycle. If the submission is accepted for substantive review, FDA will typically communicate any questions to the applicant within 45 to 60 days of receipt of the 510(k), via a request for additional information. The applicant then has up to 180 days to respond, during which time the submission is "on-hold." Upon receipt of the response to all of the reviewer's questions, the review cycle will resume with the balance of the 90 days being used to complete the review and make a final substantial equivalence determination.

De Novo

In some cases where a class II device has no legally marketed predicate, but where general and special controls provide a reasonable assurance of safety and effectiveness, the De Novo request can be an effective regulatory strategy.[r] Although a presubmission meeting is not a requirement for submitting a De Novo request, meeting with the FDA beforehand is highly recommended. Once a De Novo request is granted, a classification regulation for the type of device is established, and the device can be marketed immediately. Moreover, the new device can serve as a predicate device.

The information required for a De Novo request is more extensive than the information required for a 510(k). The information that is similar to a 510(k) is the device information, indications for use, nonclinical testing, and labeling. Information specific to the De Novo request includes a regulatory history that comprises any presubmission meetings related to the De Novo request, a classification summary that details the search for legally marketed devices of the same type, a classification

---

[q]FDA Guidance Document. FDA and Industry Actions on Premarket Notification (510(k)) Submissions: Effect on FDA Review Clock and Goals. https://www.fda.gov/ucm/groups/fdagov-public/@fdagov-meddev-gen/documents/document/ucm089738.pdf.

[r]FDA Guidance Document. De Novo Classification Process (Evaluation of Automatic Class III Designation). https://www.fda.gov/ucm/groups/fdagov-public/@fdagov-meddev-gen/documents/document/ucm080197.pdf.

recommendation, summary of benefits (information supporting the effectiveness of the device), summary of identified risks to health, and possibly clinical data.

Review times are highly dependent upon the branch reviewing the request. Although the statutory time frame for review is 120 days, the time to De Novo decisions can be significantly longer. The De Novo process can be challenging as FDA needs to consider many factors for making a risk determination for whether a particular device can be placed into class I or II. A well-planned presubmission meeting is vital for obtaining the FDA's position on the specific device and sets the groundwork for future interactions with the FDA review team.

The PMA Process

A PMA application, also referred to as a PMA, is generally required for class III devices. In order to obtain FDA approval, a PMA must contain sufficient valid scientific evidence to assure that the device is safe and effective for its intended use(s). Unlike a 510(k) submission in which the review standard is substantial equivalence to a predicate device, the review standard for a PMA submission relies upon an independent demonstration of safety and effectiveness.

Much of the nonclinical testing required for a PMA submission is the same as the testing described above for a 510(k) submission, including biomechanical testing, biocompatibility testing, sterilization testing, packaging testing, shelf-life testing, and any additional relevant performance testing. Depending upon the device and availability of relevant animal models, testing in animals may be necessary. Animal testing should either be performed according to good laboratory practices (GLPs) or if there are any deviations from GLPs, a justification should be provided, which explains why any deviations were necessary and why it does not affect the scientific validity of the testing and results.

In addition to a section addressing the nonclinical testing described above (with test reports and protocols providing in appendices), the PMA submission is also required to include the following key information: name and address of the applicant, FDA-required forms, a cover letter, table of contents, a detailed device description, a statement regarding the intended use of the device, reference to any standards, labeling, bibliography and other information, financial certification/disclosure, detailed design and manufacturing information, and a section on clinical investigations (with study protocols, reports, tabulations of data from all individual subjects, and results of statistical analyses attached). The inclusion of detailed design and manufacturing information, including quality procedures from the device manufacturer, and potentially contract manufacturers, is a key difference between the content of a PMA and 510(k) submission. The PMA must also include a summary section (called the SSED that will become publicly available and must contain certain required elements but should not include any confidential or proprietary information.

As specified by regulation, the review time for a PMA is 180 days; however, in reality, the time is longer. The PMA review process begins with a 15-day administrative, RTA, review to determine if all the information submitted is adequate to allow the FDA to start a more substantive review.[*] If the PMA submission passes the RTA review, it moves on to a limited scientific review (termed a filing review), whereby the FDA makes a threshold determination that the application is sufficiently complete to begin an in-depth review. Within 45 days after a PMA is received, the FDA will notify the applicant whether the application has been filed. If so, the 180-day period for review starts on the date that the PMA accepted for filing was received. During the in-depth review process, FDA will notify the PMA applicant via interactive review or major/minor deficiency letters of any information needed by FDA to complete the review of the application. The applicant may request to meet with FDA within 100 days (termed the 100-day meeting) of the filing of the PMA to discuss the review status of the application. If during review, the applicant submits a PMA amendment that contains significant new or updated information, the review period may be extended up to 180 days.

In addition to the review of the supportive data and information in the PMA application, the FDA Office of Compliance reviews the provided manufacturing information for compliance with FDA's Quality System Regulations (21 CFR 820) in preparation for a preapproval inspection, which is conducted for almost all original PMA submissions. In addition to inspection of the device manufacturer and/or contract manufacturer, the FDA may also perform a bioresearch monitoring (BIMO) audit of any clinical study sites that contributed clinical study data to support the PMA. Finally, based upon the novelty, benefit/risk considerations or public health concerns related to the subject device, the FDA may also hold a public panel meeting (also known as a FDA Advisory Committee). At completion of review, if approved, the approval order for the PMA is based upon the outcome of the panel meeting, the outcome of any manufacturing or

---

[*]Acceptance and Filing Reviews for Premarket Approval Applications (PMAs)— Guidance for Industry and Food and Drug Administration Staff. https://www.fda. gov/downloads/MedicalDevices/DeviceRegulationandGuidance/GuidanceDocuments/ UCM313368.pdf.

clinical site audits or inspections, and the final review decision memo of the PMA application. The approval order consists of the approval letter (including conditions of approval), the SSED, and final draft labeling.

Alternatively, if the FDA believes that it can approve the application, but still needs additional information to do so, the FDA may issue an approvable letter describing the information that is needed as a condition of approval. However, if the FDA believes that the application has a more significant lack of information, it will issue a not approvable letter describing the deficiencies. Finally, if the FDA determines that the applicant has a more significant inability to meet the requirements for PMA, an order denying the approval may be issued.

The Investigational Device Exemption Process

Usually clinical data is not required to support FDA marketing authorization of class I and II devices. However, as PMAs require valid scientific evidence for a reasonable assurance of safety and effectiveness, class III devices typically require inclusion of clinical data in the marketing application. If a clinical study is required to collect the data necessary to support approval, an IDE allows an investigational device (a device that does not have marketing authorization in the United States) to be used in a clinical investigation in order to determine safety and effectiveness. An IDE is not only required for devices that are not yet initially approved or cleared by the FDA but also for approved products that are being studied outside of their label indications. All clinical evaluations of investigational devices, unless exempt, must have an approved IDE before the study is initiated.

PMAs require at least one and often multiple clinical studies to support approval. Depending upon the complexity of the device, its benefit/risk ratio, and clinical findings and results, additional studies may be necessary. There are generally two types of clinical studies of investigational devices.

- A feasibility study is an initial limited study in humans to confirm design aspects, such as, but not limited to, design, operating specifications, safety, dose range, and side effects. This initial study may indicate that the device does or does not meet expectations, or that minor or major changes in the device, its manufacture, or clinical study parameters are necessary before proceeding.
- A pivotal study is a key, larger clinical study performed to collect definitive evidence on safety and effectiveness, typically in a statistically justified number of subjects.

All IDEs require a sponsor, which is a person or other entity (can be a company, university, hospital, or one individual) who takes responsibility for and initiates a clinical investigation but that does not actually conduct the investigation. The "sponsor" for the FDA submission may be different from the "sponsor" of the study who is providing financial support, who is responsible for any grant funding, or who may eventually bring the device to market. Whereas an investigator is an individual who actually conducts the clinical investigation. In some cases, if an individual both initiates and actually conducts, alone or with others, a clinical investigation, that person is considered a sponsor-investigator. This situation most commonly occurs in the university setting if a physician initiates a clinical study.

As defined by the IDE regulations (21 CFR 812), IDE sponsors and investigators have defined responsibilities associated with performance of the IDE. The sponsor:

- Selects investigators
- Ensures proper monitoring (securing compliance to the protocol) and IRB review and approval
- Serves as the official contact for the FDA
- Maintains records (for example: FDA and investigator correspondence, shipment and device disposition, investigator agreements, study records), provides reports to the FDA and investigators (if a multicenter study), and ensures proper labeling

The investigator:

- Conducts the study in compliance with the protocol only after it is approved
- Obtains informed consent
- Actually communicates with the IRB and obtains review and approval
- Supervises use of the device
- Maintains records and provides reports to the sponsor and the IRB.
- Returns the device to the sponsor at the end of the study

When performing a clinical study under an IDE, in addition to the IDE regulations, sponsors and investigators must also comply with the good clinical practice (GCP) requirements listed in Table 13.2

The IDE regulations do exempt certain premarket clinical studies from complying with IDE requirements. These exempted clinical studies are listed in Table 13.3. Although the types of studies listed in this table do not require an IDE to be performed, they must still comply with the GCP regulations listed in Table 13.2.

Requirements applicable to studies performed under IDE are also grouped into two categories by risk. Therefore, once it is determined that the planned study does not meet an exemption from the IDE requirements, the next step in preparing an IDE is determining whether the planned study

Table 13.2 Good Clinical Practice (GCP) Requirements

Good Clinical Practice Requirement	Regulation
Informed Consent Requirements[a]	21 CFR 50
Financial Disclosure of Investigators	21 CFR 54
Review and continuing approval by an Institutional Review Board	21 CFR 56

[a]Guidance for Sponsors, Investigators, and Institutional Review Boards—Questions and Answers on Informed Consent Elements 21 CFR 50.25(c). https://www.fda.gov/downloads/RegulatoryInformation/Guidances/UCM291085.pdf.

Table 13.3 Clinical Studies Exempted From Investigational Device Exemption (IDE) Regulations

Clinical Studies Exempted From IDE Regulations
A legally marketed device when used in accordance with its labeling.
A diagnostic device, if the testing is: • Noninvasive • Does not require an invasive sampling procedure that presents significant risk • Does not by design or intention introduce energy into a subject • Is not used as a diagnostic procedure without confirmation of the diagnosis by another medically established diagnostic product or procedure
A device undergoing consumer preference testing, testing of a modification, or testing of a combination of two or more devices in commercial distribution, if the testing is not for the purpose of determining safety or effectiveness and does not put subjects at risk.
A device intended solely for veterinary use.
A device shipped solely for research on or with laboratory animals.

is considered an SR device study that presents potential for serious risk and is implanted, supports or sustains life, or is of substantial importance in diagnosing, curing, mitigating, or treating disease.[t] If this is the case, the IDE must be submitted to the FDA for review and approval prior to

---

[t]Significant Risk and Nonsignficant Risk Medical Device Studies—Information Sheet. https://www.fda.gov/MedicalDevices/DeviceRegulationandGuidance/HowtoMarket YourDevice/InvestigationalDeviceExemptionIDE/ucm162453.htm.

initiation. Any study that does not meet the definition of SR is considered an NSR device study, and the FDA allows abbreviated requirements, such that the IDE is not submitted to the FDA and is deemed approved with IRB approval. IRB review and approval, informed consent, record keeping, and monitoring are all still required. The IDE sponsor makes the first determination regarding NSR vs. SR, and the IRB reviews this determination based upon the device description, prior investigations, protocol, subjects, and risk assessment. If IRB disagrees, they must inform the investigator and a SR IDE will be required. The FDA is the final arbiter and can help make the determination if needed.

SR IDEs that require submission to the FDA must include the following items. SR IDEs also undergo an RTA review, and if these items are not included in the submission, FDA review will not proceed.[u](https://www.fda.gov/downloads/MedicalDevices/DeviceRegulationandGuidance/GuidanceDocuments/UCM081312.pdf)

- Sponsor information
- Report of prior investigations
- Investigational plan
- Manufacturing information
- Informed consent materials
- An example of the investigator agreements and a list of names and addresses of all investigators
- List of name, address and chairperson of all IRBs.
- Name and address of all institutional sites.
- Labeling, including a statement that the device is for investigational use only

IDE submissions do not have user fees associated with the submission. The review time for SR IDEs is 30 days, at which time the IDE is either approved, conditionally approved (in which case the sponsor has 45 days to address the conditions of approval), or disapproved by the FDA. Once an SR IDE study is initiated, supplements or reports may need to be submitted to the FDA for changes/modifications,[v] unanticipated adverse device effects/adverse events, withdrawal of IRB approval, yearly progress reports, additional information, protocol deviations, and completion of the study.

---

[u]Center for Devices and Radiological Health's Investigational Device Exemption (IDE) Refuse to Accept Policy. https://www.fda.gov/downloads/MedicalDevices/DeviceRegulationandGuidance/GuidanceDocuments/UCM081312.pdf.
[v]Changes or Modifications During the Conduct of a Clinical Investigation, Final Guidance for Industry and CDRH Staff. https://www.fda.gov/MedicalDevices/DeviceRegulationandGuidance/GuidanceDocuments/ucm082145.htm.

Table 13.4 User Fees for 2018		
Submission Type	Standard User Fee	Small Business User Fee
513(g)	$4,185	$2,098
510(k)	$10,566	$2,642
De Novo	$93,229	$23,307
PMA	$310,764	$77,691[a]

[a]Small businesses with gross receipts or sales of $30 million or less are also eligible to have the fee waived for their first PMA.

Finally, in addition to compliance with IDE regulations, sponsors of IDE studies (both SR and NSR) may not:

- Charge for an investigational product if the price is larger than that necessary to recover costs of manufacture, research, development, and handling.
- Promote or test market for an investigational product
- Unduly prolong a study
- Represent that an investigational product is safe or effective for the purposes for which it is being investigated; however, scientific findings about studies may be distributed.

User Fees

FDA charges user fees for some types of submissions. User fees must be paid in advance of submitting the documentation, and the specific user fee is dependent upon the type of submission and whether the sponsor has been granted a small business designation (SBD). An SBD qualifies a company with gross receipts or sales of no more than $100 million for the most recent tax year,[x] for reduced user fees. The user fees are evaluated and change each year. Table 13.4 shows the 2018 user fees for the submission types discussed in this chapter.[x]

Electronic Copy (eCopy)

FDA requires submission of an electronic copy (eCopy) for the submission types discussed in this chapter, with the exception of the 513(g). The eCopy must be an exact duplicate of the paper copy and must comply with

---

[x]FDA Guidance Document. FY 2018 Medical Device User Fee Small Business Qualification and Certification.
[x]Medical Device User Fee Amendments (MDUFA). https://www.fda.gov/ForIndustry/UserFees/MedicalDeviceUserFee/default.htm.

specific technical standards and requirements. FDA will not accept a submission for review if the eCopy is not compliant. Information on eCopy requirements is found in FDA's eCopy guidance document.[y]

KEY TAKEAWAY POINTS

• ▶ Understand your device classification and likely regulatory pathway early, as the effort, cost, and time to market authorization differ *significantly* based on device classification.

• ▶ The intended use and indications for use of the device are as important as the device itself in determining risk class.

• ▶ The Pre-submission process is available to get FDA input, if needed, early in the device or study development process.

• ▶ The FDA website provides information about device classification and the various regulatory pathways and provides issue- and device-specific guidance documents that provide detailed advice about related marketing submission requirements and regulatory expectations.

• ▶ Regulatory submissions for performance of clinical studies and market authorization are complex documents, and the FDA review process is very challenging for those unfamiliar with the regulations, pathways, administrative requirements, and regulatory precedents. An experienced medical device regulatory consultant can provide valuable guidance navigating the FDA submission process.

BIBLIOGRAPHY

1. Humanitarian Device Exemption. FDA U.S. Food & Drug Administration website. https://www.fda.gov/medicaldevices/deviceregulationandguidance/howtomarketyourdevice/premarketsubmissions/humanitariandeviceexemption/default.htm. Updated March 3, 2018.
2. Expanded Access: Information for Physicians. FDA U.S. Food & Drug Administration website. https://www.fda.gov/NewsEvents/PublicHealthFocus/ExpandedAccessCompassionateUse/ucm429624.htm. Updated April 12, 2018.
3. Custom Device Exemption: Guidance for Industry and Food and Drug Administration Staff. U.S. Department of Health and Human Services. https://www.fda.gov/downloads/medicaldevices/deviceregulationandguidance/guidancedocuments/ucm415799.pdf. Published September 24, 2014.
4. Product Classification. FDA U.S. Food & Drug Administration website. https://www.accessdata.fda.gov/scripts/cdrh/cfdocs/cfPCD/classification.cfm. Updated May 7, 2018.

[y]FDA Guidance document: eCopy Program for Medical Device Submissions: Guidance for Industry and Food and Drug Administration Staff", issued on December 3, 2015. https://www.fda.gov/downloads/medicaldevices/deviceregulationandguidance/guidancedocuments/ucm313794.pdf.

5. 510(k) Premarket Notification. FDA U.S. Food & Drug Administration website. https://www.accessdata.fda.gov/scripts/cdrh/cfdocs/cfpmn/pmn.cfm. Updated May 7, 2018.

6. Premarket Approval (PMA). FDA U.S. Food & Drug Administration website. https://www.accessdata.fda.gov/scripts/cdrh/cfdocs/cfPMA/pma.cfm.   Updated May 7, 2018.

7. CDRH Management Directory by Organization. FDA U.S. Food & Drug Administration   website.   https://www.fda.gov/AboutFDA/CentersOffices/ OfficeofMedicalProductsandTobacco/CDRH/CDRHOffices/ucm127854.htm. Updated May 9, 2018.

8. FDA and Industry Procedures for Section 513(g) Requests for Information Under the Federal Food, Drug, and Cosmetic Act: Guidance for Industry and Food and Drug Administration Staff. U.S. Department of Health and Human Services. https://www.fda.gov/downloads/medicaldevices/deviceregulationandguidance/ guidancedocuments/ucm209851.pdf. Published April 6, 2012. Updated December 21, 2015.

9. Requests for Feedback on Medical Device Submissions: The Pre-Submission Program and Meetings With Food and Drug Administration Staff: Guidance for Industry and Food and Drug Administration Staff. U.S. Department of Health and Human Services. https://www.fda.gov/downloads/medicaldevices/deviceregulation-andguidance/guidancedocuments/ucm311176.pdf. Published February 18, 2014. Updated September 29, 2017.

10. The 510(k) Program: Evaluating Substantial Equivalence in Premarket Notifications [510(k)]: Guidance for Industry and Food and Drug Administration Staff. U.S. Department of Health and Human Services. https://www.fda.gov/ucm/groups/ fdagov-public/@fdagov-meddev-gen/documents/document/ucm284443.pdf. Published July 28, 2014.

11. Search for FDA Guidance Documents. FDA U.S. Food & Drug Administration Website.   https://www.fda.gov/RegulatoryInformation/Guidances/default.htm. Updated May 8, 2018.

12. Use of International Standard ISO 10993-1, "Biological Evaluation of Medical Devices – Part 1: Evaluation and Testing Within A Risk Management Process": Guidance for Industry and Food and Drug Administration Staff. U.S. Department of Health and Human Services. https://www.fda.gov/ucm/groups/fdagov-public/@fdagov-meddev-gen/documents/document/ucm348890.pdf. Published June 16, 2016.

13. Submission and Review of Sterility Information in Premarket Notification (510(k)) Submissions for Devices Labeled as Sterile: Guidance for Industry and Food and Drug Administration Staff. U.S. Department of Health and Human Services. https://www.fda.gov/ucm/groups/fdagov-public/@fdagov-meddev-gen/documents/ document/ucm109897.pdf. Published January 21, 2016.

14. Format for Traditional and Abbreviated 510(k)s – Guidance for Industry and FDA Staff. FDA U.S. Food & Drug Administration Website. https://www. fda.gov/MedicalDevices/DeviceRegulationandGuidance/GuidanceDocuments/ ucm084365.htm. Published August 12, 2005. Updated February 7, 2018.

15. FDA and Industry Actions on Premarket Notification (510(k)) Submissions: Effect on FDA Review Clock and Goals: Guidance for Industry and Food and Drug Administration Staff. U.S. Department of Health and Human Services. https:// www.fda.gov/ucm/groups/fdagov-public/@fdagov-meddev-gen/documents/docu-ment/ucm089738.pdf. Published May 21, 2004. Updated October 2, 2017.

16. De Novo Classification Process (Evaluation of Automatic Class III Designation): Guidance for Industry and Food and Drug Administration Staff. U.S. Department of Health and Human Services. https://www.fda.gov/ucm/groups/fdagov-public/@fdagov-meddev-gen/documents/document/ucm080197.pdf. Published October 30, 2017.

17. Acceptance and Filing Reviews for Premarket Approval Applications (PMAs): Guidance for Industry and Food and Drug Administration Staff. U.S. Department of Health and Human Services. https://www.fda.gov/downloads/MedicalDevices/DeviceRegulationandGuidance/GuidanceDocuments/UCM313368.pdf. Published May 1, 2003. Updated January 30, 2018.

18. Guidance for Sponsors, Investigators, and Institutional Review Boards: Questions and Answers on Informed Consent Elements, 21 CFR § 50.25(c): (Small Entity Compliance Guide). U.S. Department of Health and Human Services. https://www.fda.gov/downloads/RegulatoryInformation/Guidances/UCM291085.pdf. Published February 2012.

19. IDE Guidance. FDA U.S. Food & Drug Administration website. https://www.fda.gov/MedicalDevices/DeviceRegulationandGuidance/HowtoMarketYourDevice/InvestigationalDeviceExemptionIDE/ucm162453.htm. Updated May 2, 2018.

20. Changes or Modifications During the Conduct of a Clinical Investigation; Final Guidance for Industry and CDRH Staff. FDA U.S. Food & Drug Administration Website. https://www.fda.gov/MedicalDevices/DeviceRegulationandGuidance/GuidanceDocuments/ucm082145.htm. Published May 29, 2001. Updated March 12, 2018.

21. Medical Device User Fee Amendments (MDUFA). FDA U.S. Food & Drug Administration website. https://www.fda.gov/ForIndustry/UserFees/MedicalDeviceUserFee/default.htm. Updated May 7, 2018.

22. eCopy Program for Medical Device Submissions: Guidance for Industry and Food and Drug Administration Staff. U.S. Department of Health and Human Services. https://www.fda.gov/downloads/medicaldevices/deviceregulationandguidance/guidancedocuments/ucm313794.pdf. Published December 3, 2015.

MEDICAL DEVICE REGULATORY CONSULTING RESOURCES

1. M Squared Associates, Inc., 575 Eighth Avenue, Suite 1212, New York, NY 10018 www.msquaredassociates.com.
2. Biologics Consulting, 1555 King Street, Suite 300, Alexandria, VA 22314. www.biologicsconsulting.com.
3. Greenleaf Health, LLC, 1055 Thomas Jefferson Street, NW, Suite 450 Washington, DC 20007 http://www.greenleafhealth.com/.
4. Regulatory Strategies, Inc., http://www.regulatorystrategies.net/.
5. Hyman Phelps McNamara, http://hpm.com/.
6. King & Spalding, https://www.kslaw.com/practices/fda-and-life-sciences?locale=en.
7. Hogan Lovells, https://www.hoganlovells.com/en/aof/medical-devices.

CHAPTER 14

Reimbursement Basics: Who Is the Customer and How Will You Profit?

ROBIN R. YOUNG

ABOUT THE AUTHOR

Robin R. Young is the publisher of *Orthopedics This Week* and CEO of the PearlDiver health care data mining service. Mr Young was also founder of the annual New York Stem Cell Summit. Mr Young is the author of six books and thousands of articles on a wide variety of medical and technology subjects. Over his career, he has been a member of the faculty of the University of Minnesota, University of St. Thomas, and a Director of Life Science Research for various Wall Street firms. Mr Young resides in Wayne, Pennsylvania, US.

Introduction

That question "Who is the Customer?" is a multilayered problem for anyone trying to commercialize a medical device or pharma product. At various times and under certain circumstances, the customer could be the patient, the physician, the clinic, the hospital system, the third-party payer, or a combination of any two or more of the above.

Indeed, for anyone starting out to sell a medical device or a pharmaceutical product, the definition of "customer" and how to "sell" them has become ever more complex since the turn of the century.

In this chapter, we will provide you with a few key mile markers so that you will always know where you are on your journey to reimbursement and routine payment for your products.

The United States Model

In the United States, the customer for medical devices or pharmaceutical products has, essentially, three heads. One is the physician user—whose ability to drive a purchase decision is declining. The second head is the hospital or clinic purchasing manager—whose ability to drive a purchase decision is also declining. The third head is, appropriately enough, the third-party payer—and their ability to drive the purchase decision is rising.

The third-party payer is, for 90%[1] of the cases, a gatekeeper to the other two purchase decision makers.

In order to successfully commercialize a medical device or pharmaceutical product in the United States (with the notable $7 billion exception of the medical marijuana market[2]), the logical answer to "Who is the customer?" is the third-party payer.

Once a third-party payer has agreed to pay for a new device or pharma product, then the physician, who is motivated by pathology relevance, and the purchasing manager, who is motivated by economic relevance, become the customer.

To lapse into cliché, anything worthwhile is hard. And earning a profit, which necessarily requires revenues, by selling medical devices or pharmaceutical products in the United States is hard.

This tortuous journey starts with the third-party payers.

Your New Best Friend: Third-Party Payers

In the United States, three third-party payers—private insurance companies, state governments, and the federal government—pay physicians, clinics, and hospitals for the services and products required to treat patients.

The Patient Protection and Affordable Care Act, which was enacted in 2010,[3] is a federal program, which provides funding to private insurers to provide basic health care insurance services.

Private insurers provide insurance coverage through three basic types of programs:
- Private pay organizations (PPOs)
- Health maintenance organizations (HMOs)
- The Patient Protection and Affordable Care Act

Within these three basic archetypes of private health insurance, there are programs, which combine elements of a PPO with an HMO (such as point of service plans) or a PPO with a savings account (such as high deductible health plans). But these permutations are relevant to the patient or the patient's employer, not a device or pharma company.

Medicare provides health insurance coverage to US citizens who are either over the age of 65 years or disabled and both, of course. The coverage is provided through four programs[4]:
- Part A: Hospital Inpatient
- Part B: Outpatient, Physician, Diagnostics, Home Health, Administered Drugs

- Part C: Managed Care
- Part D: New Drug program

Medicaid is the state-run reimbursement system, which provides insurance coverage for low-income state residents and is one of the primary sources of coverage for long-term nursing home care in the United States.

2016 Actuarial Statistics on Payments to Health Care Providers

In 2016, health care spending in the United States reached $3.3 trillion dollars. Of that total, patients paid $353 million out of their own pocket, while public and private health insurance programs covered $2.5 trillion or 75% of the total and other third-party payers and public health programs accounted for $466 million or 14% of the total (Table 14.1).

How to Qualify Your Product for Third-Party Reimbursement

Rules governing third-party reimbursement programs (private health insurance, Medicare, and Medicaid) come under three broad categories:

1. Coverage
2. Coding
3. Payment

In this chapter, we will explain each of these concepts and how you can navigate them to successfully get past "no."

COVERAGE

In order for a medical device to be eligible for coverage, it must be approved for commercialization in the United States by the Food and Drug Administration (FDA).

Once that is in place, then a device is eligible for coverage, coding, and, eventually, payment from third-party payers.

But there is no guarantee of coverage following FDA clearance, approval, or license.

Third-party health care payers, such as Medicare or Blue Cross Blue Shield, are not required to cover every medical device that has been cleared or approved by the FDA.

Many FDA-approved/-cleared/-licensed devices are not reimbursed by third-party payers in the United States.

Health care providers—doctors, clinics, and hospitals—generally require that every product they purchase be eligible for reimbursement.

Table 14.1 Total US Health Care Spending, Aggregate and per Capita Amounts, Share of Gross Domestic Product (GDP) by Source for Calendar Years 2010-2016

	2010	2011	2012	2013	2014	2015	2016	2015 vs 2016	
								2014	2015
Spending Amounts									
Total U.S. health care spending, billions	$ 2,599	$ 2,689	$ 2,797	$ 2,879	$ 3,026	$ 3,201	$ 3,337	5.77%	4.24%
Out of pocket spending	300	310	318	325	330	339	353	2.79%	3.89%
Health insurance spending	1,877	1,950	2,023	2,088	2,228	2,383	2,487	6.94%	4.36%
Private health insurance	864	899	928	946	1,000	1,069	1,123	6.89%	5.11%
Medicare	520	545	570	590	619	649	672	4.83%	3.59%
Medicaid	397	407	423	445	497	544	566	9.57%	3.93%
Federal contributions	266	247	243	257	305	343	358	12.45%	4.37%
State and local spending	131	160	179	189	192	201	208	4.96%	3.23%
Other health insurance programs	96	100	102	106	113	121	126	7.45%	3.88%
Other third-party payers and programs and public health activity	279	280	303	313	318	325	341	2.14%	4.77%
Investment	143	150	153	153	150	154	157	2.67%	2.41%
U.S. Populations (millions)	309	311	313	316	318	320	323	0.72%	0.69%
Gross Domestic Product, billions	$ 14,964	$ 15,518	$ 16,155	$ 16,692	$ 17,428	$ 18,121	$ 18,625	3.98%	2.78%
Health care spending per capita	8,412	8,644	8,924	9,121	9,515	9,994	10,348	5.03%	3.54%
GDP per capita	48,436	49,879	51,542	52,880	54,779	56,580	57,751	3.29%	2.07%
Health care spending as percent of GDP	17.4%	17.3%	17.3%	17.2%	17.4%	17.7%	17.9%	n/a	n/a

Callout boxes:
- $3.3 trillion in annual healthcare expenditures.
- $353 million are out-of-pocket expenditures.
- 75% of annual healthcare spending is paid by public or private insurance

From Office of the Actuary, Centers for Medicaid and Medicare Services, Baltimore, Maryland.

Occasionally, health care providers will use products that are billed directly to patients. Overall, patients pay about 10% of their health care costs with personal funds.

Ensuring that every device has coverage and payment is critical pacing items for every medical product supplier.

MEDICARE COVERAGE

Medicare is the starting point for most companies seeking payer coverage for their products.

Medicare's coverage decisions are often a prerequisite for coverage by private health insurers.

Medical device companies can apply for Medicare coverage of new devices that do not fit into an existing service code by requesting either a national coverage determination (NCD) from the Centers for Medicaid and Medicare Services (CMS) or a local coverage determination (LCD) from a Medicare administrative contractor (MAC) for the procedure that involves the device.

NCDs apply nationwide, while an LCD applies only to the states within the jurisdiction of the MAC that issued it. CMS and the MACs make coverage decisions by determining whether the available evidence for a device supports the requested coverage. The processes for developing both NCDs and LCDs include opening up the discussion to external stakeholders. They are invited to share their views about the product. The public is also allowed to review and comment on draft coverage determinations.

In recent years, third-party insurers have required companies to provide more evidence of clinical benefit and cost analysis. These information requests are over and above the FDA requirements.

Many new devices receive FDA approval but remain un- or under-reimbursed as "investigational devices" for years post approval.

Eventually, with sufficient clinical and cost analysis data, third-party reimbursors will designate an approved novel device as reimbursable.

CODING

In the United States, every device and pharma product is paid according to a usage code. Those codes were developed and are maintained by the American Medical Association (AMA) or CMS.

There are five basic categories of reimbursement codes, which, in theory, cover all services and products used to treat patients.

Table 14.2 describes this multitied coding system and its various inpatient and outpatient diagnosis and procedure billing codes.[5]

Table 14.2 US Health care Code Category Outline—Inpatient and Outpatient Services and Procedures

	DRG	HCPCS HCSPCS I	HCPCS HCSPCS II	ASC	HOPPS	ICD-10
Definition	Diagnostic Related Group (DRG). The DRG code covers all hospital services and associated costs incurred during a patient stay EXCEPT physician charges. Those are billed under CPT. Only one DRG code is used per admission. The DRG is determined by the patient's reported ICD-10 code(s).	Healthcare Common Procedure Coding System (HCPCS). These codes are used to bill procedures and health care products as well as to track performance. Level I HCPCS codes are Current Procedural Terminology (CPT) codes and have three subcategories. Physicians bill for procedures or services using Level I HCPCS. Payments go directly to the physician.	Healthcare Common Procedure Coding System (HCPCS). Level II HCPCS codes represent over 4,000 categories of items. It is used primarily to identify products, supplies, and services not included in the CPT code.	Ambulatory Surgical Center (ASC) Payment System. ASCs are standalone centers that perform same-day discharge services only. There are no specific ASC billing codes; CPT codes are used to bill for procedures. Payment goes to the facility.	Hospital Outpatient Prospective Payment System (HOPPS), also referred to as APC. The HOPPS system provides Ambulatory Payment Classification (APC) codes, which are used by facilities to bill for outpatient procedures and services. CPT codes typically are used to 'crosswalk' to the APC fee schedule.	International Classification of Diseases, 10th edition. (ICD-10). Defined in ICD-10-CM manual for identifying patient diagnosis in either the inpatient or outpatient setting. Defined in ICD-10-PCS manual for reporting surgeries or procedures performed in the inpatient setting.
Issuer	CMS	American Medical Association (AMA)	American Medical Association (AMA)	CMS	CMS	CMS
Updated	Annually	Annually	Annually	Quarterly	Quarterly	Annually
Setting	Inpatient billing only	All facilities	All facilities	Outpatient only	Outpatient	Inpatient

Examples					
DRG code 470. Major hip and knee joint replacement or reattachment of lower extremity without major complications.	CPT code 27197—closed treatment of posterior pelvic ring fracture(s), dislocation(s), diastasis or subluxation of the ilium, sacroiliac joint, and/or sacrum, with or without anterior pelvic ring fracture(s) and/or dis location(s) of the pubic symphysis and/or superior/inferior rami, unilateral or bilateral without manipulation.	**C codes**—items and services for outpatient use, pass-through devices, drugs, and biologicals, new technology, and other services. **G codes**—professional health care procedures and series, which currently lack a CPT code. **Q codes**—used to identify drugs, biologics, and other medical equity or services, which are not identified by national level II codes but which need coding for claims processing. **S codes**—used by private insurers to report drugs, services, and supplies for which there are no permanent national codes, but for which codes are needed to implement policies, programs, or claims processing.	CPT code 20610—Arthrocentesis, aspiration, and/or injection, major joint or bursa (e.g., shoulder, hip, knee or subacromial bursa) without ultrasound guidance.	APC code 5116—level 6. CPT code 22867—Insertion of interlaminar interspinous process stabilization/distraction device, without fusion, including image guidance when performed with open decompression, lumbar, single level.	Diagnosis code M25.519—pain in unspecified shoulder.

Coding is the first step in a journey to eventual payment coverage. It does not, by itself, assure payment for either the procedure or an FDA-approved device.

When a new procedure billing code has been assigned by an insurer, actual payment decisions are based on a variety of factors. The payer will typically conduct an independent health technology assessment (in which a payer medical director will evaluate available technical and scientific evidence regarding the device or pharma product and the associated intervention), peer-reviewed published clinical data, real-world evidence of clinical efficacy (outside a clinical trial environment), and practice guidelines, which have been published by relevant professional societies.

If the assessment finds that the evidence supports the products safety and efficacy and it is beyond the "investigational" stage, then payers will typically pay.

Most companies apply to CMS first for a coverage code, in part because it covers all adults age 65 and over in the United States but also because commercial insurers frequently follow CMS's lead when it comes to coverage decisions.

Rather than trying to obtain coverage from the hundreds of US commercial insurers, companies who successfully obtain a code from CMS can then pivot to apply to small number of large payers—based on member enrollment, their receptiveness to new medical technologies, and the stringency of their review policies—to fairly quickly obtain insurance coverage for most of the country.

Gradually, over time, companies expand their applications to other payers as adoption of the new device or pharma product spreads.

If a device or procedure receives an "investigational" designation from a payer, it will not be covered. In those cases, the patient will typically assume financial liability for the device.

When a payer tags a device with the "investigational" label, it means that the payer has determined it lacks sufficient evidence to justify the product's use. The scope of clinical evidence required by payers often exceeds FDA requirements, which focus on the device's safety and efficacy.

Successful companies design their clinical studies to meet the FDA's safety and efficacy requirements and then also conduct a cost and value analysis to answer payer questions about the comparative value of the product as compared to current standards of care.

New Technologies

New technologies face several unique challenges when applying for payment codes from CMS or other payers. If the new technology costs more than existing standard of care, then it may receive a payment based on an older standard of care, which is inadequate to pay for the new technology. Hospitals and providers will usually not accept a new technology without a billing code.

Companies seeking reimbursement for new technologies must apply for either a new billing code, additional coverage under existing codes, and ask for a temporary pass-through payment.

For example, CMS has a rule, which provides companies with the option of applying for a new-technology add-on payment (NTAP)[6] to cover the cost of new medical technologies deployed in the inpatient setting. If approved, CMS pays 50% of the cost of the new device or technology or 50% of the overall incremental costs associated with the new technology, in addition to the full diagnostic related group (DRG) payment.

To avoid penalizing technologies simply because they are new, CMS will, during the period between the introduction of a new device and the availability of suitable cost report data, increase payment rates for devices that satisfy three criteria:

1. They have received FDA approval or clearance within the past 3 years.
2. They are sufficiently expensive that existing payment rates are inadequate.
3. They have a clear clinical benefit.

These new-technology payments remain in effect for no more than 3 years; by that time, hospitals would have submitted cost reports that include the costs of the new technology, and CMS can use its regular methodology to set payment rates.

For inpatient services, as was described above, new-technology payments are capped at 50% of the difference between the estimated cost of the inpatient stay and the regular Medicare payment rate, or 50% of the cost of the new device, whichever is less.

For outpatient services, the new-technology payment equals the estimated cost of the device, which CMS calculates using the hospital's cost-to-charge ratio. Hospitals identify the services that qualify for new-technology payments by including specific procedure or service codes on their claims.

Relatively few devices have qualified for these new-technology payments. Between 2001 and 2015, CMS approved only 19 of 53 applications (from both device and drug manufacturers) for new-technology payments under the inpatient prospective payment system (IPPS).

Medicare spending for new-technology payments has also been relatively low; between fiscal years 2002 and 2013, the program spent about $200 million on new-technology payments under the IPPS.

The medical device industry has argued that CMS should make it easier to qualify for new-technology payments and that the IPPS should pay 80% of the cost of a new device or drug instead of 50% to more strongly encourage the use of new technology (Advanced Medical Technology Association—AdvaMed— in 2016).[7]

However, the existing criteria encourage hospitals to negotiate discounts on new devices, which limits the ability of device companies to introduce new devices at higher prices and helps to contain program spending.

Work-Arounds

If the new-technology pathway is too onerous, CMS also allows companies to apply for pass-through Ambulatory Payment Classification (APC) payments for hospital outpatient procedures.[8] These payments are reserved for new, expensive-but-highly-beneficial devices that are used in procedures with existing APC codes. The pass-through typically is calculated as the cost of the device minus the cost of the device already included in the APC that is being replaced.

Finally, companies can apply for a category III (temporary)[9] code while they await issuance of a category I Current Procedural Terminology (CPT) code for their new medical technology or procedure. This provision allows companies to build a history of widespread usage with the AMA that will support establishment of a CPT I code. However, no set payment fee will be established, and it can take years to transition to a category I code. Furthermore, companies run the risk that their device or procedure will be labeled experimental, potentially disqualifying it from coverage by some payers.

Occasionally, though rarely, companies can avail themselves of the miscellaneous CPT code while they wait for a category I code.[10] Miscellaneous codes provide a mechanism for providers to submit claims for a service or item as soon as it is FDA-approved. Miscellaneous codes exist for most organs or body systems (e.g. CPT 38999—Unlisted procedure, hemic or lymphatic system).

To go this route, health care providers will be asked to provide additional documentation justifying use of the device as part of their attempt to obtain coverage. This typically involves writing a lengthy procedure note describing the patient's medical condition, the procedure itself, a list of all supplies used, rationale for using the new procedure or technology, and supporting clinical data. Payers then decide whether to provide any coverage for the procedure.

Accounting for the Cost of Medical Devices in Payment Rates

In recent years, third-party payers have increased their efforts to control the rising costs of health care in the United States. As part of that process, payers are scrutinizing the costs of medical devices and pharmaceutical products in new ways and adjusting their reimbursement policies accordingly. Here, for example, are ways that third-party payers—governmental and private—are calculating costs for inpatient and outpatient hospital services, clinician services, and durable medical equipment (DME).

INPATIENT AND OUTPATIENT HOSPITAL SERVICES

CMS has the most comprehensive system for collecting and analyzing the costs of medical devices in the United States, using data that hospitals submit each year in their cost reports.

The cost reports have information on both costs and charges, which CMS uses to calculate cost-to-charge ratios for major categories of hospital activity known as cost centers. The cost of medical devices is reported in several different cost centers, such as one for medical supplies and another for implantable devices.

CMS uses the cost-to-charge ratios to convert charges that hospitals submit on claims to an estimated cost of providing services. CMS calculates the average cost for each service across all hospitals and uses that as the basis for its payment rates under both the IPPS[11] and the outpatient prospective payment system (OPPS).[12]

As a result, Medicare's payment rates for an inpatient or outpatient service include an amount that approximates the average amount that hospitals pay for the medical devices used in that service.

DOCTOR OR CLINICIAN SERVICES

CMS accounts for the cost of medical devices using information collected from surveys fielded by specialty societies. These surveys ask about the time and intensity involved in providing a service and the associated practice costs, such as nonphysician clinical staff and the specific medical devices used in each procedure.

A group of health care professionals known as the AMA/Specialty Society Relative Value Scale Update Committee[13] then recommends clinician payment rates to CMS based on the survey information and their professional judgment.

CMS converts information on the types of devices used for a given service into an overall cost estimate using price data that it collects. CMS then calculates weights that measure the relative costliness of each physician service. However, the amount included for medical devices can often be inaccurate because the information on the number and type of medical devices used in a procedure is based on a small number of surveys, and CMS has not thoroughly updated the information on prices since 2004. In some cases, the price of a device is based on only one or two invoices.

DURABLE MEDICAL EQUIPMENT

Unlike hospital and physician services, DME (as well as prosthetics and orthotics) is an area where medical devices such as wheelchairs and home oxygen equipment are considered services in their own right. CMS traditionally used a fee schedule to pay for these products, but the Congress required the agency to begin using competitive DME products and has expanded its use since then.

Under competitive bidding, DME suppliers submit bids to provide certain products in selected metropolitan areas and indicate how much of each product they can supply. CMS selects suppliers who offer the best price and meet applicable quality and financial standards and then uses the median bid from the winning suppliers as its payment rate.

The DME competitive bidding program has substantially reduced DME payment rates, thereby saving Medicare and beneficiaries billions of dollars since its inception.[14]

CMS has also reported that the implementation of the DME competitive bidding program has not resulted in widespread beneficiary access issues.

Payment Bundling

A new strategy for containing the costs of medical products and services is to bundle the costs of a particular episode of care into a single number and then leave it to the health care provider to sort out who gets what.

Medicare's general strategy for imposing bundling payment approach is that it gives providers an incentive to more carefully monitor and limit their spending on specific episodes of care—for example, a knee replacement surgery.[15] Under the current system, providers who use more expensive devices or perform more expensive tests or services will not receive any additional reimbursement to pay for those decisions and may lose money if their costs exceed the Medicare payment rate.

This incentive is particularly strong for implantable medical devices (IMDs), which can make up a significant share of the overall costs of an inpatient stay or outpatient procedure.

Conversely, providers that can keep their costs below the Medicare payment rate keep the difference. They are incentivized to keep costs low, therefore.

Private third-party health insurers are also implementing bundling program. One difference between the Medicare programs and private insurer programs is that private insurers often force health care providers to pay for IMDs separately, instead of bundling them with other inputs.[16]

Some hospitals can also add a significant markup to their purchase price when they negotiate IMD payment rates with private insurers. This arrangement allows some hospitals to turn IMDs into a significant source of profit and (since the markups are usually calculated on a percentage basis) gives them an incentive to use more expensive devices.

In 2014, hospitals spent about $14 billion on implantable devices and almost $10 billion on medical supplies. Between 2011 and 2014, spending on implantable devices grew at an average annual rate of 4.7%, compared with 2.0% for total hospital costs. During this period, implantable devices also grew as a share of total hospital costs, rising from 8.0% to 8.7%, while spending on medical supplies increased slightly faster than total hospital costs.[17]

The higher growth in spending on implantable devices relative to total hospital spending could be because of higher prices for IMDs, higher utilization rates for procedures that use IMDs, and sluggish growth in inpatient stays that do not involve IMDs. Another concern about bundling medical devices with other inputs is that CMS's IPPS and OPPS rates are ultimately based on historical data from cost reports.

There is a 2-year delay before cost reports for a given year are available, and this lag discourages hospitals from using new devices that benefit patients but are more expensive than existing technology.

Integrated Systems

The largest hospital system in the United States is the Veterans Administration (VA) system. It manages 1,240 health care facilities (including 150 hospitals and 820 outpatient clinics) and cares for more than 6 million patients annually.[18]

And it does not accept third-party payer reimbursement.

The VA system is a government-run system, which, like the other major category of payer, the HMO, has integrated the payer function into its health care provider function. It is all one integrated system.

HMOs (such as Kaiser Permanente, UnitedHealthcare, or Blue Cross Blue Shield's HMOs) are also integrated health care providers. In total, there are about 850 integrated health care providers in the United States.

Many companies have found that selling into integrated systems such as the VA or Kaiser is more efficient than running the gauntlet of independent third-party insurers.

If an FDA-cleared/-approved/-licensed product is approved for use at the VA, it will automatically be paid for if the doctor orders it and that approval will be in place for the entire VA system.

The same is true for all integrated care systems.

Each integrated system has its own processes for evaluating new devices or pharmaceutical products. Although working with integrated systems may be simpler, it is not necessarily easier.

Trends in Reimbursement

One trend, above all, is changing how devices and pharmaceutical products are paid for and that trend is cost reduction.

Payers, in particular, have put the squeeze on hospitals and care providers who have, in turn, put the squeeze on suppliers of medical products.

This "squeeze" has come in five basic ways:

1. Denying requests for reimbursement on the basis of medical necessity.
2. Making the process of receiving payment more difficult.
3. Reducing reimbursement rates across the board.
4. Using advanced data analytics to refine or, as it seems to many providers, "second-guess" medical protocols.
5. Reducing the number of vendors approved to sell into a health care system.

The squeeze has had an effect. Health care spending growth dropped in 2016 to the lowest level in nearly 2 years, and hospital spending growth lags behind all other health care sectors. Hospital spending increased by only 0.8% year-over-year in June 2016, which was the slowest growth rate since January 1989.[19]

This cost containment wave is changing the market for medical and pharma products in a number of critical ways for suppliers. The most public example of health insurers cutting costs over the past year was Anthem's policies to not pay for unnecessary emergency department visits or imaging services at hospitals. Anthem's policies looked to nudge patients to less costly outpatient facilities, including urgent care centers and freestanding imaging centers.[20]

Increasingly, payers are combining fee-for-service payments with value-based contracts—like the bundling approach described earlier in this chapter.

Hospitals, clinics, and other health care providers are increasingly teaming up with insurers in partnerships that look more and more like integrated systems.

Finally, both payers and providers are experimenting with community-based, outpatient, strip mall medicine. By moving out of the big box, acute care, infrastructure-heavy system and into a low rent, simplified, walk-in style center, providers have been able to cut costs significantly.[21]

Those moves, in turn, will affect which products are approved for payment and find acceptance in the modern clinic or hospital.

KEY TAKEAWAY POINTS

- ▶ The third-party payer is the most critical "customer" for the company hoping to generate sales from a device or pharma product.

- ▶ Third-party payers account for 75% of all device and pharma reimbursement in the United States. Patients account for 10% of the cost of their care. The remainder is public health programs and the military.

- ▶ Obtaining reimbursement from third-party payers for specific devices or pharmaceutical products is a three-step process.

  - ▶ Step One—Get Coverage: Third-party payers need to evaluate each device or pharmaceutical product in order to determine whether reimbursement is justified and, if so, at what level.

  - ▶ Step Two—Get a Code: Once a payer decides to provide reimbursement coverage, then a code needs to be assigned. There are several types of codes.

  - ▶ Step Three—Get Paid: Once a product has earned coverage and a code, then payment is likely although not entirely assured. Occasionally more work at the provider level is required.

- ▶ The best place to start the process of obtaining reimbursement and payment is the CMS because most private payers follow CMS's lead.

- ▶ The US health care system is undergoing a long-term process of cost containment and a shift of emphasis to outcome-based economics. As a result, there are often additional steps required in order to ultimately receive payment.

- ▶ Companies who hope to navigate the reimbursement and payment gauntlet in the United States need to come armed with well-documented cost benefit data. In today's health care world, establishing clinical relevance is only the beginning. To become commercially successful, each product must also be economically relevant.

REFERENCES AND RESOURCES

1. National Health Care Spending in 2016; Office of the Actuary; National Health Statistics Group. https://www.medicalmarijuanainc.com/company/.
2. Medical Marijuana Inc, https://www.medicalmarijuanainc.com/company/.
3. Wikipedia.com; Patient Protection and Affordable Care Act. https://en.wikipedia.org/wiki/Patient_Protection_and_Affordable_Care_Act.
4. Medicare Program – General Information. https://www.cms.gov/Medicare/Medicare-General-Information/MedicareGenInfo/index.html.
5. Robin Young Consulting.
6. New Medical Services and New Technologies, Application Information for FY 2019 https://www.cms.gov/Medicare/Medicare-Fee-for-Service-Payment/AcuteInpatientPPS/newtech.html.
7. Letter to Centers for Medicare and Medicaid Services from Andy Slavitt, Acting Administrator of AdvaMed. https://www.advamed.org/sites/default/files/resource/966_advamed_comment_letter_opps_proposed_rule_cy_2016.pdf.
8. Pass-Through Payment Status and New Technology Ambulatory Classification (APC). https://www.cms.gov/Medicare/Medicare-Fee-for-Service-Payment/HospitalOutpatientPPS/passthrough_payment.html.
9. HCPCS Coding Questions. https://www.cms.gov/Medicare/Coding/MedHCPCSGenInfo/HCPCS_Coding_Questions.html.
10. HCPCS – General Information. https://www.cms.gov/Medicare/Coding/MedHCPCSGenInfo/index.html.
11. Acute Care Hospital Inpatient Prospective Payment System. https://www.cms.gov/Outreach-and-Education/Medicare-Learning-Network-MLN/MLNProducts/downloads/acutepaymtsysfctsht.pdf.
12. Medicare CY 2018 Outpatient Prospective Payment System (OPPS) Final Rule Claims Accounting. https://www.cms.gov/Medicare/Medicare-Fee-for-Service-Payment/HospitalOutpatientPPS/Downloads/CMS-1678-FC-2018-OPPS-FR-Claims-Accounting.pdf.
13. RVS Update Process: American Medical Association; 2018; https://www.ama-assn.org/sites/default/files/media-browser/public/rbrvs/ruc-update-booklet_0.pdf.
14. CMS Awards Contracts for the DMEPOS Competitive Bidding. https://www.cms.gov/Newsroom/MediaReleaseDatabase/Fact-sheets/2016-Fact-sheets-items/2016-11-01-2.html.
15. Bundled Payments for Care Improvement (BPCI) Initiative. https://innovation.cms.gov/initiatives/bundled-payments/.
16. Episode of Care or Bundled Payments – Health Cost Containment. National Conference of State Legislators; http://www.ncsl.org/research/health/episode-of-care-payments-health.aspx.
17. Report to Congress: Medicare and the Health Care Delivery System; Medpac; An Overview of the Medical Device Industry; Table 7-4. http://medpac.gov/docs/default-source/reports/jun17_ch7.pdf?sfvrsn=0.
18. U.S. Department of Veterans Affairs. https://www.va.gov/health/.
19. *Hospital Spending Growth Falls to 28-Year Low*". HealthExec; September 8, 2017. http://www.healthexec.com/topics/finance/hospital-spending-growth-falls-28-year-low.

20. *Anthem ER Denial Policy Has Insurance Industry on Edge.* insurancenews-net.com; February 21, 2018. https://insurancenewsnet.com/oarticle/anthem-er-denial-policy-insurance-industry-edge
21. Report: Healthcare Clinics Replacing Retailers in Many US Malls." RetailDive.com. https://www.retaildive.com/news/report-healthcare-clinics-replacing-retailers-in-many-us-malls/423272/.

CHAPTER 15

Business Models

HAIM MENDELSON

ABOUT THE AUTHOR

Haim Mendelson is the Kleiner Perkins Caufield & Byers Professor of Electronic Business and Commerce, and Management at the Stanford Business School, and Codirector of the Value Chain Innovation Initiative. Professor Mendelson leads the Stanford Business School's efforts in studying business models that are enabled by new technologies and their interaction with organizations, markets, and value chains. His research interests include business model innovation, electronic business, electronic platforms, and market microstructure. He was elected Distinguished Fellow of the Information Systems Society in recognition of outstanding intellectual contributions to the information systems discipline. He has published more than a hundred papers in leading journals in the areas of management science, technology-enabled business models, information systems, and finance and has served as advisor and consultant to start-ups and established companies in these areas.

Introduction

Any business organization invariably creates and delivers value for its customers and in turn extracts some of that value as its revenue. People often associate the term *business model* with the financial dimension of the process, i.e., how the organization extracts revenues and makes a profit. The actual definition of the term is, however, broader. A business model is a model of the business that describes, in stylized form, how management intends to both create and deliver value to its customers (the *value-creation model*) as well as make a profit (the *profit model*): the value-creation model and the profit model are interrelated elements of the business model. The business model encompasses the product or service, the market, and the economic engine that drives the business. The business model thus reflects management's thinking on how (and at what cost) the business will create value and deliver it to its customers, how it will get paid, and what is the logic that will enable it to meet its profitability and growth objectives.

The business model is a blueprint, which needs to be tested by an early-stage start-up or executed by an established company. As British philosopher Alfred Whitehead put it, "the art of progress is to preserve order amid change and to preserve change amid order."[1] Business models attempt to bring order and discipline to the chaotic process of building, growing, and operating a business. In a start-up that builds its business from scratch, reality tests often reject the business model, but as Whitehead put it, "in formal logic, a contradiction is the signal of defeat, but in the evolution of real knowledge, it marks the first step in progress toward a victory."[1] Established companies revisit their business models at a lower frequency, but change is inevitable as new technology, demand shocks, competition, and regulatory change call for an evolution or reinvention of their business models.

In this Chapter, I present the business model concept from the perspective of Silicon Valley, where it has been developed and used most extensively. Some authors define the business model concept even more broadly,[2] which I think reduces its utility. My view of business models focuses on the way the business *creates* value and *extracts* revenues and profits, which is defined by three core elements: a *value-creation model*, a *profit model*, and the *logic* of the business. Each of these elements is specified by answering a few basic questions, which together define the architecture of the business model.

A. *Value-creation model:*
   1. Who are your customers, and what is your product or service offering?
   2. How does the offering create differentiated value for these customers (value proposition)?
   3. What is the value chain for the offering, and what parts of the value chain does your business participate in?
   4. What are your go-to-market and market development strategies?

B. *Profit model:*
   1. What are your sources of revenue?
   2. What is your cost structure?
   3. What is your unit economics?
   4. What are your key drivers of profitability?

C. *Logic:*
   1. What is your business goal?
   2. Why (and how) will your business meet this goal?

There are a few additional subcomponents under this architectural framework. I describe the key elements of the business model architecture below.

The Value-Creation Model

GENERAL CONSIDERATIONS

The first step in business model analysis is the identification of the target customers (as well as other stakeholders) and the offering that will create differentiated value for them. Differentiation is important to attract customers and make a profit; the offering has to be better than the competition on some distinct dimensions. The dimensions of differentiation vary across companies. In the retail industry, Walmart creates differentiated value for price-sensitive consumers by selling a large variety of products at low prices. In the computer and consumer electronics industry, Apple creates differentiated value for consumers who are willing to pay for well-designed, "cool," innovative products. In financial services, the United Services Automobile Association (USAA) provides US military personnel and their families a host of financial services at superior quality by targeting their specific needs; for example, it was the first to accept check deposits from soldiers' smartphone cameras—a practice that was later adopted by all major banks, and it heavily discounts customers' auto insurance premiums when they are deployed overseas. USAA hires veterans and spouses so its employees truly understand and empathize with its customers.

Although the value-creation model is focused on customer benefits, differentiation necessarily required a comparison to the competition.

The source of differentiated value for a business, sometimes called its *value discipline*,[3] drives not only its business model but also its strategy and culture. A number of value disciplines, which can be found repeatedly across industries, deserve special attention. They include operational excellence, product/service innovation, and customer intimacy.[3,4]

OPERATIONAL EXCELLENCE

Operationally excellent businesses minimize the delivered cost of the products or services they offer to customers. They price their products or services competitively, but they also strive to reduce the intangible costs borne by their customers as the product or service is delivered to them. Thus, operational excellence is not about price alone—consider, for example, FedEx, which attempts to differentiate its offering on timeliness and reliability ("when it absolutely, positively, has to be there overnight").

Walmart's tagline has changed from "Always Low Prices" in the 1960s to "Save Money. Live Better" in more recent years, but its value-creation model remains essentially the same. Customers consistently cite low prices as the key reason for shopping at Walmart. In the United States, more than a quarter of Walmart customers earn less than $25,000 a year (the median is about $50,000),[5] and many of them still do not have a bank account (which creates an opportunity for Walmart to provide financial services to the unbanked). Walmart is positioned at the inbound logistics and retailing end of a standard product value chain (although it designs some "white label" products and sells some services). It sells a large variety of quality merchandise at lower prices than most competitors, and its stores are characterized by high availability and friendly customer service. Walmart illustrates what operational excellence is all about.[6]

As the medical device industry is undergoing consolidation and health care providers are increasingly being evaluated on both the efficiency and the effectiveness of their services, operational excellence is becoming increasingly important.

PRODUCT/SERVICE INNOVATION

Product/service innovators seek to invent and deliver the best products or services for customers, focusing on product performance. Established product/service innovators strive to create continuous, systemic innovation by delivering a stream of state-of-the-art products or services with innovative features that are appealing to their customers.[3]

Many orthopedic device start-ups have their roots in a technological innovation, which is wrapped in a product or service. They often focus on the development and commercialization of a single device. They may then broaden their reach to a wider product family or they may be acquired by established companies with scale, distribution power, and reach. Established life sciences companies put together processes that are aimed at systematically developing new products or services, and they use acquisitions to close gaps in their product pipelines. Financial analysts view these companies essentially as portfolios of products, with their market values being driven by product mix, new product flows (which drive market value up), and patent expirations (driving market value down). Valuation focuses on the prospects of products in the development pipeline, the probability they will be approved, their expected launch times, the size of the potential markets, and the product life cycles.

CUSTOMER INTIMACY

Customer-intimate businesses deliver best total solutions by tailoring their products or services to satisfy unique, or highly targeted, customer needs. Customer intimacy calls for the creation of a continuous learning relationship with customers, which means that the business has to initiate explicit or implicit dialogues with them, capture information about their behaviors and preferences, and use that information to customize products, services, content, and context to increasingly fine definitions of segments, sometimes to the point of 1:1.

First consider a traditional industrial company—Snap-on, headquartered in Kenosha, Wisconsin, which is the largest seller of premium tools to auto repair mechanics in the world. Snap-on is a Business-to-Business (B2B) provider within the auto repair value chain. Founded in 1920, the company started selling sockets that "snapped-on" to interchangeable handles, which enabled the mechanic to customize the tool to the job at hand. The company's sales force (made up of experienced auto mechanics) sells its tools by bringing them directly to customers at their workshops and demonstrating the product benefits on-site. In the 1930s, Snap-on capitalized on its customer knowledge by extending credit to selected customers. Starting in the 1950s, the company went a step further: once a week, a fully stocked walk-in Snap-on van comes to the workshop to help mechanics with products they bought previously, teach them new tricks, and showcase the benefits of new product offerings right at their repair shops. As cars became increasingly complex, Snap-on added diagnostics products, electronic parts catalogs, and systems to manage auto repair shops. Snap-on became a total solutions provider to repair shops, selling tools, systems, technology, and training support. It then expanded its scope to other complex industrial businesses requiring close support.

As discussed below, the processes that led Snap-on's evolution from a pure product innovator to one whose value proposition starts from customer intimacy are similar to those at play in the medical device industry.

CHOOSING A VALUE-CREATION MODEL

The selection of a value-creation model is a key decision that shapes organizational architecture, business processes, and technology directions. *Operational excellence* implies an emphasis on supporting the firm's operations and improving the delivery of products or services on dimensions of cost, reliability, timeliness, etc. It calls for systems and processes that increase efficiency, reliability, and speed, streamline operations, and reduce inventory throughout the value chain. *Product/service innovation* hinges on time-to-market and development speed, requiring systems and processes that speed up information flows both inside the organization and across organizational boundaries.[7] *Customer intimacy* calls for a customer-centric view of the business, which in turn emphasizes the collection, management, and use of customer data across channels, functions, and products or services.

Can a business support multiple value-creation models or value disciplines? Some researchers argue that businesses can only win by focusing on a single value discipline and by shaping their organization to excel in its execution.[3] This is true for almost all start-ups but is less commonly the case for large, established companies. I think it is useful to embark on an effort to identify a *primary* value-creation model and value discipline for a large company, but in reality, the benefits of focus should be traded off against customer requirements. Today's dynamic marketplace often raises the bar to the point where more than a single value discipline is both required (due to competitive pressures or customer demand) and achievable (e.g., thanks to new technology). Indeed, most large organizations will end up mixing multiple value disciplines. However, a company will find it difficult to focus on *improving* its performance on more than a single value discipline at a time. So, a company may well have to excel on multiple dimensions to achieve competitive differentiation, but its capacity for change is usually limited to improving a single one at a time.[8]

DIFFERENTIATION AND INNOVATION

The firm's primary value-creation model should be tied to its leading source of differentiation in the marketplace. It is well-established that differentiation (either on the value side or on the cost side) is key to profitability: if a company produces the same product or service as its competitors at the same cost, its profits will deteriorate. And, differentiation will inevitably be eroded over time because of emulation and patent expirations. Innovation enables a company to stay ahead as competitors try to narrow down or eliminate its advantage, allowing it to both create and capture incremental value.

Thus, leaders in a product market can sustain their market advantage through continuous product innovation. Consider Apple, for example: by the time its competitors catch up with its past innovations, Apple comes up with new and improved ones.[9] *Process innovation* may be equally important. Operationally excellent companies such as FedEx and Walmart illustrate how a cost advantage can result from a series of innovations, which lead to the implementation of business processes that create competitive advantage.[6] Similarly, customer intimacy can be achieved by implementing systems and processes that enable the company to build and enhance an interactive learning relationship with its customers. Hence, innovation is not limited to products, and it plays a central role under all value-creation models.

Another form of innovation is *business model innovation*. Start-ups go through an iterative process of business model discovery. They formulate a tentative business model, test it in the marketplace, and change or replace it based on what they learn. As a result, business model innovation is part of what start-ups are all about. Established companies have more stable business models, which may be used as high-level playbooks, but as these companies and their environments change, their business models may change as well. Evolving customer tastes, adoption life cycles, regulation, new technologies, or competitive dynamics ultimately lead to business model innovation, which often starts with a new value-creation model. This form of innovation can be traumatic (and sometimes fatal), as the company's organization, structure, and processes are reinvented along with its value-creation model. And yet, companies that managed to make the transition are among the leaders of the 21st century.

An important form of business model innovation that is emerging in other industries and will become increasingly important in orthopedic innovation is the transition from products to services. As devices collect increasing amounts of information and are connected over the "cloud," some vendors become service providers. The reason is that the data continuously generated through the use of the device are an increasingly important source of value. Initially, the data can simply be used to monitor the device, prevent failures through preventive maintenance, and facilitate replacements, upgrades, and repairs.

The next step is outcome-based revenue models whereby a hospital pays for the productive use of the device rather than for the device itself. "Power by the hour" revenue models whereby airlines pay for the hours of flight enabled by an engine rather than for the engine itself have been common in aviation for years. The next step is to offer a host of services based on the data generated by the engines, moving the value discipline from product leadership to customer intimacy as has been the case for Snap-on.

In health care, a key driver is the shift to outcome-based reimbursements and the increasing focus on accountable health care. The result is a shift to services that use data from multiple sources to increase the effectiveness and reduce the cost of health care, just as had been the case for mechanics and Snap-on. Major vendors such as Johnson & Johnson and GE are already offering such services and are increasingly moving toward outcome-based payment schemes for medical equipment. For example, the Comprehensive Care for Joint Replacement and Surgical Hip and Femur Fracture Treatment models introduced by the Centers for Medicare and Medicaid Services (CMS) induced these vendors to offer information and management services to hospitals as well as forms of gainsharing, which are limited today but are likely to grow in the future. The use of 3-D printing for implants will accelerate this trend as products become increasingly information-based.

VALUE CHAIN

Companies have to choose which parts of the value chain they want to participate in. For example, a company that develops new technology may choose to license its technology to an established player without being involved in either production or distribution. Or, the company may manufacture the product in-house and sell it as a component to a better-known company that embeds it as its own branded product. Another alternative is to manufacture and market the product under the company's own brand name. As we proceed from the first option to the third, the company covers an increasing portion of the value chain for the final product.

The general structure of the value chain for medical devices is shown in Figure 15.1. Large, integrated firms such as J&J, Stryker, and GE typically control most of their value chains from R&D on to customer service, as well as some of the components. The complexity of regulatory approval, which is product-specific, does not directly extend to suppliers, creating an advantage for a firm that benefits from economies of scale and integration along the value chain. In addition, innovative firms often prefer to maintain their intellectual property in-house to protect it, and branding and distribution are characterized by economies of scale. However, innovation often comes from more focused start-ups that enjoy an R&D advantage and are product-focused. Start-ups may then either license their technology or be acquired outright by a large, integrated firm, although some prefer to extend their operations into other parts of the value chain.

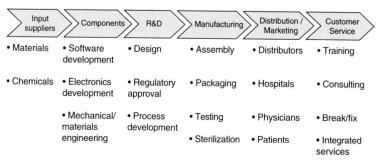

Figure 15.1 Schematic value chain structure for medical devices.

MARKET INITIATION AND DEVELOPMENT

Having a product or service that truly solves a significant problem for a well-defined customer segment is a good start, but it is not enough. "If you build it, they will come" requires an exceptional product—as well as tenacity and superior marketing skills. The adoption of almost any innovation requires an effective go-to-market strategy that focuses on getting the product or service through regulatory approval and on to market.

The go-to-market strategy must be designed in conjunction with the other dimensions of the value-creation model and in particular, the choice of product (or service) and its customers and stakeholders. Throughout the process, product development, marketing, and sales evolve dynamically and interact with one another. This dynamic interaction translates into evolving choices of customers (or customer segments), offerings, and sales channels. A new orthopedic device has to be "sold" to regulators, physicians, and procurement executives, each focusing on different dimensions of the product's value proposition.

In general, a product's sales and distribution channels may be classified into three groups:

- **Direct physician sales,** where the company uses its own sales force or sells the product directly to doctors. Direct sales may take the form of field sales, phone sales, or online sales, with the former being most common.
- **Institutional sales,** where the company has to first persuade physicians of the general efficacy and effectiveness of the product and then go through a procurement officer who focuses on the device's total cost of ownership, effectiveness, adherence to various standards, and management complexity.
- **Indirect channels,** where the company uses independent resellers or sales agents to market and sell the product and collect a commission or markup. These channels may also provide consulting, financing, and other services. To induce them to create additional value for the customer, some form of partnership is often called for.
- **Partnerships,** where a channel relationship is used to gain access to end markets and to provide customers a more attractive or integrated solution. The partner may be an integrated device maker or an integrator who wraps the product with other components to create a more complete, integrated solution. Or, it may be an original equipment manufacturer (OEM) who is looking to sell your product or service along with its own.

The Profit Model

The profit model of a business starts with an identification of its revenue streams and the associated costs. Since revenue = price × quantity and price is a key dimension of the value created for customers, it links the value-creation model to the company's profit model.

REVENUE MODELS

In general, the most common revenue models are:
- **Transactional:** Customers pay a fixed price per unit of the product or service. Transactional revenues often incorporate fixed fees and quantity (as well as other) discounts. For services, prices may be negotiated in advance based on the attributes of the transaction or they may be variable, based on either inputs or outcomes.

As discussed above, transactional revenue models may be outcome-based, where some output or outcome variables are measured and a payment formula is used to calculate a price, or payment is based on the achievement of a measurable outcome, which is relevant to the customer. For example, since 2017, Medtronic signed contracts that require it to reimburse hospitals if its product Tyrx, an antibacterial sleeve, does not protect against infections in patients receiving cardiac-device implants. Medtronic CEO Omar Ishrak explained the motivation for moving to outcome-based revenue models as follows:

Medtronic is focused on technologies to improve outcomes. We use biomedical engineering to alleviate pain, restore health and extend life. Historically we've done that by creating credible evidence that our technologies do change outcomes. But at the end of the day, we and the industry get paid on the technology itself and a promise that those outcomes will actually be changed. We are moving, just like the rest of healthcare, to a value-based model, where we get paid in some fashion for actually achieving the outcome. It's a step we have to take to make sure that the value we create with our technologies is truly realized. And when it gets realized, we will get paid fairly for it... My aspiration would be that all of our revenue gets paid through, or is at least tied in some fashion to, some kind of outcome-based measurement.[10]

As discussed above, this revenue model is tied to the gradual transition from product-based business models to service-based business models, which are often subscription-based.
- **Subscription:** Customers pay a fixed fee per unit of time, and they receive in return a fixed number of units of the product or service (e.g, one issue of a magazine monthly or up to three DVDs out at

Netflix) or unlimited, "all-you-can-eat" use over the subscription period (e.g., a monthly cable TV subscription or membership at a club). For medical devices, the customer may make a fixed payment per unit per month or a payment per hour of use.

Subscriptions are often associated with customer intimacy, as they are naturally based on a relationship between the service provider and the customer. Moreover, the subscription revenue model creates an incentive to invest in customer loyalty and to collect information that will help the business to better serve and retain the customer.

- **Licensing:** Under this revenue model, the customer pays a royalty or license fee, which allows it to use, sell, or copy the product within a given period of time (unlimited in time if the license is perpetual), subject to limits on the scope of use based on geography, nature of use, etc. An orthopedic innovator who is most interested in the invention process and less interested in the commercialization of the technology may license her patent to a commercial medical device vendor, collecting a fixed royalty on each unit sold. Although the royalty is only a small fraction of the final product's price, the vendor will likely sell many more units than the inventor, and the inventor can spend all of her time on her passion: invention.

Businesses often receive multiple revenue streams, where different customers pay according to different formulas or revenue models, or hybrid revenue streams, where a given customer's payments combine different revenue models.

COST STRUCTURE

The cost structure specifies the activities that drive the different costs of the business and how they add up to total cost. Fixed costs are costs that are independent of the level of activitye.g., R&D costs, rent, fixed licensing costs, etc. Variable costs are costs that depend on the level of activity. For example, in a device manufacturing operation, materials costs are proportional to the volume of units produced; delivery costs may depend on both shipping distance and volume; and installation and training costs are driven by the number of buyers. Variable costs may be proportional to volume or they may exhibit economies of scale e.g., purchased materials with a quantity discount. In some cases, they exhibit diseconomies of scale, e.g., when an operation approaches its capacity limit or when key resources are so scarce that their marginal costs are increasing. The breakdown of costs between fixed and variable is an important driver of the business model. Other things being equal, lowering the ratio of variable to fixed costs makes the business more scalable.

Business model analysis focuses on revenue and cost *flows*, whereas some costs are incurred on a one-time basis or infrequently, e.g., the purchase of capital equipment. These costs are typically converted to economically equivalent flows using the firm's cost of capital or by examining, for example, equivalent lease rates for purchased equipment.

UNIT ECONOMICS AND DRIVERS OF PROFITABILITY

Once the revenue and cost structure have been specified, the next step in business model analysis is to break the business into meaningful recurring units and to analyze the associated "unit economics." A "unit" is simply an important driver of scale, which is replicated in the overall business; in the case of medical devices, it is the number of units sold. Once the relevant units have been identified, the analysis proceeds by examining one unit's profitability given the revenue and cost structures. The analysis takes into account the revenues and costs associated with the unit itself without allocating any fixed costs from higher levels. For a medical device business where the unit is one device, the analysis amounts to estimating the gross margin on the sale of one (average) unit (the difference between its sale price and the sum of the purchase price and all other variable costs associated with the unit). Indeed, for many businesses, the gross margin is a key driver of profitability, and a central question is what is the *break-even point*—the volume that would allow the business to recover its fixed-costs given its gross margin.

When the revenues are subscription-based, a natural unit of analysis is a single customer over her subscription period. Consider, for example, a business that is based on monthly subscriptions. Then, we track the cash flows associated with the average subscriber, which may include:
- Customer acquisition costs that lead to the start of a subscription;
- The monthly subscription payment received as revenue;
- The cost of serving the subscriber during the month; and
- Costs incurred to induce customer retention (e.g., special incentives, phone calls, etc.).

An important driver in this case is the *churn rate*the percent of customers who terminate their subscriptions in any given month. With these parameters, the analysis of unit economics will examine the net present value of the cash flows received from the average subscriber, which may then be used to analyze the key drivers of profitability and how they may be improved.

An important by-product of the analysis of unit economics is that it helps to determine the venture's key drivers of profitability. This is obtained either by exercising a spreadsheet model or by examining the structural relationships among the revenue and cost drivers.

Unlike the other business model elements, the unit economics and the drivers of profitability are not choice variables. Rather, they are *derived* from the choices made for the other elements of the business model.

Logic of the Business

The logic of the business comprises two elements. First, what is your business goal? Second, why do you believe you will meet this goal, and how? To set your business goal, you need to first define your planning horizon and then identify your business priorities over that horizon. For example, a social entrepreneur may set as her goal the alleviation of a specific social problem, whereas a for-profit venture may need to prioritize profitability vs. growth. Early-stage ventures typically define directional rather than specific goals as they evolve their business model.

Second, you need to explain why and how your business will meet this goal. The explanation may be quite intricate, elaborating on the business strategy, key processes, resources and capabilities, partnerships, and other factors. The starting point, however, is a single-page argument showing how the business will achieve its goals, e.g., how it will attract customers, be competitive and profitable, and grow. This is often done by depicting a "virtuous cycle" showing how the elements of the business model will reinforce one another.

Concluding Remarks

Would you build a house without putting together a blueprint first? No. A business model is in essence a blueprint for your business. For established businesses, the business model documents the key business choices and provides a platform for change. When innovators develop a new idea to create a new business and bring it to market, the evolving blueprint of the business—its business model—helps them to guide the innovation and commercialization process.

The business model architecture provides an actionable logical structure that defines the basic elements of the economic blueprint for a business. It can help:

- Entrepreneurs to design new ventures and iterate on the choices they make;
- Managers to execute on, as well as rethink and transform, existing businesses;
- Innovators to put together and evaluate new ideas; and
- Investors to make better investment decisions.

The business model architecture comprises three core elements:
- The value-creation model;
- The profit model; and
- The logic of the business.

This architectural framework, however, is only a starting point. It imposes some structure on an inherently unstructured process, where innovation, initiative, and nonlinear thinking are key drivers. It is designed to better align the creative process with customers, markets, and economic realities, increasing the likelihood that great ideas will see the light of day and may even become great businesses.

KEY TAKEAWAY POINTS

- ▶ Business models are the blueprints of the business. Just as you would not build a house without putting together a blueprint first, business model design is a key first step in putting together a new business.

- ▶ A business model comprises three components: a value-creation model, a profit model, and the logic of the business.

- ▶ The process of business model development is iterative and experimental. In each stage, you should develop a tentative business model, identify its key hypotheses, test the model, and iterate until you reach a viable business model.

- ▶ Think of your entire business model as a prototype that requires testing and revisions.

- ▶ There are three major value-creation model archetypes: operational excellence, product leadership, and customer intimacy. Each archetype has its own logic.

- ▶ Orthopedic innovations tend to migrate from product leadership to customer intimacy. Plan for the migration and be aware of the difficulties it may entail.

- ▶ Once your value proposition is clear, focus on your go-to-market strategy.

REFERENCES AND RESOURCES

1. Bayer H. *Great Ideas of Western Man*; 1964.
2. See Zott C, Amit R and Massa L. *The Business Model: Theoretical Roots, Recent Developments, and Future Research*. IESE Working Paper. September 2010.
3. See Treacy M, Wiersema F. *The Discipline of Market Leaders: Choose Your Customers, Narrow Your Focus, Dominate Your Market*. Addison-Wesley; 1995.
4. See Porter ME. *On Competition*. Harvard Business School Press, 2008; Treacy M, Wiersema F. *The Discipline of Market Leaders: Choose Your Customers, Narrow Your Focus, Dominate Your Market*. Addison-Wesley; 1995.

5. Source: Kantar Retail.
6. This Is Described in More Detail in the Case Study *Walmart* by Mendelson H, Graduate School of Business, Stanford University.
7. See, Mendelson H and Ziegler J. *Survival of the Smartest*. Wiley; 1999.
8. A Company's Capacity to Change Depends on its Organizational IQ. See, Mendelson H and Ziegler J. *Survival of the Smartest*. Wiley; 1999.
9. This Is Described in Detail in Three Case Studies by Mendelson H, Graduate School of Business, Stanford University: *Apple and The Music Wars, The iPhone: Apple's Third Act*, and *Apple in 2018*.
10. "*Medtronic Moves to a New Health-Care Model: Pay Only If it Works.*" The Wall Street Journal; February 20, 2018.

CHAPTER 16

Marketing, Sales, and Distribution

NANCY PATTERSON

ABOUT THE AUTHOR

Nancy Patterson, MBA, is a Venture Analyst and the President and CEO of Strategy Inc., www.strategyinc.net, a life science marketing and financial due diligence company founded in 2000. Strategy Inc. provides market and business analysis services for emerging life science technology entities to inform the probability for successful commercialization. Clients include emerging entrepreneurs, enterprise companies, and financiers with technologies in all product lifecycle stages; however, over half of the innovations where clients seek Strategy Inc. insight are preclinical. Global Reach: Nearly 46% of entities seeking Strategy Inc. services over the last 10 years have been international from Europe (especially France, Spain, and Germany), Israel, Asia, and South America.

Marketing, Sales, and Distribution

The orthopedic devices industry will continue to be a promising area in the global medical technology space and is expected to rank third in sales after cardiology and in vitro diagnostics by 2020. According to Frost & Sullivan, the industry generated revenue of $39.40 billion in 2016; revenue is expected to grow at a compound annual growth rate (CAGR) of 3.3% to reach $44.82 billion in 2020.[1]

The emergence of advanced technologies, the rise in orthopedic disorders, and the desire for joint replacement at a younger age along with other changes will drive industry growth. In addition to the promise of revenue and market growth, life science innovation entrepreneurs are driven by the desire to deliver improved clinical outcomes for patients and also for their technology to be acquired for an enviable price, as has been enjoyed historically by many.

The development cycle of an orthopedic innovation requires that management prepare a strategic plan that includes the eventual marketing, sales, and distribution of the innovation. Once an entrepreneur develops an innovative technology and it is validated through clinical studies along with achievement of regulatory approval, the path to marketing and sales is opened. However, significant hurdles still exist to successfully commercialize an innovative life science technology. To introduce a new technology, especially a paradigm-changing technology, steps to successful commercialization include educate the target market about the value proposition, persuade customers to make a purchasing decision, deliver the offering, and lastly ensure that the user and support infrastructure are fully and properly trained on the product use. A review of the top ten US orthopedic companies by revenue highlights recent acquisitions of technology to enhance their product portfolios. Table 16.1 shows the orthopedic clinical areas where each company has product offerings, confirming that most of these larger companies include broad and ever-expanding portfolios.

Successful commercialization of an innovative technology requires a sales, marketing, and distribution organization plan that effectively communicates the value proposition of the offering to the target market. In an effective value proposition, improvement-cost equation compels key decision makers to modify their behavior and adopt the technology (Figure 16.1). Because there are many stakeholders in the orthopedic innovation field who can influence the adoption decision, the effective strategy must be multidimensional and tailored to the needs of each primary stakeholder group. The most innovative technologies deliver breakthrough improvements in the practice of medicine; however, the conservative culture of clinical leadership moves cautiously to adopt change.

The desired for successful commercialization dictates the need for a well-designed marketing, sales, and distribution plan and effective collaboration between the two departments to communicate the value of the innovation. The sales and marketing activities included are shared between departments and often fluctuate during the sales process; however, the tasks listed below outline the different activities required.

MARKETING: BUILDING EXPONENTIAL LEADS

A **Marketing plan** is the organizational framework, built on the foundation of sound market research, that strategically identifies, defines, and quantifies marketing objectives to achieve financial goals and maximize profit potential. The plan describes target markets, outlines marketing strategies and the operational steps to execute, and includes the required cost of goods for the product to be competitive and the budget needed to allocate usually scarce corporate resources, both human and fiscal. The marketing plan is one component of the overall business plan required to secure investment funds to develop the technology. This clearly outlined strategy becomes

Table 16.1 Top 10 Orthopedic Companies by Annual Revenue 2018/2017

Company	Revenue (2017, 2018)	Orthopedic/Spine Product Categories	Example Companies Acquired Over Time
1	Stryker (SYK) www.stryker.com, founded 1941, HQ: Kalamazoo, Michigan, 33,000 employees Sales in 100 countries, 38 y of growth	2017—$12.4B, net earnings $1.02B 38% Orthopedics 6% Spine 9.9% Sales growth 27% from acquisition Net earnings ↓38.1% due to US tax reform	Craniomaxillofacial Sports Medicine Foot and Ankle Joint Replacement Trauma Extremities Spine	K2M $1.4B, August 2018 HyperBranch—Adherus Dural Sealant $220M, October 2018, Mako Novadaq fluorescence imaging $701M, June 2017 Physio-Control, February 2015, $1.28B
2	DePuy Synthes www.depuysynthes.com, a Johnson & Johnson company, acquired 1998, founded 1895, 18,200 employees Comprehensive portfolio of orthopedic and neuro products and services	2018—$9.3B 38.1% Joint reconstruction 17.6% Knee 16.1% Hip 4.4% Extremities 28.3% Trauma 8.1% Arthroscopy 17.0% Spine 4.6% Orthobiologics	Knee Trauma Hip Shoulder Craniomaxillofacial Sports Medicine Spine	Emerging Implant Technologies, $ undisclosed, September 2018, 3-D-printed spinal implant maker

Continued

Table 16.1 Top 10 Orthopedic Companies by Annual Revenue 2018/2017—Cont'd

	Company	Revenue (2017, 2018)	Orthopedic/Spine Product Categories	Example Companies Acquired Over Time
3	Zimmer Biomet www.zimmerbiomet.com, founded 1927, 18,200 employees Operations in >25 countries Sales in >100 countries	2018—$7.8B Net income $1.75B 35.0% Knees 24.0% Hips 21.8% SET (Surgical, Sports Medicine, Foot and Ankle, Extremities and Trauma) 9.7% Spine and craniomaxillofacial (CMF)	Knee Hip Sports Medicine Biologics Foot and Ankle Trauma Extremities Craniomaxillofacial Spine	Medtech SAS $132M, July 2016, robotic assistance LDR Holding Corporation, $1B June 2016, cervical disk Cayenne Medical, June 2016, Compression Therapy Concepts
4	Smith & Nephew www.smith-nephew.com, founded 1856, 16,000 employees Sales in >100 countries, United States represents 48% of global revenue	2018—$4.8 20.7% Knees 12.6% Hips 10.4% Trauma and extremities 13.2% Sports Medicine Joint Repair 12.9% Arthroscopic Enabling Tech	Knee Hip Trauma Extremities Sports Medicine	Rotation Medical $210M, October 2017, tissue regeneration for rotator cuff repair Blue Belt Technologies, $275M, January 2016, Navio system (robot-assisted surgery) Arthrocare, $1.7B, February 2014, sports medicine
5	Medtronic (Spine Div) www.medtronic.com, 86,000 total employees, founded 1949, operates from >370 locations in ~160 countries, >46,00 patents, United States represents 53% of global revenue	2018—$2.7B 8.9% Spine	Spine (under restorative therapies group)	Mazor Robotics $1.6B, September 2018, Covidien, $42B, January 2015, Responsive Orthopedics, $ undisclosed, June 2016, low-cost hip and knee replacements

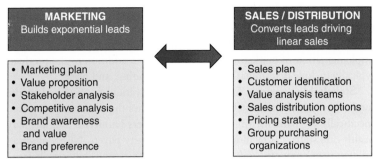

Figure 16.1 Marketing and sales activities for successful commercialization.

a road map followed and continually updated to allow both the marketing and sales organization to pivot in their selling activities as necessary to ensure success. The marketing plan further allows the organization to position the technology in a crowded environment and to highlight the specific benefits of interest to purchasers such as improved outcomes, operative speed, consistency of outcome, reduced cost, ease of use, quality results, and more.

Marketing efforts should be focused on developing demand in defined market segments, such as in selected geographical areas or with certain hospitals or physicians' groups. In developing this demand, the device manufacturer may gain important insight into marketing to broader segments. Once demand is established in the defined areas, it is easier to expand by citing the earlier customer relationships as success stories.

For a new entrepreneur, especially for clinicians who have made the transition from clinical care to business, outlining the scope of activities required can seem overwhelming; however, it is critical to develop this multiyear document and modify as necessary. This activity can be outsourced to a part-time marketing resource before full-time marketing leadership has been added to staffing.

An orthopedic innovation **value proposition** is a clear statement that explains how the innovation solves a current clinical challenge or improves clinical care by delivering specific benefits. The orthopedic innovation value proposition should include the improvement threshold that any new solution would have to meet to cause key stakeholders to change their behavior and adopt. A device must provide value for the user, the payer, and the provider. However, the idea of value is not simply limited to cost versus utility. Value is created when the care pathway is easier and more intuitive to execute. When done effectively, a company can capitalize on the total value a technology provides to all its stakeholders. For example, Stryker (Mako) value proposition claims that its robotic-arm–assisted technology—used in partial knee, total hip, and total knee procedures—has reduced overall readmission costs by 66%. Once defined, the value proposition drives the implementation of marketing activities, which in addition to the product, typically include determination of price, positioning, and place.

Stakeholder analysis for orthopedic innovation, as discussed in the market analysis chapter, includes the four entities that influence adoption, specifically (1) patients, (2) health care providers (clinicians and ancillary health care staff), (3) facilities, and (4) third-party payers. Needs of stakeholders may compete, and it is the innovator's responsibility to balance requirements. Each party's anticipated willingness to pay for innovation is affected by peer-reviewed clinical outcomes, value analysis data, price of current technology solution including bundling with other products, competitive dynamics, procedure volumes, sales channel purchasing relationships, acquisition sales cycle, and more.

Competitive analysis (also covered in Chapter 4), is a comprehensive competitive landscape analysis to ensure that an entrepreneur can accurately benchmark their technology against other solutions available to the target market. Competitive analysis is not just market research, but an objective market assessment including both direct and indirect competitors currently available and, as discernible, innovation in development at competitive companies, universities, think tanks, or technology accelerators. As development decisions are prioritized, it is critical to lead market preferences and trends by understanding emerging engineering solutions, including, for example, in orthopedic innovation, sensor technology, that should be included in product development. To be effective, the process must be dynamic not static, as new market entrants and enhancements of existing products to address market needs are continually emerging.

Orthopedic products include a strong movement toward smart implants with embedded sensors that measure loads, joint stability, temperature, motion, enzymes, bacteria levels, pH, particulate matter, and more to detect early clinical adverse events and proactively treat. Most of this innovation is coming from small, risk-taking start-ups, rather than the top 10 orthopedic companies such as Stryker, DePuy Synthes, Zimmer Biomet, Smith & Nephew, etc. An example is innovation that can deliver information during surgery such as positioning of the hip during surgery, the Intellijoint HIP.[2]

Sensors in orthopedic innovation can measure bone ingrowth measurements or spinal fusion to detect loosening based on the use of magnetic sensor oscillators. Current technology to monitor fusion and provide a fusion status is shown in Intellirod Spine's LOADPRO. Future innovation may be able to both diagnose and treat the patient without surgical intervention by delivering drug therapies such as antibiotics or growth factors or stimulation locally remaining dormant until activated.

Understanding innovation is critical to ensure that the product being developed moving toward product sales will be perceived as leading-edge technology.

Brand awareness and brand value is important to ensure that stakeholders are aware of the value proposition that your innovation offers creating a level of customer demand. Methods to increase brand awareness include traditional avenues such as journal advertising and brochures, results of clinical trials presented by key opinion leaders at peer-reviewed forums that have been enhanced with the shift to social media, online presence through web-based partnerships with orthopedic societies, trade shows, Facebook, Twitter and You Tube testimonials of product performance, and more. Professional societies can be especially valuable advocates for new technologies that address both patient and clinician concerns with specific diseases.

For a comprehensive understanding of the current landscape against which to position a developing technology, attendance at one of the nearly one hundred orthopedic trade shows on a local, regional, national, or international level is recommended. As a health care professional, this forum provides the opportunity to directly view competitive products, and as a clinician/target customer, secure information not available to marketing and sales professionals. It is important to remember that **exhibition** at these meetings is not only undesirable early in development cycle, in some instances is strictly prohibited by regulatory agencies. In addition, no matter how proud you are of your development accomplishments, revealing your innovation strategy is not recommended, as larger organizations with increased resources may attempt to circumvent your patent protection and initiate parallel development, reducing your market advantages.

Attendance as a participant at these meeting will rapidly advance expanded understanding of the landscape. It is also a desirable and cost-effective method to meet with potential key opinion leaders, who will be eager to understand emerging market entrants and may be interested in becoming advisors to your development. Seek the assistance of market research organizations to identify possible formats to organize such cost-effective meetings.

A list of >20 US-based orthopedic trade shows by month is shown below, with two of the larger European meetings included (Figure 16.2). A link to each website and separately the page of each respective annual meeting is available in the electronic version of this book, included with book purchase. Note that the participation can range from a smaller meeting with 500 to 1,000 attendees, to the largest meeting, the American Academy of Orthopedic Surgeons (AAOS) with 28,000 attendees. A smaller meeting can provide a more intimate venue for dialogue, possibly reduce registration and travel costs, where a larger meeting can deliver the full scope

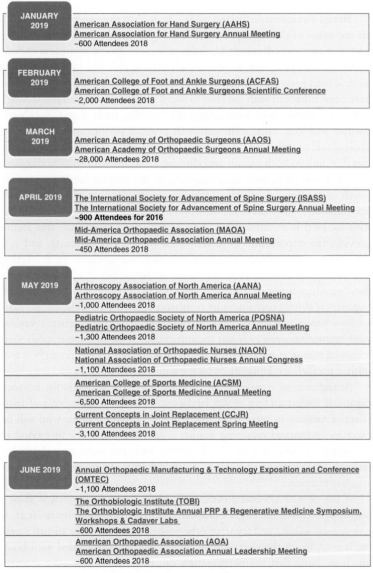

Figure 16.2 Orthopedic Trade Shows by Month.

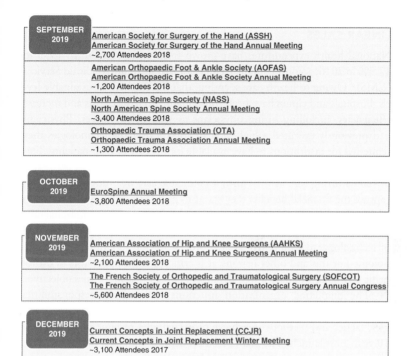

Figure 16.2 Cont'd

of competitive technology and afford the opportunity to meet with an increased scope of key opinion leaders, often presenting at the trade show, and may be available to set up a private meeting with minimal costs.

Costs to attend these meetings are not inconsequential with registration, travel, and the lost opportunity costs of reduced surgical time. However, attendance at one or more of these events early in the developmental process will provide incremental insight into the competitive landscape, provide an opportunity to develop contacts that can be leveraged, and also possibly redirect a product development decision to align with lead industry trends.

Brand preference requires market research of your target market on an iterative basis, through individual surveys, in-person meetings with key customers and purchasing functions, and targeted, metric-based market research that clarifies buying decisions. It is important not only to include the decision makers in the research but also the influencers, such as orthopedic nurses, imaging technicians, value analysis committee leadership members, purchasing department, and of course hospital administrators, all of whom are included in the purchase decisions.

SALES/DISTRIBUTION: CONVERTING LEADS DRIVING LINEAR SALES

National health expenditures have grown from 6.9% of GDP in 1970 to 17.9% in 2016, according to the Centers for Medicare and Medicaid Services (CMS).[3] Owing to health care spending that has reached unsustainable levels, hospitals and clinics have been consolidating to reduce costs and increase efficiencies, including hiring physicians as salaried employees. Physicians had previously executed a high level of control over the technologies they requested for institutions to have available for the care of their patients. This process has changed through health care institutions taking a more active role in standardizing care as they form accountable care institutions (ACOs) to capture the financial benefits they stand to gain from Medicare in the form of shared savings. Such changes have caused modifications in traditional sales models, where physicians preferences were nearly the only hurdle for the sale of technology, to a more regimented process for the adoption of new technology. For this and other reasons, it is critical for the innovators of orthopedic technology to have a well-defined sales plan to achieve sales objectives.

The marketing organization functions outlined the responsibilities required to generate the leads for sales. **A Sales plan** is the specific strategies, tactics and methods to achieve projected sales revenue objectives 5 to 10 years post launch. The plan, based on defined sales targets, outlines sales tactics anticipated to secure market share, describes measurement metrics to determine performance, and includes a budget for estimated expenses. Innovators seeking investments are strongly motivated to structure the sales model that will deliver the maximum revenue, as projected sales volumes ultimately drive investments and eventually a higher exit acquisition price.

Valuation

Integral to investment strategy is determination of a technology's value. A defensible financial valuation steeped in sound assumptions is critical to resonate credibility with potential investors. Traditional financial valuation methods are inadequate for development stage life science technologies. The challenge is to deliver a justifiable financial valuation for an emerging medical technology that may be preclinical, and where comparables may not enjoy the value proposition of the emerging innovation. This effort requires a team experienced with the nuances of Medtech, able to accurately capture the value. An accurate and defensible company valuation is critical to secure the highest level of potential investments. This requires quantification of the value proposition through market projections, company comparables when possible, the range of potential exit values, and probability of achieving a successful exit.

The sales plan includes the outline of the number and types of sales representatives that are required to achieve sales targets based on the anticipated sales cycle. More complex products, such as robotic guidance systems, high-definition arthroscope/videoarthroscopes, with costs well above $5,000 to $10,000 capital equipment threshold, require a longer sales cycle and direct sales representatives to support the sales process, as do higher cost joint surgery and spinal implants. Other smaller hand-held orthopedic instrumentation such as that used for arthroscopic procedures may be able to be sold through alternative sales channels.

Sales leadership is responsible for determining the customer identification through customer relationships of seasoned sales representatives. In addition, there are databases to support standardized selling processes to orthopedic and health care facility leadership. Journal clubs and membership societies are also sources of potential leads. Web-based social media such as Facebook, Twitter, and LinkedIn are all current outreach media for conveying positioning and product messaging.

Bundled Pricing

Sales strategy to drive sales volume by grouping similar or complimentary products or services together at reduced prices than they would command individually. Bundled pricing benefits the seller as it affords the simplicity of a single-priced bundled product, which reduces the costs for marketing and sales as a unit. In addition, bundling affords the opportunity to capture market share in an allied product category that may be currently serviced by a competitive product. Bundled pricing has a tendency to decrease transparency of single-line itemized pricing, which can provide sales organizations the ability to increase pricing on specific products for internal accounting and initiate price balancing for ones where there is greater margin. Bundled pricing aligns with the shift to bundled payments initiated by the Affordable Care Act. Under a bundled payment model, providers and/or health care facilities are paid a single payment for all the services performed to treat a patient undergoing a specific episode of care. An "episode of care" is the care delivery process for a certain condition or care delivered within a defined period of time.

Differential Pricing

A strategy of selling the same product or service to different customers at different prices, based on factors such as sales agreements, volume commitments, delivery requirements, customer segments, and other market segmentation. A differential pricing strategy allows a company to adjust pricing based on various situations or circumstances. The United States requires reduced pricing for military and veteran's health care facilities; however, in an era of cost containment, most all institutions align themselves for price reductions.

Gainsharing

A new business management strategy is being adopted by some health care facilities to increase profitability by motivating health care staff to reduce cost of care through inclusion in financial profit-sharing incentives. This process is aligned with the cost of life science technology, because higher physician preference items can significantly impact profitability; however, the organization's actual performance is compared to baseline performance (often a historical standard) to determine the amount of the gain. Because gains are measured in relationship to a historical baseline, employees and the organization must change in order to generate a gain.

Sales Distribution Channels

For innovation that is targeted primarily at physicians and facilities, one of the critical questions is determining the best sales strategy. There are a number of options for distribution of an orthopedic innovation to choose from or potentially the option of a hybrid model, which is becoming a market trend in selling orthopedic products. The different options listed are explained in expanded detail below: (1) direct sales force, (2) independent sales representatives (also called distributors or manufacturers' representatives), (3) stocking distributor who purchases the products for a reduced price, stocks the product, and then resells, and (4) partnering with a well-established company with an aligned and proven sales force.

For a product with a long technical sales process, a direct sales force is often the best selection. After preparing a well thought out job description, hiring a **direct sales force** can be accomplished in several ways. The company can select to source their own sales representatives using a range of outreach methods such as posting the position on online job search websites, job posting on the company website, outreach during trade shows, using a rep-matching service or database, take advantage of LinkedIn, or, although expensive, ($10,000 − $20,000 + in addition to fees per hire) recruit through an executive search service. These processes can take up to 6 months to identify an aligned direct sales force of any size; however, the resulting team is 100% focused on the company's sales mission. Such an undertaking is expensive and thus resources must be allocated accordingly.

An alternate option is to use **independent sales representatives** (also called a distributor or manufacturer's sales representatives) as a key part of the sales strategy. Independent representatives (distributors) are independent contractors who have existing relationships with target clinicians and usually the purchasing organizations of key institutions. They are paid on a commission basis to sell product lines in a specific region. Independent reps serve as a company's field sales and customer service. These independent reps usually have their own companies or work for a rep firm that employs a group of salespeople. They work as independent contractors on commission only (generally resulting in higher commissions on each sale, which can be up to 10% of the sale) and may represent other brands, but hiring an independent rep requires minimal/no up-front risk. Independent sales representatives usually sell several related, noncompetitive products for a well-defined territory and possess the depth of the existing networks and relationships, which can expedite the achievement of sales objectives and can also open up new business opportunities in existing markets.

Management of an independent sales organization relies on an internal company-based sales management team to ensure these independent representatives are well trained and will allocate sufficient time and effort to convert leads to sales. Table 16.2 includes examples of companies that provide independent sales representatives that are included below with a link to their respective websites incorporated in the electronic version of the book that is provided with book purchase.

Stocking Distributor

A supply chain entity that purchases life science technology at a significant discount (often 25%-30%) warehouses the products and then resells the products to health care facilities and providers, often within a defined territory or region. Stocking distributors are generally different from independent representatives, as they actually purchase the inventory. Stocking distributors commit to specific minimum orders, which allow a medical device company to project revenue. The representative from a distributor needs to have high-level training and manufacturers technical support available to ensure that committed sales levels will be achieved. Table 16.3 shows a list of orthopedic device distributors, outlined by the regions they serve, with the links to their websites active in the electronic version of this book included with book purchase.

Table 16.2 Independent Sales Representative Companies and Membership Organizations
Independent Sales Representative Companies
• RepHunter   • MedCepts   • RepRight   • Global Edge Recruiting   • Manufacturers' Agents National Association   • Sales and Marketing Network
Medical Sales Representative Membership Organizations
Health Industry Representative Association: An online directory that is one of the most-used sources by manufacturers seeking independent sales representatives. All sales representative agencies and manufacturers agencies who are a member are listed in the directory.
Independent Medical Specialty Dealers Association: IMDA members are a premier provider of Specialty Medical Sales, Service, and Education. IMDA's dealer members are typically dealers that have relationships with the key opinion leaders in their regional coverage area.

Partnering With a Well-Established Company

To provide a measure of security, manufacturers regularly enter into distribution and marketing arrangements with large, well-established companies, with an aligned and proven sales force. Such manufacturers prefer to concentrate on their core strengths such as product conception, research and development, and production. They select to outsource the sales process to proven professionals, with appropriate distribution networks in place, to sell their products. Although device manufacturers will earn less by entering into these arrangements compared with distributing their products themselves, in certain situations is maybe advantageous to guarantee distribution with a proven entity versus risk failure, attempting to execute in an area that is unknown on one's specialty. Such agreements can be structured to cover some regional markets or customer categories and not others. The partnering company may also be a target entity to purchase the technology.

PRICING STRATEGIES

Setting the price for an emerging orthopedic technology is based on a number of factors including the perceived value of the technology, pricing of comparable technologies, and what the market will support. Value-based pricing is the method that is the most effective to support. When the price of new innovation can be directly linked to the value of the improvements

Table 16.3 Orthopedic Device Distributors

	Company Headquarters	Areas Served	Product Market Segments
1.	American Medical Concepts (AMC) Wilsonville, OR	OR, WA	Joint Reconstruction, Spine, Trauma
2.	Biosystems Waltham, MA	ME, VT, NH, RI, MA, NY	Spine, Orthobiologics, Orthopedic Braces
3.	Cal Med Orthopedics, Inc. Lake Forest, CA	CA	Joint Reconstruction, Orthobiologics, Soft Tissue/ Arthroscopic
4.	Chesapeake Surgical Laurel, MD	MD, DE, DC, VA	Joint Reconstruction, Orthobiologics, Soft Tissue/ Arthroscopic
5.	Medinc of Texas Houston, TX	TX	Joint Reconstruction, Trauma, Orthobiologics, Soft Tissue/Arthroscopic
6.	CrossLink Orthopaedics Norcross, GA	FL, GA, NC	Joint Reconstruction, Spine, Trauma, Orthobiologics
7.	Innotek Medical Products, Inc. Oak Brook, IL	IL, IN, OH, WI	Spine, Trauma, Orthobiologics
8.	RSW Medical Dunes, SD	ND, SD, NE, IA, MT	Joint Reconstruction, Trauma, Orthobiologics, Soft Tissue/Arthroscopic
9.	Source Surgical, Inc. San Francisco, CA	CA, NV	Spine, Trauma, Orthobiologics
10.	SouthTech Orthopedics, Inc. Raleigh, NC	NC	Joint Reconstruction, Trauma, Orthobiologics, Soft Tissue/Arthroscopic

Continued

Table 16.3 Orthopedic Device Distributors—Cont'd

	Company Headquarters	Areas Served	Product Market Segments
11.	Spartan Medical Silver Spring, MD	ALL US	Spine, Trauma, Orthobiologics, Orthopedic Braces
12.	Supreme Orthopedic Systems Marriottsville, MD	MD, VA, DC, DE	Joint Reconstruction, Trauma, Orthobiologics, Soft Tissue/Arthroscopic
13.	Surgi-Care Inc. Waltham, MA	NH, VT, RI, ME, MA, CT	Joint Reconstruction, Orthobiologics, Soft Tissue/Arthroscopic, Orthopedic Braces
14.	Synergy Medical Systems (an AMC company) Eugene, OR	OR, WA, AK, CA, NV, ID	Orthopedic Braces, Orthopedic Prosthetics
15.	Three Rivers Orthopaedic & Spine Products, Inc. Latrobe, PA	PA, OH, WV	Joint Reconstruction, Spine, Trauma, Orthobiologics
16.	West Coast Medical Resources, LLC (WestCMR) Clearwater, FL	ALL US	Joint Reconstruction, Spine, Trauma, Orthobiologics, Soft Tissue/Arthroscopic

it will deliver, purchasers and payers have a higher probability to support adoption. With documentation to confirm the value delivered by the technology, this will support both value analysis scrutiny and the most expedited adoption. When it is possible to document improved clinical outcomes and a payer or provider can save money on follow-up care with the use of a technology, these provide a compelling argument for adoption.

Although development costs cannot be the driving force behind pricing strategies, there is value in reviewing development costs of innovation. The report "FDA Impact on U.S. Medical Technology Innovation,"[4] includes the results of more than 200 medical technology companies who were surveyed about the US medical device regulatory process. The Stanford University report states that average cost to bring a low-to-moderate complexity product from concept to market is $31 million with more than 77% of that, $24 million, spent on Food and Drug Administration (FDA)-dependent or related activities. High-risk more complex products, that follow a PMA regulatory path, costs averaged $94 million, with $75 million spent on FDA-linked stages, nearly 80% of the total cost of bringing devices to market. The survey was sponsored by the Medical Device Manufacturers Assn., the National Venture Capital Assn., and "multiple state medical industry organizations."

Group Purchasing Organizations (GPOs) aggregate the purchasing volume of health care providers such as hospitals, surgery centers, and clinics and home health agencies to realize savings by negotiating discounts from manufacturers, distributors, and other vendors. The largest GPO, Vizient, founded in 2015, is a member-driven alliance of not-for-profit hospitals, academic medical centers, ambulatory care facilities, physician practices, nursing homes, and home health agencies. Vizient members work with their GPOs to save more than $1.8 billion annually on required supplies and services to deliver patient care. A 2010 study from the US Government Accountability Office found that an estimated 98% of America's 5,000+ hospitals use GPOs voluntarily to purchase approximately 73% of hospital purchases where the institutions claim between 10% and 15% savings through participation.

Device manufacturers preparing to move into sales should stay in contact with GPOs and apply periodically for inclusion within their networks. Manufacturers should track competitive products that are included and respectfully convey the advantages of their product line to the key decision makers of the GPOs. Often, a buying group considering a contract with one medical device manufacturer will entertain competitive products that are presented in a timely manner. With persistence, a device manufacturer may, over time, gain access to these large-scale networks.

If a manufacturer is losing out on buying-group relationships because its product line is not yet diverse enough, it should consider teaming up with other manufacturers selling complementary (noncompetitive) products that fill out the line. Together, manufacturers with this kind of relationship can often present a compelling package to organized buying groups.[5,6]

Orthopedic Group Purchasing Organizations Plus

ExperTech Surgical is a new category of orthopedic services that is a GPO plus service. ExperTech provides case support and technicians for any manufacturer's orthopedic implant requested by the hospital or surgeons. This combination of product acquisition and a lower case management service cost can reduce the overall implant costs (~10%-25%), reduce the number of staff in the operating room, and provide a single contact point for hospital and surgeon staff regardless of the manufacturer. ExperTech manages all case logistics, including ordering instruments and implants. They are agnostic to the manufacturer and simply obtain the desired products. They assist operating room staff by confirming all needed instruments are pulled, sterilized, and properly assembled. As they are technically trained and certified by each manufacturer, technicians assist the surgeon and hospital staff as requested to answer questions regarding the use of available technology during a case. Currently their footprint is the Eastern Seaboard; however, with the high level of interest, they are expanding nationwide for certain markets. They manage the documentation, tracking and security of products, all while reducing overall costs by as much as 10% to 25%.

VALUE ANALYSIS TEAMS

In recent years, health care facilities and GPOs have added value analysis teams to the purchasing process to compare the features and cost-effectiveness of any new product being considered for inclusion. Members of these diverse, professional, and experienced teams execute a rigorous analysis as a component of the purchasing cycle and have gained influence in purchasing decisions. Understanding that a health care facility value analysis team will audit an innovation as a component of the technology assessment process and as a hurdle to adoption confirms the importance of competitive analysis in the product development market analysis process. In addition, it is important for the sales and marketing staff to prepare value analysis support materials addressing the anticipated questions to assist with the value analysis review. Such information should include at least: (1) indications for use, (2) mechanism for use, (3) clinical trial data, (4) validation of regulatory review, (5) instructions for use, (6) validation of economic value, (7) competitive product comparison, (8) product ordering information, (9) company insurance validation, and (10) references. Value analysis teams include medical/surgical physicians and nurses, purchasing professionals, C-suite involvement, pharmacy, clinical laboratory, facilities, and more to include a representation of all stakeholders. Sales professionals will need to present documentation to address the value analysis process and verify the value of the technology being offered.[7-9]

KEY TAKEAWAY POINTS

- ▶ Steps to successful commercialization include educate the target market about the value proposition, persuade customers to make a purchasing decision, deliver the offering, and lastly ensure that the user and support infrastructure are fully and properly trained on the product use.

- ▶ The top 10 orthopedic companies acquire innovative orthopedic technology every year to enhance and expand their product offerings.

- ▶ There is the need for a well-designed marketing, sales, and distribution plan to communicate the value of the innovation.

- ▶ Marketing is responsible for building leads; sales is responsible for converting leads into sales.

- ▶ The orthopedic innovation value proposition should include the improvement threshold that any new solution would have to meet to cause key stakeholders to change their behavior and adopt.

- ▶ It is important to select a sales distribution channel that will best support the types of technology and sales strategy.

- ▶ A marketing plan is the organizational framework and strategic road map that identifies, defines, and quantifies marketing objectives to achieve financial goals and maximize profit potential.

- ▶ The marketing plan should be continually updated: market dynamics, competitive landscape and changes in clinical care change the environment where the product is positioned.

- ▶ Need to ensure that the value analysis materials that include product features, cost-effectiveness, clinical validation, and competitive product comparisons are prepared to support acceptance of any new product being considered by the Value Analysis Teams.

REFERENCES AND RESOURCES

1. *Alliance of Advanced BioMedical Engineering*. Frost and Sullivan; 2017. https://aabme.asme.org/posts/innovations-in-orthopedic-devices-and-procedure-improvement-solutions-to-transform-the-industry.

2. Buford T. Disruptive Trends in Orthopedics. https://orthostreams.com/wpcontent/uploads/2017/12/7_Disruptive_Trends_in_Orthopedics.pdf.

3. https://www.cms.gov/Research-Statistics-Data-and-Systems/Statistics-Trends-and-Reports/NationalHealthExpendData/NationalHealthAccountsHistorical.html.

4. Makower J. *FDA Impact on U.S. Medical Technology Innovation (A Survey of Over 200 Medtech Companies)*. November, 2010.

5. The Narrowing Distribution Funnel: How to Get Your Medical Device to Market MDDI. Medical Device and Diagnostic Industry. https://www.mddionline.com/narrowing-distribution-funnel-how-get-your-medical-device-market.

6. Group Purchasing Organizations: How GPOs Reduce Healthcare Costs and Why Changing Their Funding Mechanism Would Raise Costs. https://www.ftc.gov/system/files/documents/public_comments/2017/12/00222-142618.pdf.

7. *The New Rules of Clinical Supply Chain Management*. Lumere Enlightened Healthcare; 2016. https://insights.lumere.com/hubfs/Lumere.

8. Gina Thomas RN. *Value Analysis and Utilization Tools: Healthcare Can't Afford to Not Look at Inappropriate Utilization, April 17, 2018*. https://www.lumere.com/blog/value-analysis-utilization-tools-healthcare-cant-afford-not-look-inappropriate-utilization/.

9. Montgomery K, Schneller ES. Hospitals' strategies for orchestrating selection of physician preference items. *Milbank Q.* 2007;85(2):307-335.

CHAPTER 17

Business Operations: What Is Needed for Sustainable Revenues

CHRISTOPHER K. WEST

ABOUT THE AUTHOR

Chris West serves as president of the ZeroTo510 medical device innovation program. Chris is a former executive in the pharmaceutical/biotech industry with over 20 years of experience in sales leadership as well as tactical and strategic marketing on industry-leading brands such as Advair, Valtrex, and Avodart. Chris moved to Memphis as Vice President of Sales (and Company Officer) for the biotech start-up, GTx, Inc. Chris has overall responsibility for the direction of the ZeroTo510 program and recruitment of cohort companies. With demonstrated expertise in launching new products, Chris acts as a business mentor and commercialization advisor for start-up companies with the goal of helping them translate their innovations into commercial products.

Introduction: Scope and Assumptions

A sound regulatory strategy lays out a new product's development plan and associated activities for a start-up company. Although tedious, this road map can offer comfort to the start-up team in knowing that it is on the right path to Food and Drug Administration (FDA) submission, with clear markers of progress and definitions for success.

No such road map exists to teams for the commercialization plan, however, and there are multiple routes to success—and failure. The pressure and anxiety to build a winning commercialization plan can mount as teams move through their development plan and toward FDA submission. Inexperienced Founders know they need to launch their product and get to the elusive "sustainable revenues" but are not sure how or when.

This chapter outlines our preferred launch strategies to reach sustainable revenues. As background, ZeroTo510 is a Medical Device **Accelerator**[1] based in Memphis, TN and is an affiliate of the Memphis Bioworks Foundation.[2] ZeroTo510 has been nationally ranked by the Seed Accelerator

Project in 2014, 2015,[3] 2016,[4] and 2017.[5] ZeroTo510 has accelerated 29 teams through 2018, covering a wide span of inventions and markets, helping early-stage inventors to craft the development plan necessary for FDA clearance (typically a 510(k) pathway) as well as the commercial plan to successfully launch the product into their respective marketplaces.

Many of our inventors are physicians, staff members, engineers, and researchers and have never sold a medical product before joining our program. We commonly hear questions from Founders such as:

- What do I need to do to demonstrate success to potential investors and/or acquirers?
- Should I build a national sales network or focus on a regional plan?
- How can I grow my company without running out of money?

Most importantly, we hear an overarching question of "How do I get my product out as fast as possible to as many customers as possible?"

We believe, based on our experience, that this is usually the wrong approach. Instead we advocate a "make haste, slowly" approach that values repeat sales from customers with low acquisition costs due to proximity to corporate Headquarters and supported by the company's efficient, internally managed operations. The company grows to introduce the product to new customers in high-potential territories in concert with its ability to support them operationally.

The advice in this chapter comes from CEO interviews of several start-ups in the Memphis ecosystem, as well as the experiences from our investment partner, Innova Memphis. Innova is a leading early-stage medical device investor, with capital investments in more than 50 medical device companies to date.[6]

Our bias is that Memphis is not as capital rich as other markets, which has forced a discipline in both the product development and commercialization plans for our start-ups. As a general rule, both of these plans are subject to stage-gate funding, with demonstrated success necessary to merit further investment. To that end, we have written this chapter to the entrepreneur who has boot-strapped his or her way through the development plan and has a limited commercialization budget.

Finally, while we use examples from both within and outside the orthopedic industry, we believe these learnings transcend industry.

"Festina lente" ("make haste, slowly")   CAESAR AUGUSTUS

Our Commercialization Road map

Many entrepreneurs believe that the definition of launch success is for their product to "go viral" and become an overnight success. In our experience, this approach is more likely to lead to a disjointed launch with overtaxed operational efforts, skyrocketing expenses, frustrated customers, and a dispirited sales force.

How does this happen? In an effort to quickly ramp up revenues, companies can push sales activities too fast and too far. Customers are "interested in learning more," so the Headquarters personnel find themselves frequently flying to appointments to answer questions about the product, train staff, and discuss pilot studies necessary to get approval by the institution's **Value Analysis Committee**. Inventories balloon in anticipation of a quick uptake, only to be sacrificed after an early adopter suggests a clever "tweak" to the device to improve its functionality. Pilot studies languish as Headquarters staff are so distracted that they never finalize study protocols or recruit patients. Subsequently the product is never approved by the hospital or facility, and the customers who tried it once go back to their "tried and true" products. The team, exhausted and quickly burning through cash, go back to their venture capital partners to ask for another round of financing.

In our ecosystem, a "winning launch plan" is one that values repeat sales from core customers in a cost-effective manner. We propose a three-step process to achieve these goals:

PRECLEARANCE: PREPARE FOR A LOCAL PILOT

Brian Austin is the former CEO of ExtraOrtho, which was acquired by Zimmer Biomet in 2011.[7] A serial entrepreneur, Austin has since launched several other medical device companies, applying the lessons learned from ExtraOrtho. He believes that this is a critically important period for companies; not only should they be focused on clearance activities but also planning to introduce the product to customers ready to use it, supporting the launch with internal operations, and building a launch cash flow model. His advice:

a. *Identify a local product champion to assist in prototype development and pilot your product.* A local orthopedic surgeon took an interest in ExtraOrtho's lead trauma product. This surgeon invited Austin to frequently observe surgeries during the prototype iteration phase, pointing out deficiencies with competitor products and providing suggestions on the optimal solution. He was also a rapid adopter of the product post clearance and provided critical feedback on a series of small product improvements for maximum benefit to the patient and surgical team once he was able to use the product daily. Austin now counts on three rounds of preclearance product iterations and then one postclearance iteration of small improvements that can only be uncovered through frequent product usage. Austin accordingly keeps a lean launch inventory to minimize waste.

b. *Model anticipated customer onboarding activities and costs.* Gaining physician or surgeon product recommendation is only half the battle—the other half is getting the hospital or facility to approve, and pay for, your product. Ryan Ramkhelawan,[8] another serial start-up founder turned venture development professional, advises teams to model out in great detail what this process looks like and how long it will take. Key questions include:

- Who from the hospital's financial system can approve the product? Is this a Value Committee decision?
- Will a formalized pilot study be required by the facility to evaluate the product? If so, how many patients will be required, what are the end points, and how does the customer define success?
- How does procurement get the product into their system? What will be required to generate a purchase order?
- How much inventory does the hospital keep on hand, and what is the process for getting a product or device out of inventory and into the surgery or procedure as required?
- What staff will need to be trained on the product? Can the sales representative conduct this training or will it be someone from the home office?
- Will the hospital or facility require dedicated customer service capabilities? If so, can the existing home office personnel provide these services or will it require hiring additional staff?

Ramkhelawan's lesson learned: this process will take far longer with your first customer than you think, which obviously impacts how quickly the management team can expect revenues. He advises leaders to spend significant time understanding and documenting this process, which will not only inform the cash flow model for when to expect revenues but also provides a target for improving the time to uptake for the next hospital or customer.

c. *Build as many internal operations processes as possible.* One important way to minimize costs and keep a pulse on customer feedback is by fulfilling as many key functions as possible internally. Examples:

  i. Inventory management system: Austin has manufacturing partners ship parts to his company, and the management team assembles anything that does not require clean room assembly. This allows the team to minimize assembly costs as well as prevent excessive inventory levels on parts and products, particularly during the early launch phase when one final round of iteration may be required.

    ii. Shipping: As soon as a product sale comes through, a team member sends out the replacement product via a standard shipping software platform.

    iii. Billing: Rather than outsourcing all billing to a certified public accountant (CPA), one member of the management team is responsible for billing, and a CPA firm performs a quarterly audit. Not only does this minimize these costs, it also provides the management team with immediate feedback on their cash flow model and comparisons with previous time periods.

d. *Cash is King*! Another revelation for Austin was the importance of the on-hand cash during the launch phase. He advises teams to "keep your powder dry" for as long as possible by understanding your cash flow model and using it to make cost-effective decisions. There are two essential components to this cash flow model:

    i. *Have a deep understanding of the static cash flows to run your business*. Business owners should know their "burn rate" of being in business, regardless of any other activities. These ongoing overhead costs include such things as salaries, rent, patent fees, insurance, systems, etc. This burn rate is usually the largest expenditure for a start-up, and spending decisions should be weighed against this burn rate. Austin described an example where he was able to negotiate better pricing with his vendor on each round of prototype iterations—but would take weeks longer to deliver. He finally realized that the small amount of money he was saving on development costs was outweighed by several weeks of cash burn, while the rest of the company was idle, waiting for the next prototype. Now his largest consideration is how quickly he can get to FDA clearance and cash flow.

    ii. *Model the dynamic cash flows to achieve sales*. Cash outflows will likely increase in the short term after a sales activity:

       1. As described above, there can be a lengthy sales cycle to get a product introduced to a customer and then approved by the hospital or facility. Understanding this time gap is crucial to managing cash flows.

       2. Think through the costs for instrument sets. If your product requires an instrument set to be used in the procedure, you will be required to manufacture a certain number of sets to get started, and these are most likely not reimbursable expenses during the procedure.

       3. Finally, expenses will likely increase in the short term when a sale is made to pay commissions to the sales representative, order additional inventory (if necessary), and ship replacement

product to the sales representative or customer. There may be a 60 to 90 day gap between when the device is used and when the facility remits payment. Entrepreneurs often fail to appreciate the difference in timing between cash outflows on a sale and the resulting cash inflows months later.

POSTCLEARANCE PILOT: FAIL FAST—AND LOCAL

Most CEOs spoke to the need to resist the urge to scale before their product and systems were ready. Instead they recommend a small pilot launch with a local product champion in order to perfect their product and pressure test their internal processes. The local pilot provided the management team the opportunity to work through the onboarding activities necessary to get the product approved and into the hospital or facility and game-plan how to shrink that time for the next customer or hospital.

Finally, a local pilot allows the company to build personal relationships with key stakeholders within the system, which can help the company overcome the inevitable mistakes in a cost-effective manner.

Keys for This Stage

a. *Count on at least one more round of product iteration postclearance.* According to Austin, no matter how robust the product development process is, customers will usually identify improvements through frequent use. These are often minor improvements, such as color-coding pins, providing depth marks on drills and pins, or staff suggestions on improvements to packaging to make it easier to access the product during surgery, but to the end customer, these improvements can make the procedure easier and more efficient. Despite the myriad postclearance activities for his company, Austin made it a priority to observe as many procedures with his new product as possible to validate his product before expanding beyond these local product champions.

Importantly, consult with your regulatory team on any proposed postclearance product changes. Be sure to always adequately follow your design control procedures and assess the impact of these changes. Some small changes to the product may be possible with only a letter to file explaining the changes, while more significant changes may require another submission. Your regulatory team can help you remain FDA compliant.

b. *Minimize inventory.* With the assumption that changes will be made to the launch product, manufacture as few units as possible. This will minimize scrap inventory (and expenses) as well as returns of outdated units from customer inventories. This also minimizes customer confusion and prevents older models from being used in procedures.

c. *Work relentlessly to compress the product onboarding process.* It is critically important to compress the time between a physician stating a desire to use your product and the company being reimbursed. To that end, days matter in the onboarding process, and every effort should be made to master this process. Ramkhelawan spoke to the diligence that the management team of Restore Medical Solutions[9] spent documenting each step of the onboarding process and then making plans to compress the times for the next customers. For example, the team built financial models based upon actual data from early hospital adopters. Subsequently, in lieu of a pilot study for each new hospital, Restore Medical offered pro forma financials along with a promise to track actual results post adoption. Not all customers agreed to this tactic, but for some, it enabled the team to get their product approved (and to revenues) more quickly.

d. *Pressure test internal systems in a cost-effective manner.* Mistakes will likely occur as the management team learns the inventory management system, billing, and shipping. Developing a personal relationship with an understanding local partner can help smooth over any damage from early launch mistakes and can minimize the costs to meet face to face with key stakeholders to resolve issues, rush in product replacements, etc. As an example, Austin remembers driving inventory from his office directly to the hospital and into surgery.

e. *Update cash flow models.* Although static costs may not change during this phase, previous assumptions can be updated on the costs associated with bringing a new customer on-board as well as the lag between sales and revenues. Document any hidden costs, such as:

   i. Expenses associated with training staff members;
   ii. Inventory needed to conduct pilot studies;
   iii. Customer service requirements by the facility; and
   iv. On-hand inventory needed at the facility.

Understanding these expense and revenue assumptions is critical to the next phase: scaling the product regionally.

POSTPILOT: EXPAND REGIONALLY

Once your product has been in the hands of your local champion and staff for weeks without further suggestions for improvement, internal operational systems have been tested and improved, and sufficient inventories have been established, it is time to consider expanding beyond the local market to ramp up revenues. Anxiety can build as teams think through the seemingly limitless customer engagement options, ranging from approaching prestigious academic institutions all the way to selling into small community hospitals that have expressed an interest in your product. All of these options provide opportunities as well as limitations, and a limited budget can punish bad decisions for cash-strapped start-ups.

The key to sustainable revenues in this phase is to invest the company's early sales cycles and resources targeted to a narrowly focused set of high-potential customers. Steven King, CEO of Restore Medical Solutions, advocates a system he calls "strategic planning and precision selling" to direct sales efforts to a select group of high-potential customers meeting a specific target profile. He then implements a "rope limits" policy to further segment customers within driving distance of the Headquarters to make this strategy as cost-effective as possible. King opines that focusing efforts on these high-potential customers gives the sales team the best opportunity to generate initial revenue while validating valuable information with respect to the company's sale cycle, product/market messaging, and pricing. He also understands that the Headquarters team will likely be highly involved, pulling through this sale with presentations to the Value Committee, conducting pilot studies, training staff members, and other onboarding activities. This "strategic planning and precision selling" philosophy within the "rope limits" constraints helps the company to quickly gain revenues from high-potential customers while minimizing expenses. Here is the plan:

a. *Strategic planning*: Plan sales territories with the highest probability of success because of a mixture of disease prevalence, access to key customers, and profitable reimbursement. As an example, PATH EX, Inc.[10] has developed a technology to speed the diagnosis and treatment of **sepsis**, an overwhelming and potentially fatal inflammatory response that develops, following severe infection. Although a patient may potentially develop sepsis in any hospital across the country, previous research from published medical literature indicates that people living in impoverished areas are at an increased risk of developing infections, and high sepsis mortality clusters range from the southeast to mid-Atlantic United States (Figure 17.1).[11]

For a regional expansion, the obvious choice is to place new territories in areas with deep red, signifying strongly clustered cases of sepsis infections. One can assume that in these hard-hit areas customers will be more receptive to learning about and

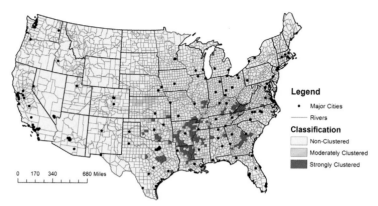

Figure 17.1 Moderately and strongly clustered sepsis mortality groups within different regions of the United States.[11] (Reproduced with permission from Moore JX, Donnelly JP, Griffin R, Howard G, Safford MM, Wang HE. Defining sepsis mortality clusters in the United States. *Crit Care Med.* 2016;44(7):1380-1387.)

possibly adopting a new solution to this problem and also easier for the team to build the financial case for a new product with hospitals' Value Committees.

b. *Initially establish "rope limits" for new territories to minimize customer acquisition costs.* This philosophy, espoused by Steven King of Restore Medical Solutions, was borne from a previous start-up experience, where the company was rapidly burning through cash while desperately attempting to gain traction. The company had sponsored a booth at a national convention and met several potential customers who were "interested in learning more" about their product. In support of that objective, senior management spent the next several months on planes flying around the country to meet with these prospective customers in person. It proved to be a very costly endeavor to qualify, sell, and support the customers on a long-distance basis. In an effort to minimize expenses and focus sales efforts, the company's CEO instituted a "rope limits" policy whereby all customer-selling activities had to meet the following criteria: (1) prospective customer had to be within a 4-hour drive from the home office and (2) had to be a large hospital of a specific size (which matched the customer profile where the company experienced success in early evaluations). Contrary to everyone's expectation, the smaller, drivable territories reduced the cost of the sales cycle, improved the support level for the implementation process, and gave senior management and technical support the opportunity to interact with the customers during the acquisition phase and the customer onboarding phase.

c. *Precision selling with an emphasis on building adopters.* All CEOs spoke to the need for the company to build a solid base of revenues based on repeat sales from loyal customers. CEO Buck Brown of iScreen Vision, Inc.[12] said, "This is the most important metric that we track, and we review our progress on a monthly basis." CEO King opined that during this phase "It's imperative to identify key customers and pull them through to full adoption before you prospect for new customers." To that end, King works with his sales teams to identify and focus efforts on a "Top 10 Customer" list. King meets frequently with sales representatives to discuss sales strategies and results with these top customers and then acts as a personal conduit back to the operations team to resolve any customer service issues. Finally, King advocates instituting a balanced compensation system, which rewards the higher profitability of repeat sales to existing customers while continuing to incentivizing transactions with new customers.

d. *Support sales efforts with efficient operational support.* Another key theme among start-up CEOs was the constant struggle between allocating scarce resources to revenue generating activities versus additional operational capabilities. CEO Brown spoke to the need to "run yourself lean" from an operations standpoint but also acknowledged that the primary reason most customers stop using their product was a failure to "take care of me" on the operations side, rather than a product failure. Here are key considerations for cash-strapped start-ups:

   i. *Standardize the onboarding process for new customers.* In order to gain product approval by the hospital or facility and to realize revenues as quickly as possible, seek to anticipate and standardize the steps of the onboarding process as much as possible. Designate a standard "customer training" team of home office personnel with prepared curriculum. If the hospital requires a pilot study, have established study protocols available for immediate approval and get to implementation as soon as possible. Understand what information is needed to get your product into the procurement system and generate a purchasing order. Have sufficient inventory ready to generate and sustain sales.

   ii. *Stage-gate operational spending with sales activity.* Eventually small companies can encounter a time where operational demands outpace staffing and resources. To address those circumstances when operational demands exceed current capacity,

CEO King advocates implementing a backlog calendar and engaging customers (using the calendar) to manage expectations and to orchestrate implementation and delivery of products/services when the resources are available. Admittedly, this will result in a short-term delay or push of some revenue; however, King believes the short-term delay of revenue is preferred over significantly increasing fixed expenses, while the company's revenue ramp is still maturing and/or until such time the company has a healthy sales backlog.

iii. *Keep your pulse on customer satisfaction metrics.* CEO Brown works diligently to track customer loyalty metrics. Brown frequently either meets with or sends short surveys to his top customers to gauge their satisfaction with his products and services and pays particular attention to areas of dissatisfaction. In his experience, the reason most often cited by loyal customers who stopped using his products was a lack of operational support rather than a product failure. These surveys help him to uncover and correct areas where top customers are dissatisfied with their service before they lose that customer forever.

Summary: Make Haste, Slowly

Start-up CEOs understand that they need to get their company to sustainable revenues as quickly as possible but often make the mistake of trying to "go viral" with disastrous consequences. This approach can lead to companies pushing sales efforts further and faster than their operations can support, while the increased expenses and lack of revenues can quickly drain cash reserves. Instead we advocate a "make haste, slowly" approach that values repeat sales from customers with low acquisition costs because of proximity to corporate Headquarters and supported by the company's efficient, internally managed operations. The company grows to introduce the product to new customers in high-potential territories in concert with its ability to support them operationally and a healthy cash flow position.

KEY TAKEAWAY POINTS

- ▶ Cash is King! Create a monthly cash flow model of the company's static (day-to-day) cash burn as well as the anticipated timing of expenses and revenues from a product sale.

- ▶ Identify a local product champion to assist with prototype development and then pilot the product post clearance. Count on three rounds of prototype development prior to FDA submission and one more round post clearance when it is used on a frequent basis.

- ▶ Keep inventory levels low until ready to scale the product regionally and build the internal operation systems to support product sales in a cost-effective manner.

- ▶ Become an expert on the hospital approval and onboarding process. This will likely take longer than anticipated and delay revenues.

- ▶ When ready, expand sales efforts strategically to areas with high-potential return on investment (ROI) because of disease prevalence and unmet patient needs.

- ▶ Confine sales efforts to "rope limits" within driving distance of Headquarters to enable senior management to assist in the customer acquisition and onboarding processes in a cost-effective manner.

- ▶ Above all, value repeat sales from top customers and align your organization's incentive systems to reward sales efforts accordingly!

REFERENCES AND RESOURCES

1. Zero to 510 Medical Device Accelerator. Available at http://zeroto510.com/.
2. Memphis Bioworks Foundation. Available at http://www.memphisbioworks.org/.
3. Seed Accelerator Project Ranking for 2015. Available at at http://seedrankings.com/2015-rankings.html.
4. Seed Accelerator Project Ranking for 2016. Available at http://seedrankings.com/2016-rankings.html.
5. Seed Accelerator Project Ranking for 2016. Available at http://seedrankings.com/2017-rankings.html.
6. Venture Nashville. VC Innova Memphis ignites $31MM RBIC fund, projects 20 transactions by year-end 2018. Milt Capps. Available at http://www.venturenashville.com/vc-innova-memphis-ignites-31mm-rbic-fund-br-projects-20-transactions-by-year-end-2018-cms-1563. www.innovamemphis.com.
7. Memphis Daily News. Zimmer Acquires Memphis-Based ExtraOrtho. Aisling Maki. Available at https://www.memphisdailynews.com/news/2011/nov/22/zimmer-acquires-memphis-based-extraortho/.
8. Ramkhelawan R. Available at http://www.ryanram.com/. https://www.linkedin.com/in/ryanramkhelawan/.
9. Restore Medical. Available at http://www.restore-med.com/.
10. PATH EX, Inc. Available at https://pathex.co/.
11. Moore JX, Donnelly JP, Griffin R, Howard G, Safford MM, Wang HE. Defining sepsis mortality clusters in the United States. *Crit Care Med*. 2016;44(7):1380-1387.
12. iScreen Technologies. Available at http://www.iscreenvision.com/.

CHAPTER 18

Funding Approaches: Who, When, Why, and in Exchange for What?

LARRY YOST, KATHARINA BARTA

ABOUT THE AUTHORS

Larry Yost has over 30 years of combined experience with domestic and international medical device, pharmaceutical, and molecular diagnostic companies. He is the Founder and Managing Partner of The Atticus Group, a full-service consulting firm which specializes in supporting strategic and tactical pre- and post-commercialization activities for early-stage companies who are developing innovative medical technologies. This includes companies developing devices targeted toward the orthopedic and spine markets. He received a Bachelor of Science from the Purdue University School of Pharmacy.

Katharina Barta is currently studying International Business and Economics and Marketing at the University of New Hampshire. Her role with The Atticus Group is to support the discovery and compilation of market data and business research. Originally from Salzburg, Austria, Katherina's professional interest is the identification of how U.S. companies can best interact with companies outside the United States from an international business perspective in order to facilitate the development and implementation of cooperative projects.

Money never starts an idea; it is the idea that starts the money

W. J. CAMERON

The process of pursuing and maintaining adequate funding for an early-stage medical technology company is similar to the training and endurance required to run a long-distance race. You will need to complete the fundamental groundwork prior to the initial pursuit of funding, tackle the fundraising process using an appropriate strategy, and then top off the funds as the company accomplishes its milestones in order to achieve a recurring revenue ramp or progress to a potential liquidity event.

The typical stages of a "race," as it applies to the fundraising process, can be divided into obtaining seed capital or non-dilutive funding, attracting angel investors, receiving venture capital (VC) financing, and then achieving a liquidity event. There may be a need to obtain bridge funding in between some of these stages, mezzanine financing, or even account receivable financing prior to a liquidity event, such as an initial public offering (IPO) or acquisition by a company whose strategic business interests align with your technology.

Preparing for the Initial Fund Raise

While the initial groundwork associated with the development of a new orthopedic technology can occur anywhere from an inventor's garage to a fully equipped biomedical engineering laboratory, at some point additional resources will be required to further develop this idea into a working prototype or a device that can be used for the next phase of the development process. The above also includes conducting a thorough patent search and submitting a patent application for your invention along with creating a legal entity for your company. The time, effort, and oftentimes cash you and potential co-inventor(s) have personally invested in taking an idea to this stage can be thought of as the required upfront training needed to get you to the starting line.

Now is the time to prepare the initial "pitch" deck which will be used to sell your idea and the associated technology to early investors. A pitch deck should be a short slide presentation geared toward potential investors which provides an overview of the company, its technology, and the business plan for providing a return on their investment (Table 18.1).

Your pitch to potential investors and responses to their questions will aid them in having an initial understanding of the potential opportunity and risks associated with investing in your company. This will set the stage for making a decision relative to conducting a more thorough review as a part of a comprehensive due diligence process.

In addition to your pitch deck, you also need to have a data locker full of supporting documents in case your pitch garners serious interest from a prospective investor. At a minimum, the data locker should include your pitch deck, documents you reference in your pitch deck which support your assumptions for medical need, market size, and competitors, an executive summary, all of your legal agreements your intellectual property (i.p.), pro forma financials, and term sheets, if applicable. Not having a data locker is like showing up for a race without realizing you need to register as an entrant.

Table 18.1 Contents of a "Pitch" Deck	
Topic	**Description**
Your idea	What is your invention and the associated intellectual property?
Market need	What is the medical need for your technology? How will it help patients?
Market opportunity	What is the market size as it relates to either procedure volume or revenue?
Business model	How will you commercialize and sell your product?
Competitive threats	Who are your potential competitors and what are the anticipated barriers to market entry? How is your technology better than the competition?
The team	Who are the individuals who work for the company or are supporting the company's efforts on a consultative basis? What expertise and experience do they bring to the table?
Milestones	What are your development and commercialization timelines and associated deliverables?
Financials	What is the projected spend to achieve the above milestones? What are your estimated revenue projections?
The investment "ask"	How much money are you looking to raise?

With your initial pitch deck in hand and a full data locker, you are now ready to approach the starting line and begin your early fundraising efforts.

Raising Seed Capital

Seed capital is the initial investment funds received are used to assist with the next stage of product development and to support initial exploration of the market. The objective of these funds is to better establish the viability of your technology and its role in the marketplace in advance of pursuing incrementally larger amounts of funding. This funding can be obtained as either dilutive or non-dilutive financing. Dilutive financing is any kind of funding where you and your co-founders give up ownership in a part of your company. Non-dilutive financing means the funding you receive that does not require you to give up any equity or ownership in the company. Non-dilutive funding is typically in the form of a grant from the government, a foundation, or an organization. While your personal assets can be source of seed capital (otherwise known as "bootstrapping"), the following are alternative funding options.

FRIENDS, FAMILY, AND BUSINESS COLLEAGUES

Obtaining a loan or direct investment from your friends, family, or individuals within your business network could be an early source of seed capital for your company. While loans might be perceived as a somewhat less risky option, you will need to draw up a formal "promissory note" that sets forth the terms of the loan, including the repayment schedule. This approach is often a good alternative since obtaining a loan from a bank or other lender can be difficult at this stage of your company's history due to the inherent development risks.

Another option is a direct investment in your company in return for an equity stake. This type of investment can be arranged with less paperwork, documentation, and diligence compared with more formal financing options. The downside of this option is that it will force you to set an enterprise value, which can be difficult to do during the early stages of a company's existence. Setting a valuation too high at this point can potentially sink the company's prospects for successfully obtaining financing or a potential liquidity event in the future.

As there is a potential for loss of the entire investment due to the risks associated with an early-stage medical device company, the impact of the above on your personal relationships with the parties involved needs to be considered.

SBIR/STTR GRANTS

A common source of non-dilutive seed capital for early-stage orthopedic technology companies is the U.S. Government's Small Business Innovation Research (SBIR) program.[1] Closely related to this is the Small Business Technology Transfer (STTR) program, a sister program which is designed to provide seed capital for cooperative technology development initiatives between small companies and academic or nonprofit research institutions in the United States.[2] These highly competitive awards-based programs are intended to assist small business in the early development of their technology. The objectives for the SBIR/STIR program are listed in Table 18.2.

The SBIR/STIR programs are divided into three phases. Phase I, or the start-up phase, is designed to provide companies with awards up to $150,000 to support efforts to establish the proof of concept for their technology, including feasibility studies, the determination of technical merit, and identification/establishment of commercial potential for the

Table 18.2 Objectives for the SBIR Program[1,2]

- Stimulate technological innovation;
- Meet federal research and development needs;
- Increase private sector commercialization of innovations developed through federal R&D funding; and
- Foster and encourage participation in innovation and entrepreneurship by socially and economically disadvantaged persons and women-owned small businesses.

SBIR, Small Business Innovation Research.

technology. This phase is also intended to enable the government to assess the company's organization and its ability to achieve predetermined milestones prior to consideration for future federal grant support. Research and development work associated with Phase I awards typically have a duration of 6 months for SBIR grants and 12 months for STTR grants.

Phase II SBIR/STTR grants are designed to enable the continuation of R&D efforts which were initiated in line with Phase I funding. These grants of up to $1,000,000 over a 2-year time period are awarded based on the results achieved during Phase I along with the scientific and technical merit and commercial potential of the technology, as defined in the company's Phase II project proposal. It is important to note that only companies who have received a Phase I grant are eligible for a Phase II award.

Phase III of the SBIR/STTR grant programs is defined as the actual commercialization of the technology following the completion of the milestones outlined in the company's Phase I and II project plans. The government does not provide funding for Phase III with the intent that companies obtain any additional funding from either the private sector or non-SBIR/STTR governmental funding sources. Table 18.3 lists the requirements for companies to be eligible to apply for grants awards via the SBIR/STTR programs.

While the SBIR and STTR programs are similar objectives, they have two basic differences. For SBIR, the Program Director/Principle Investigator must be primarily employed (over 50% of their time) by the small business submitting the grant request at the time of award and for the duration of the project period, unless a waiver is granted by the National Institutes of Health (NIH). For the STTR Program, there is no stipulation as to whether the Program Director/Principle Investigator is primarily employed by either the small business or the collaborating nonprofit research institution at the time of award and for the duration of the project period. Also, while the SBIR program encourages research partnerships but does not make this a requirement, STTR stipulates that small businesses

Table 18.3 SBIR/STTR Eligibility Requirements[3]

- The company's place of business must be located in the United States and it should operate primarily within the United States.
- The company must have less than 500 employees.
- The company must Be organized for profit.
- The company is a legal entity in the form of an individual proprietorship, partnership, limited liability company, corporation, joint venture, association, trust, or cooperative. If the company is a joint venture, there must Be less than 50% participation by foreign business entities in the joint venture.
- The company owns or has exclusive rights to the intellectual property associated with the technology and all associated commercialization rights.

Complete eligibility requirements can be found at: https://www.sbir.gov/sites/default/files/elig_size_compliance_guide.pdf.
SBIR, Small Business Innovation Research; SBTT, Small Business Technology Transfer.

must formally collaborate with a nonprofit research institution. Under STTR, the small business must perform a minimum of at least 40% of the work outlined in the project proposal and the nonprofit research collaborator must perform at least 30% of the work.

DEPARTMENT OF DEFENSE AWARDS

Another source of non-dilutive financing for your medical technology can be Department of Defense (DoD). The DoD offers over 100 awards designed to fund the development of new medical technologies.[4] It is important to note that DoD awards are usually legally binding contracts as opposed to being a grant. This means less flexibility in terms of utilization, a higher fiscal requirement, and more frequent reporting. Most DoD awards involve a two-step submission process which includes submitting a concept paper as a first step and then an industry submission. An advantage of DoD awards is they support high-impact, high-risk projects, that other funding sources, such as venture capitalists, may be hesitant to invest in. For most programs and awards that the DoD offers to the medical world, a multiyear budget request is required. The DoD supports the development of medical technologies with a broad range of awards and research areas, not all of which are required to be directly related to military objectives.

Oftentimes, large non-dilutive funding opportunities are fueled by Congress. An example is the Congressionally Directed Medical Research Program (CDMRP) managed by the DoD.[5] CDMRP is a collaboration between Congress and the U.S. military which funds many research areas, including military medical research and other disease- and injury-specific research. This global program administers management support for the Defense Health Program's core research areas.

FOUNDATIONS

Another source of seed financing can potentially be foundations and organizations, some of which have specific interests in the area of orthopedics your technology is addressing. The Orthopaedic Research and Education Foundation, or OREF (www.oref.org), and the Arthritis Foundation (www.arthritis.org) are examples of musculoskeletal-focused nonprofit medical and patient-focused organizations which have investigator-initiated and research-specific competitive grants. While grants from these organizations are typically limited, they can be an excellent source of early non-dilutive capital for your company and support efforts to validate your technology prior to efforts to attract larger investments.

OTHER ALTERNATIVE SOURCES OF SEED CAPITAL

While the above represent common paths to obtaining early funding, there are several additional alternative sources of funding which could represent good options for you to pursue with your technology. This includes the following:

- *Start-up competitions*

Start-up competitions, which are also known as pitch or business plan competitions, are a newer funding option. You can look at this like winning a prize for your idea after presenting it to a panel of judges and industry investors after meeting the required timeline and rules of the competition. While this may be daunting to some, there are several key benefits associated with taking part in a start-up competition, including obtaining early initial capital which can be helpful when developing a prototype, expanding your network to include potential future investors and advisors, and gaining additional exposure in the industry.

- *Incubators*

Incubators are external organizations that assist early-stage companies by offering office space, management training, monetary support, and more. The business support these organizations provide is designed to accelerate the growth of a start-up with associated guidance from an array of professionals. Incubators offer some key benefits like an inspiring work environment, higher credibility for your start-up due to the backup of an incubator business, and numerous learning and support opportunities. Most incubators focus on a specific industry and are often interested in equity, making it critical for you to do the appropriate amount of diligence on the incubator prior to electing this route for your company.

• *Accelerators*

Accelerators are very similar to incubators as they also provide services like company space, business advice, or networking opportunities. Unlike incubators, however, accelerators are highly selective and competitive. While incubators are usually more suitable for a start-up in the early stages, accelerators align more with companies that are rapidly growing. Accelerators are normally short-term options for emerging companies with their main focus of mentoring several companies and their management teams over a 6- to 12-week time period program. This leads to a creative and highly educational learning-by-doing type of environment. One of the key advantages of accelerator programs is they usually help build a network with venture capitalists which, in turn, can create an easier path to becoming part of their investment portfolio.

• *Crowdfunding*

Crowdfunding is a newer option for obtaining early seed capital to support the development of your idea. As the amount of actual individual investment is typically very small with this approach, you will need to grab the attention of many potential investors all at once, and thus your pitch must be convincing and dynamic. A great advantage of crowdfunding is that the amounts that are being raised are usually much higher than the ones coming from incubators or angel investors. Crowdfunding offers an opportunity to validate the concept and to create a demand on the market, which in turn makes your technology more attractive to future investors. This option of funding is growing and is becoming more and more applicable in the medical world with several crowdfunding opportunities now dedicated to the medical industry (Table 18.4).

Table 18.4 Examples of Crowdfunding Platforms	
Platform	**Website**
Nonspecific crowdfunding platforms	
Kickstarter	www.kickstarter.com
Indiegogo	entrepreneur.indiegogo.com
InventureX	inventurex.com
Medical device–focused crowdfunding platforms	
MedStartR	www.medstartr.com
B-a-MedFounder	www.bamedfounder.com

Obtaining sufficient seed capital to fund your company is similar to making it to the first water stop in a long-distance race. You are feeling good about what you have accomplished, you are maintaining a good pace, and you just drank some water or Gatorade to replenish your liquids in order to fuel yourself through the next part of the race. Now you need to pursue additional funding to maintain your energy stores as the race progresses.

Attracting Angel Investors

"Angel" investors are individuals who invest their own money in an entrepreneurial company. Angel investors can be affiliated individuals, like family or friends, or unaffiliated investors who you have no prior relationship with or who have no previous involvement with your company. Angel investors are typically, but not always, high net worth individuals who invest in your business with the intent of gaining a higher rate of return. These individuals are usually not professional investors, but professionals with disposable income. They can oftentimes be doctors, lawyers, accountants, or other professionals who are willing to invest in start-ups in order to obtain an equity position in your company, or individuals who have a strong personal interest in your technology based on their personal or a family member's medical history associated with the problem you are working to solve.

Obtaining funding from angel investors is an effective way to obtain financing beyond the seed capital stage. It is important, however, that the investor understands that there is a considerably high level of risk associated with their investment, as there may be no return or loss of their capital in the event of a business failure. In addition to their financial support, angel investors may also be a good source of guidance based on their business experience. The network of individuals they are connected with can also provide insight which may help accelerate your development activities. Disadvantages of obtaining financing from angel investors includes partial loss of the control of your company and the need to include them in some of the decision-making for your business along with giving them an equity stake in the company.

Angel investors usually contribute funding in amounts ranging from $25,000 to $100,000 and typically do not carry a fiduciary duty. The level of due diligence varies from one angel investor to another with the level of on-going involvement in your company ranging from coffee once a quarter to direct involvement on a week-to-week or monthly basis as a part of your business planning and decision-making process. How do you find angel investors if you decide that you want to pursue this type of funding? Table 18.5 lists several online sources for identifying potential angel investors.

Table 18.5 Examples of Online Resources for Finding Potential Angel Investors	
Name	**Website**
FundingPost	www.fundingpost.com
U.S. Angel Investment Network	www.angelinvestmentnetwork.us
Gust	gust.com
American Capital Association	www.angelcapitalassociation.org

Angel investors are often looking for inspirational founders who have an innovative technology and an impressive pitch deck. It is critical that you have an effective plan of how you will present yourself and your company and to identify the key business metrics, industry dynamics, and target audience that an angel investor is looking to get involved in. Be prepared for the individual to ask to take an active role in the company including a request to take a seat on your Board of Directors. Understanding their expectations and your level of involvement you are willing to accept are important in determining if they are the right option as an investor in your company. If you find that the individual is not an ideal fit, or they are unwilling to invest, you can still gain some possible benefit by asking them for an introduction to other individuals in their network who may be potential investors.

You are now half way through the race, and the toughest part of the race is still to come. In order to maintain your pace and push forward, you ingest an energy gel and continue to drink more liquids (and maybe eat a banana) to help maintain your endurance and avoid having your legs cramp up as you push forward.

Obtaining Venture Capital

At some point your company will require significantly more resources to move your technology forward toward commercialization. This includes, but is not limited to, funding to enhance your product offering, to complete preclinical and clinical studies required for regulatory filing, and to create a supply chain for components and the manufacturing of your device. Additionally, there will be costs associated with hiring experienced individuals who can successfully drive your efforts forward along with the associated facility and infrastructure costs. Following commercialization, additional resources will be needed to build out your commercialization team and to support incremental sales and marketing expenses. This requires significantly more energy gels than you used earlier in the race.

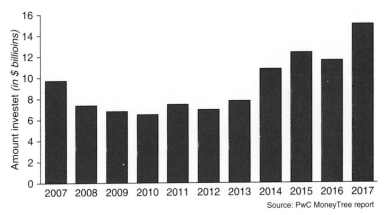

Figure 18.1 Total annual investment amount from venture capitals (VCs) in the health care sector (2007-2017).[5] (From Department of Defense. Congressionally Directed Medical Research Programs (CDMRP). http://cdmrp.army.mil/.F.)

At this point, most companies pursue VC financing in order to gain access to the level of capital required to fund all of the above-mentioned efforts. VCs are professional investment managers who utilize money raised from other sources to invest in emerging companies with the goal of receiving a high rate of return over a defined time period. The VCs consolidate money from a variety of investors and can include money received from individual investors, pension funds, charitable foundations, endowments, consolidated funds from wealthy families, and corporations.

VC investments in health care–related companies continues to be popular with over $15 billion of VC money invested in health care companies during 2017 representing 771 deals.[6] Figure 18.1 shows the trend in total annual investment amount from VCs in this same sector over the past decade. Figure 18.2 shows the distribution of total VC investments for health care–related companies in 2017 by company stage.

Typically, one VC takes the "lead" on making the investment with other VC's being "followers." The lead VC will typically provide a larger percentage of the total dollar amount compared to the other VCs. They will also take on the responsibility for most of the due diligence efforts, negotiate the terms of the deal, and assume a Board of Directors position once the financing has closed. The follower VCs often takes a less active role in the above process and with the on-going operations of the company. It is important to identify in advance whether a VC is typically a "lead" or a "follower" and their track record of investment amounts in similar type companies as yours. Some VCs tend to avoid riskier investments in early-stage

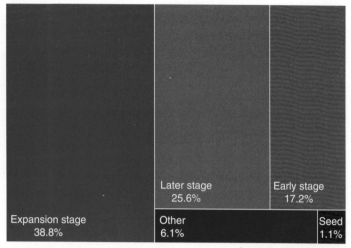

Source: PwC MoneyTree report

Figure 18.2 Distribution of total venture capital investment for health care–related company by stage of growth (2017).[5] (From Department of Defense. Congressionally Directed Medical Research Programs (CDMRP). http://cdmrp.army.mil/.)

companies, opting instead for companies who have achieved specific clinical or regulatory milestones. A good lead VC can also utilize their network to attract other VCs to be a part of your deal.

As obtaining VC financing is a highly competitive dash for cash, you need to ensure your company stands out when you are making your pitch, especially because the person you are pitching to will be hearing multiple pitches from many companies. Critical to this pitch is to excite them about how your innovation will address a large unmet medical need, that the market it addresses is large with a low number of barriers to entry, and that you and your team have the insight, experience, and skill to achieve the milestones you outline within an appropriate timeframe. You must also have a solid business model which communicates how you plan to manufacture, commercialize, and distribute the product while also overcoming any regulatory, reimbursement, or pricing barriers. Companies whose technologies have a market potential of less than $250 million will struggle to obtain VC financing while those whose market potentials exceed $500 million or over $1 billion per year will attract a lot of attention.

What are the trade-offs associated with accepting VC money? Many entrepreneurs have difficulty once they accept financing from a VC as they have lost their independence and are now reporting to someone else. Owing to the large equity stake VCs typically take, they feel it is no longer "their" company and there is sometimes a loss of decision-making ability. Another common occurrence is forced management changes when the VC pressures founders to accept new team members they believe will enhance the company or push for specific members of the current management team to be removed.

Once an interested VC has completed their full due diligence and made a decision to pursue investing in a company, they will provide a term sheet which outlines the deal structure. The term sheet will also identify a "pre-money valuation" reflecting their assessment of the value of your company prior to the investment being considered. The total investment in your company to date, the number of shares issued, the size of your potential market, the level of risk associated with your technology, and historical or current valuations of comparable companies in the market you are targeting are typically incorporated into the valuation process. Unfortunately, there is no agreed upon standard for determining the valuation of a start-up company in the medical device sector and many differing methods exist.[7-9]

In return for their investment, VCs will receive preferred stock in your company with founders and previous investors holding common stock. It is common for most start-ups to also maintain a pool of common stock for employee stock options which can be used to attract and retain experienced and high performing talent. Once you accept the term sheet and the appropriate legal documents are drawn up and signed by both parties, the VC will arrange a transfer of funds.

Typically, the money from VCs is provided over time in "tranches" and not all at once. How much and when your company receives this money (or tranche payments) depends on prenegotiated development and commercialization milestones. The amount of money a company raises is based on budgetary projections and financials calculations to achieve the identified milestones, with some leeway for unexpected delays or cost overruns.

The total amount of money agreed to is considered a "financing round" with some companies requiring more than one round of financing to sustain operations. These rounds are designated as Series A, Series B, and so on with the price of the company's stock hopefully incrementally increasing with each round. Some VCs will continue to reinvest in a company with subsequent rounds (e.g., returning investor) while new investors may be needed for future rounds in lieu of current investors or when a greater amount of financing is required. It will become much more difficult to raise money with good terms, and investors will become concerned, if there are continued delays in your company's progress. This can result in the need for unanticipated additional rounds of funding and possibly a "down round" when the company's stock is priced less than it was for a previous round. This is a warning sign for both the company and individually for the founders and management team and a potential call for a corporate shake-up by the investors.

CORPORATE VENTURE CAPITAL

Very large organizations often have their own VC arms which invest in start-up companies. Some of these VCs have an investment focus which is dictated by the business interests of their parent company while others may be independent and able to invest in companies whose focus or target markets are far afield of those of the parent company. Understanding the latitude they have in this respect is important when assessing corporate VC opportunities. As corporate VCs often invest in companies whose products are a strategic fit for their business, they often represent a path to a future acquisition of your technology or the company as a whole.

You are now three quarters through the race. While you have had to endure several challenging uphill climbs, avoid your competitors pressing your pace, and ignore the pain in your legs and your mounting exhaustion, you persevere. Now it is the critical time to ignore these distractions and focus your attention in order to make it to the end of the race.

Additional Financing Options

Sometimes companies need to top off the tank between late-stage financing and a potential liquidity event. Alternative financing options such as taking out a loan, accounts receivable financing, or mezzanine financing can be considered at this stage. When taking out a loan, you receive money from an investor and agree to repay that money at a predetermined interest rate. The rate is often based on the level of risk associated with the loan and the perceived ability to repay. Loans can come from banks, individuals, the government, or other sources. Accounts receivable financing is another way of acquiring funding and involves leveraging the company's accounts receivable balance. In other words, using that amount owed to you via outstanding invoices to obtain a loan in a manner similar to payday loans. Mezzanine financing is a combination of debt and equity financing. It takes the form of a large loan which typically has a high interest rate. The lender is willing to make a mezzanine investment because they will have the security of being able to convert this to equity if the loan is not fully paid back within the time period agreed upon. Mezzanine financing is usually more appropriate for later stage companies because a lender is typically reluctant to make an investment if the company does not have a high cash flow or steady growth rate.

The Liquidity Event

A liquidity event represents the desired exit strategy for most start-up companies. Achieving this milestone enables founders and investors to cash out their shares in the company, with investors hopefully receiving the desired return on their investments. In our long-distance race analogy, this can be considered the finish line. All the pre-race training along with your effort and perseverance during the race spent getting this point are now rewarded with a medal and a T-shirt. The liquidity event can take the form of an IPO or potentially an acquisition by a strategic company with a business focus in the same market as your technology.

INITIAL PUBLIC OFFERING

An IPO represents when a company first offers stock to the public. The proceeds from the IPO are typically used to raise capital to support on-going operations and fund the business expansion. The process for filing an IPO requires extensive preparation and paperwork, including meeting all of the requirement outlined by the Securities and Exchange Commission (SEC). As a significant amount of time, effort, and planning are required in order to successfully file and execute an IPO, this can have a tremendous impact on the ability of smaller companies to manage their day-to-day business operations. Understanding current stock market conditions and the projected valuation of your company are important considerations when deciding if and when to do an IPO. If a decision to pursue an IPO is made, you will need to identify an investment bank or underwriting firm to assist with and help facilitate this process. While a more detailed discussion of the pros and cons of filing an IPO and the steps required for the filing process would be too lengthy to include in this chapter, there are a number of sources elsewhere where this information can be found.[10–12]

STRATEGIC ACQUISITION

A very common alternative to an IPO as an exit strategy for medical technology companies is the acquisition of the company or its technology by a large company with strategic business interests which aligns with your technology. Many large medtech companies augment their internal R&D efforts by seeking out innovative technologies developed by smaller companies. Identifying potential strategic acquirers early on and maintaining on-going communication with key decisions-makers within the company as you achieve your development and commercialization milestones is critical to maintaining visibility as a potential future acquisition target.

Conclusion

There are numerous funding approaches which start-ups can pursue to assist with the financing of their efforts. These approaches typically differ based on what stage the company is at and the amount of financing required. While additional financing options beyond what are described above do exist, our hope is the information we have outlined provides entrepreneurs with a map to help plot their course as they go from the start to the finish line with their innovation.

KEY TAKEAWAY POINTS

- ▶ There are numerous potential funding options for medical technology start-up companies depending on what stage the company is at.

- ▶ Some financing options require innovators to give up equity stake in the company (dilutive funding) while others do not (non-dilutive funding).

- ▶ It is critical to be able to communicate a well-conceived and comprehensive business plan with achievable milestones when pursuing financing.

- ▶ Equity investors are looking for a high return on their investment within a reasonable time period.

- ▶ Large companies with business interests in the same market that your technology targets have the potential to be a source of VC for your company or to be a strategic acquirer.

REFERENCES AND RESOURCES

1. The SIBR Program. www.sbir.gov/about/about-sbir.
2. The STTR Program. www.sbir.gov/about/about-sttr.
3. SBIR and STTR Programs Frequently Asked Questions. www.sbir.gov/faqs/eligibility-requirements.
4. Grants.gov. https://www.grants.gov/.
5. Department of Defense. Congressionally Directed Medical Research Programs (CDMRP). http://cdmrp.army.mil/.
6. The U.S. Money Tree Report. Q2 2018. PwC. www.pwc.com/us/en/industries/technology/moneytree.html.
7. AAdvani. How to Value Your Startup: These Three Steps Will Help You Determine What Your New Business is Worth; Entrepreneur. www.entrepreneur.com/article/72384.
8. Nasser S. *The Parisoma Review. Valuation for Startups—9 Methods Explained.* Medium; 14, 2016. https://medium.com/parisoma-blog/valuation-for-startups-9-methods-explained-53771c86590e.

9. Cohn P. *How Do VC Firms Value a Start-Up?* Quora; June 14, 2016. https://www.quora.com/How-do-VC-firms-value-a-start-up.

10. Solomon G. *10 Requirements for a Successful IPO*. Fortune; March 11, 2013. http://fortune.com/2013/03/11/10-requirements-for-a-successful-ipo/.

11. The U.S. Securities and Exchange Commission. Going Public. www.sec.gov/smallbusiness/goingpublic.

12. *US IPO Guide 2018 Edition*. Latham & Watkins LLP; May 31, 2018. https://m.lw.com/thoughtLeadership/lw-us-ipo-guide.

CHAPTER 19

Alternative Pathways: Reconsidering Licensing and/or Codevelopment

SEAN MICHAEL RAGAN

ABOUT THE AUTHOR

Sean Michael Ragan is a noted popular writer on science, technology, and entrepreneurship. As a longtime editor and contributor for *MAKE: Magazine* and its online outlets, Mr Ragan has been a leading voice in the Maker Movement since its early days. In 2014, he launched Foundry Heavy Industries, a consultancy and media company dedicated to collecting, preserving, and analyzing the experiences of independent hardware entrepreneurs and capitalizing on that knowledge base to educate inventors and investors alike. His first book, *The Total Inventor's Manual,* was published in 2017.

Introduction: Scope and Assumptions

Exploiting the mature capital, infrastructure, and expertise of an established manufacturer-distributor will in most circumstances greatly reduce time-to-market over "going it alone," as well as saving considerable effort and risk. For these and other reasons, licensing is often recommended[1,2] as the first, best option for individual inventors seeking to monetize their intellectual property. In the medical equipment industries, where unit costs are typically high and regulatory burdens intensive, the incentives to opt for licensing over independent development tend to be stronger than in the general case.

This chapter focuses on the process of licensing an invention to a company interested in manufacturing and distributing it for or in cooperation with its inventor. This process is conveniently described in three phases: (1) identifying potential licensees, (2) generating interest, and (3) "sealing the deal" with an interested party. It is assumed that the invention to be licensed can be embodied as a useful physical device; that it is protected as intellectual property (IP) by one or more patents pending or issued; and that it has been reduced to practice as a looks-like and/or works-like prototype. It is also assumed that the inventor has retained competent legal counsel.

Identifying Potential Licensees

Companies that may elect to manufacture and distribute an invention under license will be described as **prospects**. It is almost always in an inventor's interest to approach as many *quality* prospects as possible. The caveat is important; as quality falls off, there comes a point of diminishing returns beyond which the chance of success does not justify the labor or political costs of making an approach that may be received as indiscriminate or inappropriate. There are a number of factors to consider when evaluating prospect quality. These may be broadly grouped under three headings: experience, amenability, and responsiveness.

EXPERIENCE

An established history of successfully manufacturing and distributing devices similar in function and construction to the preferred embodiment of an invention is the single most important factor in evaluating prospect quality.[2] A company with experience in functionally similar devices will be better positioned to distribute a product incorporating that invention; one with experience in similarly-built devices (i.e., having similar construction) will be better positioned to manufacture it. The best candidates will meet both criteria. All other factors being equal, experience distributing functionally similar products is likely to be more valuable than experience manufacturing products having similar construction, especially in the medical device industry where distribution carries higher-than-average overhead costs.

Individual inventors of orthopedic devices are likely to be practitioners also,[3] who will as a matter of professional necessity be very familiar with major manufacturers in their field and their respective product lines. Those without such expertise should invest the necessary time in market research to acquire it. Once a full picture of the market is in mind, "Whose product line does this invention seem to best fit in with?" will be a useful question to ask.

AMENABILITY

A prospect may be ideal in terms of experience and existing product lines but have little or no interest in licensing outside inventions. This may be a matter of explicit policy, or it may be simply a kind of cultural prejudice. A company that is amenable to working with outside inventors and/

or licensing intellectual property from outsiders is said to be "open"; one which is not so amenable is said to be "closed." An inverse correlation between the openness of a company and its size has often been posited, and for this reason, individual inventors are sometimes advised[2,4] to seek out "goldilocks" prospects big enough to comfortably capitalize a new product, but not so big as to have become closed.

Whether in some broad context such a correlation does exist, it is not *necessarily* true that a larger company will be less open, and in the narrower context of certain industries, it will be found that there is no discernible correlation or even that the general trend is reversed. In the case of highly specialized scientific and medical equipment and particularly implanted devices, companies that work closely with practitioners and are responsive to their feedback enjoy clear competitive advantages over those with an insular approach and are likely[3] to have a more open culture or even dedicated administrative channels in place for collecting and exploiting new ideas from their expert user bases. Note that the presence of such channels does *not* always imply amenability on the part of management to formal IP licensing arrangements, and one should be careful not to misconstrue interactions with a sales rep or support agent. These established points of customer contact will probably not have the authority to negotiate on behalf of the company they represent, but may be able to provide an introduction to someone who does.

RESPONSIVENESS

The ease of identifying, contacting, and holding the attention of the person or persons empowered to make licensing decisions on behalf of a prospect company may vary widely from organization to organization. A prospect may have the appropriate experience set and be amenable to licensing external IP, but have nonexistent or inadequate workflows for responding to outside solicitations. In the best case, one readily identified and easily contacted executive has unambiguous authority, responsibility, and incentive to receive and respond to external licensing offers, as well as available time and resources to promptly do so. In other cases, the costs in time and effort of "keeping the ball rolling" will be higher and, in the extreme, may become prohibitive.

Generating Interest

Once a set of quality prospects has been identified and prioritized, as many as practical should be approached at the same time, starting with the highest-priority group. Having multiple simultaneously interested prospects has potential advantages for a would-be licensor, and even if none of them ultimately expresses interest, it will still almost always be better to have determined that outcome sooner rather than later.

A stepwise strategy for approaching prospects is outlined in Figure 19.1. At no point in the process should technical information be discussed in writing. As a rule, written communication should at this stage be avoided if at all possible and limited in any case to scheduling and other administrative details. Note that such precautions are *not* intended primarily for the security of the inventor but as a courtesy to corporate prospects, who may be exposed to future liability if it can later be proven that they were in possession of particular technical information at a particular time.

SOCIAL NETWORKING

Because human beings naturally respond faster and with a greater degree of trust to those who are familiar than to strangers, personal networking tends to be a much more effective strategy than **cold-calling** for approaching prospects. Thus, the first point of contact with a potential licensee will ideally be located through an inventor's existing group of professional and personal acquaintances. Online social media platforms can be very effective tools for building and tracking such connections. In the event that multiple

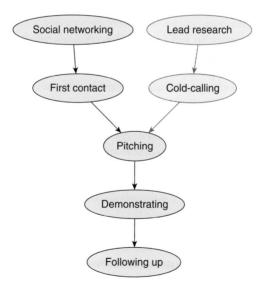

Figure 19.1 Approach process schematic, with disfavored "cold-calling" path in gray.

connections exist at a particular organization, the more familiar person is to be preferred as a first contact; where this is no clear preference in terms of familiarity, the contact highest in the management structure should be chosen.

Communications with a **first contact** will generally proceed through a sequence of four stages: (1) scheduling a face-to-face meeting or telephone conversation, (2) framing the discussion, (3) identifying the **decision-maker** within the organization with whom to discuss licensing arrangements, and (4) securing an introduction to that person. See Table 19.1 for sample phrases appropriate to each stage and correlated comments.

PITCHING

Decision-makers may be introduced through various channels, and the optimal tone and level of detail to convey will vary depending upon the medium through which they prefer to communicate. As a general rule, an in-person meeting to physically demonstrate the prototype or prototypes should be the inventor's objective. Depending on interest and availability, decision-makers may want to take a phone call or participate in a video-conference before agreeing to sit for a live demonstration, and an inventor should be prepared to "pitch" an invention in several scenarios where time and interactivity are more limited than in a scheduled face-to-face demonstration. Table 19.2 provides annotated sample language for the most common pitching contexts.

At some stage up to and including the demonstration meeting itself, a prospect company may request the signing of a **waiver**. As with all legal documents, this should be reviewed by and discussed with counsel before responding. Though it is inconsiderate to present a waiver without forewarning in a context where involving counsel would create an awkward delay (such as the beginning of the demo meeting), such a scenario may arise, and depending on the terms of the waiver in question, it may still be in an inventor's interest to sign without significant protest. For this reason, inventors should discuss with counsel the legal rationale for and common provisions of such waivers, so that they are prepared to make an informed on-the-spot decision about a particular waiver that may be put in front of them.

DEMONSTRATING

The demonstration presentation should be practiced, professional, and confident. The prototype or prototypes should themselves be compelling and persuasive in form and function. If possible, examples of prior art products should be on-hand as well so decision-makers can directly observe and

Table 19.1 Stages of Communication With Prospect First Contact

	Acceptable Channels	Sample Language	Comments
1. Scheduling	Meeting Phone call Electronic mail SMS Social media Instant messaging	• "Could I take you out to lunch sometime?" • "Could I get you on the phone for a minute?" • "I have an idea I want to bounce off you." • "I'd like to ask your help with something."	• Avoid written communications. • Be generous, friendly, and considerate. • Emphasize importance. • Enlist support.
2. Explaining	Meeting Phone call	• "I have this idea about..." • "I think it would work better than..." • "Seems like it would fit in your product line." • "We could help a lot of people."	• Go into as much technical detail as needed. • Convey excitement. • Be knowledgeable. • Ennoble the effort.
3. Assessing	Meeting Phone call	• "Do you do in-house development only?" • "Do you license IP?" • "Who'd be the best person to talk to?"	• Collect prospect background info. • Identify decision-makers(s).
4. Networking	Meeting Phone call	• "Should I contact her?" • "What's the best way?" • "Would she take a call?" • "Would you mind introducing us?" • "Thanks. I owe you one."	• Get an introduction. • Collect decision-maker background info. • Express appropriate gratitude.

Table 19.2 Contexts Short of Demo for Which an Inventor Should Prepare to "Pitch"

Context	Sample Language	Comments
Email	• "I'm a specialist in…" • "I've had this idea, and I'd like to put it in front of you." • "Do you have some time to look at my prototype?"	• Emphasize credentials. • Minimize written technical detail. • Work toward in-person demo.
Voice mail	• "I have a practice over at…" • "I specialize in…" • "Jane suggested I talk to you…" • "I have an idea I'd like to bounce off you if you have a couple minutes."	• Project confidence. • Emphasize credentials. • Make yourself familiar. • Be concise. • Work toward in-person demo.
Chance encounter ("elevator pitch")	• "Do you mind if I ask…" • "How does your product development pipeline work?" • "Do you license any IP?" • "So there's this problem with…" • "If I had an idea for a better way to do that, would you be interested in seeing it?"	• Transition gracefully. • Gather intelligence. • Frame technical problem/market opportunity. • Make your agenda clear. • Work toward in-person demo.
Phone call	• "Thanks for your time today." • "Basically, I've invented…" • "I think it could make a big difference in…" • "I designed this because I wished I could buy it myself." • "I don't know much about manufacturing." • "It seems like it would fit in with your product line."	• Be respectful. • Cut to the chase technically. • Emphasize the opportunity. • Clarify motivations. • Enlist support. • Work toward in-person demo.
Videoconference	• "I'm glad we got to do it this way…" • "Here's my prototype…" • "You can see that…" • "And here's an existing product…" • "The essential improvement is…" • "I have some slides if screen sharing will work…"	• Focus on the prototype. • Work toward in-person demo.

experience the improvements over existing technologies in the IP under consideration. The demonstration may also include an oral presentation describing the background, functioning, and advantages of the invention, as well as a discussion of how it compares to existing products and how it might be manufactured. It should *not* disclose any **confidential** information, which is any information that has not already been made public in a patent filing or other context, nor should it describe potential future developments of the technology that might be outside the scope of an inventor's existing IP. Presenters should plan to bring all media, materials, and equipment needed to give the presentation to the demonstration meeting and to take them away at its conclusion. Presenters should also be prepared to field questions up to and including planning how to respond if prompted about acceptable licensing terms. (See below.) Finally, presenters should come with enough printed copies of key presentation materials to leave one with any meeting participant who asks, though these should as a rule not be offered unless requested.

FOLLOWING UP

Demonstration meetings will usually resolve with an indication of interest and any follow-up steps that should be taken. Even if the demonstration has been successful, decision-makers will usually want some time to deliberate and may specify a time period after which the inventor should expect to be contacted. If the prospect will not offer a date, 14 days is generally considered an appropriate period to wait before making follow-up contact. Unless a prospect requests otherwise, parallel approaches should meanwhile continue.

Sealing the Deal

Once a prospect shows interest in a licensing arrangement, the process of negotiation should be considered to have begun. (From this point forward, the term **licensee** will be used to refer to the prospect, and **licensor**, to refer to the inventor, even though these terms are not technically accurate until the license is actually in effect.) When negotiations are in process, the licensor should as a rule suspend parallel discussions and not enter into negotiations with any other party. A situation in which more than one company is interested in licensing at the same time *can* work strongly in an inventor's favor but is also risky.[5] Savvy licensees may well request formal assurances that the licensor is not currently negotiating with any other party.

The advice of experienced legal counsel will be essential during the negotiating process. In the context assumed by this chapter (i.e., that the licensor is an individual inventor and the licensee is a company), it will usually be best if the parties adopt a "lawyer-back" protocol at the start of negotiations, in which licensor and licensee communicate directly with each other, by any mutually agreeable means, and confer privately with their attorneys between contacts to discuss the contents of those communications. Once the parties have come to terms, it will likely save time and reduce the possibility of miscommunication if the parties shift to a "lawyer-front" protocol in which opposing counsels communicate directly to hammer out the language of the contract. Note that it is a breach of professional ethics[6] for an attorney to attempt to contact an opposing counsel's client directly; a licensor who receives any communication from a licensee's attorney should not respond and should notify own counsel immediately.

NONDISCLOSURE AGREEMENTS

At any point during any relationship between two business entities, either party may request the signing of a nondisclosure agreement (NDA) by the other. Though NDAs are frequently discussed in the context of technology entrepreneurship, the preoccupation with them among individual inventors seeking to license IP to a manufacturer-distributor is often overemphasized. Under the modern "first to file" test in place in the United States and most English-speaking nations, an inventor who has filed a properly prepared patent application is secure against the remote possibility of "idea theft" that existed under the old "first to invent" standard, so long as that inventor is careful not to disclose anything not covered by existing filings. The circumstances under which an individual inventor might expect to benefit from an NDA are generally limited to those in which a disclosure of the confidential technical details of an invention must happen *before* a filing date has been established with the relevant patent authority, such as in the employment of a draftsperson to produce patent drawings or of a machinist or other fabricator to produce a prototype. There may still be tactical advantages to asking a licensee to sign an NDA, however, and individuals in negotiation with corporate licensees should expect to be asked to sign one themselves. Licensors should consult with counsel on the utility of drafting an NDA and on any NDA they are requested to sign.

NEGOTIATING

The negotiation of licensing terms is a domain for experts,[7] especially in a high-pressure face-to-face scenario. The process by which a negotiation unfolds can be as important in determining the outcome as the negotiation per se.[8] Though some cases may be exceptional, in the context of this chapter a low-pressure negotiating process that unfolds over the course of days or weeks by fax, e-mail, and/or phone—in which offers and counteroffers can be fully thought through and responses calmly considered—will probably be more in the licensor's interest than an in-person meeting or series of meetings. Before going into a demonstration or other meeting with a licensee alone, a licensor should discuss with counsel how best to respond if asked point-blank to negotiate terms; this might be done out of authentic enthusiasm, idle curiosity, or a desire to gain tactical advantage in subsequent negotiations,[9] for instance by inviting premature **anchoring**.

The primary objective in negotiations is for both parties to come to agreement about an informal document called a terms sheet, which simply lists the key parameters of the deal in plain language. Once a version of this document is complete that meets with both the licensor's and the licensee's approval, it can be left with the lawyers who should be able to work directly with each other to agree on the specific language that will go in the contract. For a manufacturing license, the most important parameters to be included in the terms sheet are listed in Table 19.3.

Table 19.3 Major Parameters to be Negotiated in a Manufacturing License

	Definition	Subsidiary Considerations
Term	The period of time over which the license will extend.	• When will it start? • When will it end? • Can it be renewed?
Exclusivity	The extent of the licensor's rights to license the IP to other parties.	• Exclusivity favors the licensee. • Nonexclusivity favors the licensor.
Advance	Amount to be paid by the licensee at the start of the licensing period.	• What is the amount? • Is it against royalties? • Or in addition to royalties?
Royalty	Recurring percentage of net sales to be paid by the licensee during the licensing period.	• What is the percentage? • Will it change with time? • How often will licensee pay?
Assignability	The extent of the licensee's rights to transfer the license to other parties.	• Is the license transferable? • Transferability favors the licensee. • Must licensor approve? • Approval favors the licensor.

Conclusion: On "Codevelopment"

It is a fundamental assumption of this chapter that development of the invention, as intellectual property, will be completed *before* licensing begins and that the inventor will have by that time drawn a legal bright line around the IP with well-prepared patent filings. Put differently, it is assumed the licensor intends to "walk away" from the invention once a license has been secured and leave further development, including any refinements or improvements that may occur during the process of design for manufacture, in the hands of the licensee. Any other arrangement in which the inventor participates in further development of technology based on the licensed IP should be considered **codevelopment**, which requires more complex negotiations and contracting arrangements to ensure that the parties have agreed, in advance, about how the rights to any new IP they may generate through cooperation will be shared among them.

KEY TAKEAWAY POINTS

- ▶ Experience in manufacturing and distributing similar products is the most important factor in evaluating a potential licensee.

- ▶ Social networking is a more effective strategy for approaching potential licensees, on average, than cold-calling.

- ▶ An in-person demonstration of the prototype should be the preferred objective of a licensor during the pitching process.

- ▶ The advice of an experienced attorney will be required during the negotiation phase.

- ▶ The process by which a negotiation unfolds can be as important as the negotiation in itself.

- ▶ Licensing IP already protected by patent filings is a much simpler process than codevelopment of new IP.

REFERENCES AND RESOURCES

1. Hawker C. *Why Licensing Is the Best Way to Get Your Product on Store Shelves*; 2013. [online] Entrepreneur.com. Available at https://www.entrepreneur.com/article/230557. Accessed February 2, 2018.
2. Pressman D, Tuytschaevers T. *Patent it Yourself*. Berkeley: NOLO; 2014.
3. Chatterji A, Fabrizio K, Mitchell W, et al. Physician-industry cooperation in the medical device industry. *Health Aff.* 2008;27(6):1532-1543.
4. Creane A, Konishi H. Goldilocks and the licensing firm: choosing a partner when rivals are heterogeneous. *SSRN Electronic Journal*. 2009. [online]. Available at https://dlib.bc.edu/islandora/object/bc-ir:103283/datastream/PDF/download/citation.pdf. Accessed Febeuary 2, 2018.

5. Casamatta C, Haritchabalet C. Dealing with venture capitalists: shopping around or exclusive negotiation. *Rev Finance*. 2014;18(5):1743-1773.

6. Meeker H. *Technology Licensing: A Practitioner's Guide*. Chicago: ABA Publishing; 2010.

7. Stim R. *Profit from Your Idea: How to Make Smart Licensing Deals*. Berkeley: NOLO; 2011.

8. Malhotra D. Control the negotiation before it begins. *Harv Bus Rev*. 2015;93(12):66-72.

9. Wheeler M. *Negotiation (Harvard Business Essentials Series)*. Boston: Harvard Business School Press; 2003.

CHAPTER 20

Postlaunch Physician Relationships: How You Maintain Loyalty?

MILES C. WILSON

ABOUT THE AUTHOR

Miles C. Wilson, President, Nerves & Bones, Inc. Miles has a decade of experience as a medical device marketing and sales professional. He holds a Bachelor of Science in Biotechnology (SUNY Brockport) and a Masters of Business Administration in Health Care (Cleveland State University). Prior to entering the medical device marketplace, Miles coached college basketball for 10 years for prestigious institutions like the United States Naval Academy, The Citadel, Randolph-Macon College, and Hobart College. Miles resides in Rhode Island with his beautiful wife Kristen and their four boys. He enjoys saltwater fishing and playing hoops with his boys in his free time.

Defining Surgeon Loyalty

Surgeon loyalty can best be defined as repeatable and consistent product usage. In order to achieve this status within a doctor's practice the efficacy of the technology and the outcomes for the patient will need to be safe and reliable. This will lead to loyalty.

Loyal surgeon customers allow for scalability of your technology. Being able to properly forecast growth based on loyal surgeon usage allows for a business to be more efficient in how it manages the business activities needed to scale the technology.

Gaining and maintaining market share requires a focused and well-planned strategy. Although price is becoming more important in today's health care economy, surgeons are often making device/implant decisions based on efficacy and benefits to their patients. To penetrate a market as complex as health care, you will need two key components as part of your strategy: (1) data supporting your technology and (2) people to communicate the benefits of your technology.

If a premarket approval/investigational device exemption (PMA/IDE) was needed for regulatory approval of your technology, supplying data demonstrating efficacy should already be at your fingertips. If not, investing in a well-designed postmarket study with early adopter surgeons is a sound strategy to consider. These surgeon partners will undoubtedly grasp the perceived benefits of your technology and be willing partners in ensuring that the theoretical benefits do indeed help patients. It is important to target surgeon partners who are experts in the field where your technology best fits and understand the importance of achieving perfect outcomes at the earliest stages. Another important thing to consider is the Individual Review Board (IRB) of the hospital sites where the study shall be conducted. If the IRB is convoluted and time consuming, you may want to consider a different partner. Although time consuming and costly, driving data demonstrating efficacy for your technology will be well worth it once you try to scale your market penetration. Today, most, if not all, health systems have a product approval process that requires efficacy data. Additionally, many insurers are denying patient access to technologies when there is a lack of data. The importance of this part of your commercialization strategy cannot be over-stated—data is the key to opening the flood gates.

You now have a well-designed, perfectly manufactured, FDA-approved technology with solid data proving it benefits patients. Unfortunately, it is not going to scale itself. This is because surgeons are complex decision-makers, and to make things more difficult, they are very busy human beings. This is where a well-educated and efficient sales person can benefit your technology.

A sales force can be achieved in a couple different ways, each having its own strengths and weaknesses. You can hire a direct sales force or contract with an independent sales company. Hiring your own sales force will give you unparalleled focus and control of how your technology is marketed and serviced. It comes at a big price tag. The average salary of a medical device sales person is well into the six figure range and ensuring you get the most effective people for the job will take time and resources. Add in auto allowances, insurance/benefits, and the cost mounts quickly.

Your other option is to contract with an independent sales organization. There is little upfront cost to these relationships because the contracted company pays its sales force. Depending on the willingness of the contracted company you may be able to increase focus on your technology with exclusivity clauses and increased commissions. You can ensure their effectiveness by delineating performance markers within the context of the contract.

Both types of sales forces will require a marketing and sales strategy that allows you to address a few key questions:

1. How do doctors/surgeons learn about the benefits of your technology?
2. How do doctors/surgeons get trained on your technology?
3. How do you ensure these doctors have positive reproducible outcomes using your technology?

A well-trained and educated team of professional sales people will help you answer these questions. It starts with the hiring or contracting process. Make sure the team you decide to employ are the people you want waving your technology's flag every day. They should be well-groomed, well-educated, well-mannered individuals with a competitive spirit. Most importantly, they should have a keen interest in helping doctors help their patients.

Once you have the right team of sales people in place, you need to ensure they become experts on your technology and why it exists. This involves educating them on the anatomy, disease states, and pathologies you are treating. Ensure the sales team understands all the benefits of your technology but also the potential hurdles doctors may encounter during the use of your technology. Health care sales professionals often act as consultants; not only do they promote the technology, they also ensure quality outcomes with service. A well-designed sales training program will ensure they can do both effectively.

Once trained, an effective sales team can target end-user doctors and get the face time necessary to communicate the benefits of your technology. This step is hard, and its difficulty cannot be overstated. However, with persistence and additional strategies, your message should be able to reach the market effectively. Trade shows, advertisements in scholarly journals, and peer-to-peer education events can all be effective tools to helping get your technology exposure to the market. Having early adopter doctors present the data they gathered at societal meetings is one of the best ways to supplement your sales team's efforts. The data, as mentioned earlier, are a vital component to your success.

Once interest has been demonstrated in using your technology, you need to change your focus on educating the doctor. This is best achieved with a doctor training program. Again, these can be costly events, but if a loyal customer base is your end goal then you will need to ensure reproducible positive outcomes. Doctor trainings are best done peer-to-peer. This allows for an unparalleled level of communication. Doctors can speak freely about how they best utilize the technology and how they see it helping their patients. Cadaveric laboratories are often used in the medical device marketplace to a high level of success. If capital is tight, you can consider laboratories with dummy models that replicate the anatomy in a true fashion. Also, web-based technologies for virtual trainings have been employed with success in recent years. Doctors are busy and these web-based events help save valuable time and travel for both the technology maker and doctor end user. A hands-on review of the technology is the minimum training that is suggested. Keep in mind, the pathway used for regulatory approval may determine the level of training needed. The regulatory body may have delineated how doctors are trained on your technology.

A well-trained sales consultant and a well-trained surgeon will be your best chance at having positive outcomes with your technology. Additional strategies that are often helpful include having a technology expert attend first-time user events. In the medical device market these product experts will travel to a first surgery to lend support to the local sales team and surgeon. Having a doctor consultant proctor attend first cases takes this concept a step further. The theme remains the same, however, ensuring quality reproducible outcomes.

Supporting the marketplace with high-quality data, expert consultative sales people, and quality technology training programs are the best way to ensure patients benefit from your technology. When this all comes together and patient's lives are improved you will undoubtedly develop long-lasting loyal relationships with the doctors that are in charge of their care.

KEY TAKEAWAY POINTS

- ▶ Surgeon customers are cultivated through data-driven sales.

- ▶ Sales people are a key component to the adoption of new technologies. They should be smart and clear communicators and present themselves well.

- ▶ Sales teams can take the form of two different types: direct or contracted sales teams each having their own strengths.

- ▶ Repeatable technology usage defines a loyal surgeon relationship. This is achieved when the efficacy of the technology and the service of the technology are consistent and reliable.

CHAPTER 21

Successful Exit: Acquisition Considerations

JOSH SANDBERG

ABOUT THE AUTHOR

Josh Sandberg has been consulting in the musculoskeletal industry since 2004. Throughout this time, he has had a positive impact on his clients' businesses, transforming them into the enterprises they were meant to be. Josh has keen insight into the challenges his clients face and how to navigate them successfully. This wisdom comes from a deep understanding of the industry and corporate nuance. Josh's experience as an executive in a start-up business has given him the ability to understand what it takes to thrive in a hands-on environment, where desire and dedication are paramount to success.

Starting in 2004, Josh joined The De Angelis Group and quickly ascended to a leadership role at the premier executive search firm focused exclusively in the musculoskeletal industry. In 2010, Josh cofounded Ortho Spine Companies, which is the parent company of Ortho Spine Distributors (OSD), Surg.io and Ortho Sales Partners (OSP). OSD is a searchable database that helps ease the frustration of finding orthopedic distributors throughout the country. Surg.io is a cutting edge software solution for manufacturers and hospitals to better manage their inventory in the orthopedic and spine service line. OSP is an end-to-end solution that helps companies approach the global market in a cost-efficient way. Our team has hundreds of years of experience and can help clients navigate the many challenges inherent in bringing new technologies to market through exit.

Introduction

Almost every company begins with the end in mind. It takes years and a lot of hard work to take a project from a napkin sketch to development only to have to get approved by the FDA and find surgeons willing to believe your research and that the product(s) you have produced are better for their patients. While it would be noble for that to be the only end goal, the company has shareholders that have put in considerable time and money with the hopes that proper execution will lead to an equity event of some sort. There are many possibilities for this event to take place. A list of these options include, but are not limited to, the following:

- Venture capital
- Private equity
- Initial public offering
- Merger
- Acquisition

In this chapter, we will look at the considerations that a company must consider in advance of a potential acquisition.

Preliminary Cautions

One of the most common first steps an entrepreneur makes after a successful patent or prototype development is to approach some of the large **strategics** in an effort to find a commercialization partner. The entrepreneur must be cautioned that these large companies are always more than willing to listen to innovative ideas, but rarely seriously consider a partnership or acquisition without some limited commercial success. The main risk associated with this technology reveal (even when done under NDA) is that the strategic can gain an immense amount of data about your product, idea, patent, and financing which offers them a strong competitive advantage in any eventual transaction discussions. It is critical for the entrepreneur to understand the complexity of this relationship and protect their idea and product's future by only revealing pertinent information at the appropriate times.

Understanding What an Acquirer Wants

When developing the corporate strategy, it is always a good exercise to look at recent examples of successful exits and to focus on the dynamics at play before and after the acquisition was completed. Sometimes, the circumstances are obvious, while others require some additional insight. Here are a few good questions to seek the answers to during the strategic planning process:

- Was the acquisition a pure technology play where the strategic was able to advance their entry by acquiring a platform technology? (e.g., Globus Medical purchasing Excelsius Surgical)
- Were the acquired companies' revenues **accretive** to their existing business? (e.g., Zimmer purchasing Biomet)
- Who were the surgeon champions and what involvement do they have to the acquiring entity? (e.g., NuVasive purchasing Vertera Spine)

- Was the acquired company in financial distress? (e.g., Arthrex purchasing Sonoma Orthopedics)
- Did the acquired company offer a sales channel in other countries that was attractive to the acquiring company? (e.g., Globus Medical purchasing Alphatec Spine's business outside the United States)

Every transaction happens for a reason. It is critical to understand the underlying circumstances to why a transaction happened so the business can be built in a manner that is attractive to potential strategic partners while maintaining the ability to build a sustainable business that can operate independently and quite possibly on the public market.

Building the Business

There are several dynamics that must align for a strategic to consider prior to engaging in an acquisition discussion. Many of these circumstances are outside of your control so the best course of action begins with building a strong foundation for sustainable business. There was a time in orthopedics where it seemed that companies wanted to rush a technology to the market, invest a minimal amount into operational infrastructure and inventory, and spend more time on product marketing than tracking clinical outcomes all while being able to show a strong initial growth trend. It has been said many times, "We want to be bought in 2 to 3 years." There are several issues with trying to build a business with this mindset.

First, to attract a surgeon to be an early adopter, strings are usually attached. Companies will enter into a development or consulting contract with a surgeon to help refine current products or develop future generations of products. On one hand, it is extremely necessary to have a "voice of the customer" in these development and refinement periods. However, from an acquirer's point of view, these contracts create obstacles to maintain the revenue after the change of control. There have been many examples of revenues collapsing after the acquisition has completed. Due to the significant interest displayed by the Office of the Inspector General (OIG) in recent years, it is incredibly important for the manufacturer to develop these programs delicately. They are necessary, but generally, the business that is tied to a consulting project will not count toward the revenue multiple during negotiations.

How the company establishes its sales force is also very important to the potential acquirer. For example, if one of the top five market share leaders is the potential buyer, they like to see controllable revenue. If the sales force is comprised entirely of nonexclusive independent sales agents or distributors, the probability of revenue evaporation is very high. Predictably, gaining access to sales intelligence and relationships is near impossible without a commitment from the acquiring company to allow the established agreement to survive the transaction. On the other hand, an early-stage company with limited resources cannot afford the high price of a direct or exclusive sales team. If a midcap company is the acquirer as part of a roll-up, they likely will be most interested in how much overlap there is between the two sales forces. It would be a positive for the acquiring company if during due diligence it is determined there is a low percentage of overlapping sales representatives.

In developing the sales strategy, there are several options that companies have attempted with mixed results. There is no one size fits all solution to establishing a sales force. It is critical to have a deep knowledge of where the products fit in the current landscape and how different regions can play a role in growing the business. If the company's products treat pathologies that are regionally specific, it might be wise to show a potential acquirer that the products can dominate a region that has a high volume of procedures. For example, if the product treats a condition that is most often found in elderly patients like osteoarthritis, deploying a focused effort in areas like Florida or Arizona where there is a larger population of patients can prove the model to a potential acquirer.

A third topic of interest, and possibly the most important, to the acquiring company is quality of sales. During the acquisition process, the due diligence team will examine which customers have used the product and how predictable the usage was thereafter. For example, if 10 surgeons used the technology and six of those surgeons stopped using it after a few surgeries, the acquiring company would want to know why the turnover was so significant. These data points are really important for them to know how well the suite of products will scale with their customer base and in their sales channel. Also, this information will help the company determine if there are issues they will need to deal with regarding instrumentation or implant performance.

As the company creates and executes its strategy, it is very important to consider the logic a potential acquirer will use when they evaluate the business. To experience a quality exit, it is very important that the percentage of customers that are tied to a consulting arrangement be kept to a minimum. A higher than average consultant to user ratio will dramatically decrease the value in an acquirer's eyes. It is also critical for the company to create a sales channel that can show immediate and sustainable success while also allowing the potential acquirer to feel comfortable that the products will maintain momentum during the arduous integration process. Lastly, keeping the focus on quality of sales over worrying specifically about quantity of sales will likely be well received by the acquiring company. The due diligence process is almost exclusively an exercise in risk mitigation, and the acquiring company will want to have comfort that after the integration process is complete, the revenue generated pretransaction will survive posttransaction.

Timing Is Everything

Timing is one of the most underrated elements of a successful exit. There have been countless companies that have experienced early success and have turned down offers that they would gladly accept years later. Timing affects the transaction process in two different ways.

1. When is the right time based on industry trends?
2. When is the optimal time to exit for maximum return to the shareholders?

First, it is critical that the management team and board of directors pay close attention to the trends of the industry. There have been violent shifts in the market based on a variety of reasons like political change or economic challenges. These issues can be identified as trends that take years to develop or they can happen practically overnight. It can be easy to focus so intently on the day-to-day challenges of a business that the broader perspective is completely lost. The management team must stay close to the customer and establish a culture of that is intently focused staying in the forefront of trends. It is a good idea to support and attend smaller scientific meetings to listen to what surgeons are talking about on a broader scale. These meetings offer an insight that is rarely seen in a competitive industry.

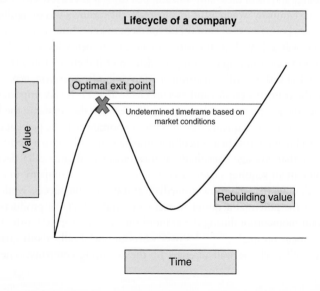

Determining the optimal time for an exit can be tricky to determine. Unlike industry trends, which are often objective, internal timing is highly subjective and contains many variables. Strategics will look at a business and determine the areas where they find value and that does not always synchronize with the target companies view on their own value. Here are a few areas that need to have a clear message and strategy prior to engaging in potential acquisition negotiations:

1. **Product development pipeline**—A good company is constantly developing updated generations of existing technologies or working to complete a product portfolio. The timelines can vary immensely but must be wisely prioritized to maximize value.

2. **Results of upcoming clinical results**—In today's climate, every company needs to be using advance analytics and traceability techniques to capture patient data. Using these data to produce peer-reviewed white papers can create tangible value to an acquirer, but if done right, the company will always be close to another milestone.

3. **Product recognition**—There are many different ways products can be recognized, but the most common are through media outlets, Congresses or Societies, and podium presence as invited faculty.

4. **Surgeon champions**—Who is using the product and the context of their relationship with the company can speak volumes to the potential acquirer.

5. **Sales force momentum**—The sales force should be consistently driving value and opportunities in the marketplace. The timing of an acquisition will always leave some potential value unrealized.

Typical Terms

Assuming the product has shown initial market success and a potential acquirer has shown interest in engaging in transaction discussions, what can the entrepreneur expect as it relates to deal structure? Deals can and will have their own character because no two deals are the same. However, the elements will have a common look and feel. You should expect a successful transaction to be a mixture of cash, equity, and milestones. Here is a quick breakdown of each of these elements:

1. **Cash**—Cash would represent the most secure component of the transaction. This is the amount of money the acquirer will pay the target entity at the close of the transaction. This is the clearest representation of how much value the acquirer has truly considered in the product or company. The cash component of the transaction

can be based on a variety of factors but the most common include revenue, profitability (earnings before interest, taxes, depreciation, and amortization [EBITDA]), and product pipeline epth.

2. **Equity**—To lighten the impact on the balance sheet, acquirers usually offer some form of equity in their company in the transaction. If the acquirer is a publically traded company, the value is pretty easy to determine and potentially liquidate. However, if the acquirer is also a privately held entity, the value is much less clear. One can expect the value to be determined on the last valuation of that business (likely their last funding event), but that could have been several years prior or determined during the mutual due diligence period. Also, it is critically important to determine what preference the shares are and if they are subject to potential dilution in later rounds. Owing to the complexities of this component, be sure to engage an experienced representative that will ensure the entrepreneur's best interests are considered.

3. **Milestones**—This is another area that can be quite difficult to evaluate. If the deal is structured to be milestone heavy, it will be certain that the acquiring company will offer dazzling spreadsheets that impress greatly. The reality, however, is that these milestones rarely come to fruition due to a variety of potential issues. Market conditions play a big part and can create unforeseen challenges. The acquirer could have a change in leadership that loses the intensity or focus of the product. Other situations that have been seen include the following:
   a. Inability of the acquirer to integrate the business or product (e.g., Zimmer Spine acquiring Abbott Spine).
   b. Sales team's inability to convert or integrate the business or product (e.g., Medtronic acquiring Kyphon and losing 50% of revenue).
   c. Ineffective operational support/product supply issues (e.g., RTI Surgical acquiring Pioneer Surgical).
   d. Acquirer ends up being purchased (e.g., Kyphon acquires St. Francis Medical Technologies in 12/2006 and is acquired by Medtronic in 7/2007).

Developing an idea or product and creating a business is an exhilarating process. The entrepreneur will experience a litany of emotions during the process: excitement, fear, anger, joy, hope, and confusion. This chapter was designed to help create some comfort as the journey is set to begin. Be objective and build the business with the end in mind to ensure the last emotion experienced is not anguish.

KEY TAKEAWAY POINTS

- ▶ It is important to build a sustainable company and not be overly focused on a quick exit. Companies that are "built to sell" with a weak foundation rarely experience an exit.

- ▶ Do not rush to the strategics in hopes of a distribution partnership. These types of relationships rarely work out the way they are envisioned.

- ▶ Guard your secrets. Even disclosure after an NDA does not fully protect you from creating a competitor.

- ▶ Be in tune with the market dynamics. There is an optimal time for a transaction, and you do not want to miss that window.

- ▶ Have a realistic value in mind so you do not miss the opportunity to exit at the optimal point. If that timing is missed, it could require your company to demonstrate the ability to scale and that can take years to achieve.

CHAPTER 22

Concept to Commercialization Case #1: Pioneering the X-Stop Interspinous Decompression Device

ALEXANDER ROSINSKI, ROMAN DIMOV,
JEREMI LEASURE, JAMES ZUCHERMAN, KEN HSU

ABOUT THE AUTHORS

Alexander Rosinski, MS

Alexander is a medical student at the University of California, Irvine. He received a bachelor's degree in biochemistry from the University of Washington and a Master of Science in global health at UCSF. He is currently a research fellow at the San Francisco Orthopaedic Residency Program.

Roman Dimov

Roman is a premedical student at Stanford University.

Jeremi Leasure, MSE

Jeremi is the San Francisco Orthopaedic Residency Program's Director of Research. He received a B.S. in mechanical engineering at Temple University and a Master of Science in mechanical engineering from Drexel University. He has conducted numerous biomechanical studies, and his work has appeared in the *Spine Journal*, *Journal of Neurosurgery*, and *Global Spine Journal*. Jeremi works closely with orthopedic surgeons to develop new surgical techniques and devices. He has invented and developed several orthopedic implants including SIMFix by Bonsano Medical and AVANCE by Originate Life Science.

James F. Zucherman, MD

Dr Jim Zucherman is a board-certified orthopedic surgeon who specializes in the surgical treatment of degenerative conditions of the spine. He graduated with honors from the University of Southern California in 1970, and he received his medical degree from the Baylor College of Medicine, Houston, Texas, in 1974. He completed his internship at Los Angeles County USC General Hospital in 1975 and a general surgery residency at Mt. Zion Medical Center in 1977. Subsequently, he completed his orthopedic surgery residency at the San Francisco Orthopaedic Residency Program in 1981 and a pediatric/orthopedic spine surgery fellowship at the Duchess of Kent Children's Orthopaedic Hospital at the University of Hong Kong in 1982.

Dr Jim Zucherman has pioneered numerous surgical techniques. He developed and performed the first laparoscopic lumbar spinal fusion as well as the first percutaneous cervical diskectomy in the United States. With his partners Dr Hsu and White, he performed the first pedicle screw instrumentation case west of the Mississippi. He has been a Principal FDA investigator for many clinical trials involving new technologies for the lumbar and cervical spine. He has been a principal investigator for Prodisc and Flexicore lumbar disk replacement FDA trials, minimally invasive X-Stop and Wallace device FDA trials, and Cervicore and Prestige cervical disk replacement trials. He has authored numerous publications in peer-reviewed journals and surgical textbooks and has presented his research at conferences worldwide. He is currently developing the Staflex motion-preservation minimally invasive spine stabilization device through Spartek, Inc. Dr Zucherman's special interests include interspinous process decompression, motion-preservation in the cervical/lumbar spine, and total disk arthroplasty.

Ken Hsu, MD

Dr Ken Hsu received his medical degree at the State University of New York Downstate Medical Center in 1976 and completed his internship at Loma Linda Medical Center. He completed a general surgery residency at Mt. Zion Hospital in San Francisco and an orthopedic surgery residency at the San Francisco Orthopaedic Residency Program, where he has continued to serve as a faculty member for nearly two and a half decades. Following his residency, Dr Hsu completed a fellowship in Spine and Pediatric Orthopaedic Surgery at the University of Hong Kong, one of the world's premiere centers of surgical spine care. He is currently a spine surgeon at St. Mary's Medical Center in San Francisco.

Ken Hsu has served as the President of San Francisco Orthopaedic Surgeons Medical Group since 2003 and as a director of spine services at St. Mary's Spine Center since 1988. Dr Hsu is world-renowned as a coinventor of the X-Stop device, a minimally invasive surgical solution for patients with symptomatic lumbar spinal stenosis and the first interspinous decompression device (IPD) to be approved by the FDA for use in the United States. He has presented at numerous national and international spine surgery conferences. Dr Hsu has also authored numerous peer-reviewed publications and book chapters in surgical textbooks. He was among the first spine surgeons to use pedicle screw fixation of the spine in the Western United States. Well-known for his astuteness and unique humor, Dr Hsu has participated in numerous clinical trials of spine surgical devices, including the X-Stop, Flexicore and Prodisc lumbar total disk replacements, and the Cervicore cervical total disk replacement.

Step 1. Patient Zero Was Studied

O! for muse of fire, that would ascend the brightest heaven of invention **WILLIAM SHAKESPEARE**

The story of X-Stop's commercialization starts with a severe adverse event during surgery and the necessity to prevent it from happening again. In 1996, an elderly man, after laminectomies for multilevel lumbar stenosis, awoke disoriented not remembering who he was or where he was from. That patient never regained his mental function, though the spinal stenosis symptoms resolved. This case served as an impetus to look for an approach that may obviate general anesthesia.

Step 2. The Reason for Treatment Was Studied

Somewhere, something incredible is waiting to be known **CARL SAGAN**

The X-Stop was invented based on a thorough understanding of a very common disease, such as lumbar spinal stenosis.

Lumbar spinal stenosis (LSS) was first described as a narrowing of the spinal canals associated with leg pain and atrophy. This was in 1803 by Portal of France.[1] Further reports from Verbiest and Kirkaldy-Willis defined our understanding of the diseases development. Starting with and completely involving degenerative changes in both facets and disk, abnormal motion and stability lead to osteophyte formation.[1] This osteophyte formation together with hypertrophy of the facets and an intervertebral disk protruding into the canal combine to restrict neural element space. The most common presenting symptom of this disease is neurogenic intermittent claudication (NIC).[1-3] The symptoms usually were well known to be **posture-dependent**, being relieved by positions of lumbar flexion such as sitting or pushing a shopping cart.[1,2,4] Further investigation revealed a link between relief of symptoms and an increase in canal diameter during this forward flexion as displayed in Figure 22.1. The goal further developed, the minimally invasive solution requiring only local anesthetic would need to alleviate the symptoms of lumbar spinal stenosis by maintaining a forward flexion at the affected level. Stephen Kuslich had shown that lumbar diskectomies could be routinely performed under local anesthesia. The postural dynamic of neurogenic intermittent claudication was consistent in many cases and explained by the spinal canal size change in lumbar extension versus flexion (noted anecdotally on myelograms). A terminal extension blocking device was conceived that could be placed outside the spinal canal under local anesthesia. As many patients had no

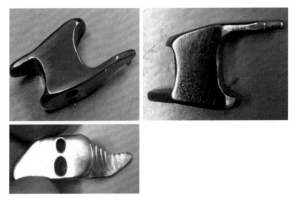

Figure 22.1 First-in-human prototype of the X-Stop implant. Single-component, stainless steel construction. This design was implanted in one patient.

symptoms in the flexed sitting position, if they were able to maintain that position in standing at the stenotic segments, the claudication symptoms should resolve.

Step 3. The Innovations That Had Come Before Were Studied

If you steal from one author it's plagiarism; if you steal from many its research   WILSON MIZNER

The posture-dependent nature of the disease suggested nonrigid fixation was required, to halt motion during extension and allow motion during flexion. At the time of X-Stop's invention, it was generally thought that metallic internal fixation would become painful in a nonfused spinal segment. This created some initial hesitation; however, there were several reports of a nonrigid fixation technique via the interspinous process space. A more thorough understanding was developed.

During the 90s, a growth in the field of orthopedic biomechanics further developed a wide variety of implant technologies.[5] During this period, the field was making giant leaps investigating nonrigid stabilization of the spine spine.[6] Interspinous spacers were an existing nonrigid stabilization concept, put into practice in the 1950s with the publication of the Knowles vertebral distraction method.[7] Next was the Wallis implant, first developed in 1986, aimed for nonrigid stabilization of lumbar spine.[8] It included a titanium interspinous blocker and an artificial dacron ligament. The implant constituted a "floating system" without bony fixation, eliminating loosening. A second generation of this implant was made of polyetheretherketone (PEEK).

Prior to X-Stop, all of these interspinous implants were used to treat disk or nucleus pulposus herniation and segmental instability. The work ahead was to develop an embodiment of this concept to treat lumbar spinal stenosis with a minimally invasive method, using local anesthesia.

Step 4. The Seed-Stage Team Members Were Assembled

Great things in business are never done by one person. They're done by a team of people STEVE JOBS

The X-Stop's journey from concept to commercialization begins with the assembly of individuals and organizations that participated in its formation. The composition of the founding X-Stop team was an entrepreneur, an engineer, and two orthopedic surgeons.

Entrepreneur Mr Henry Klyce was responsible for organizing the business and fundraising efforts. Mr Klyce was a serial entrepreneur of medical device companies, prior to the X-Stop. He had cofounded and developed several companies to acquisition. He had just sold his percutaneous diskectomy and fusion cage company, subsequently serving on the Board of the purchasing company, as Chairman.

Mechanical engineer Mr Burney Winslow was responsible for the design, production, and quality of the device. Mr Winslow was a VP-level engineer with experience in operations, research and development, and engineering management, prior to X-Stop. He worked with Mr Klyce in Surgical Dynamics to develop percutaneous disk removal systems and interbody implants.

Dr James Zucherman and Dr Ken Hsu were responsible for the design of the device, delivery of the device, and leading the clinical investigation. In 1982, Dr Zucherman started practice as an orthopedic spine surgeon at St. Mary's, a teaching hospital in San Francisco. In 1984, Dr Ken Hsu joined Dr Zucherman in practice where they performed the first United States pedicle screw fixation west of the Mississippi. They were the first to publish this new technique in the United States. Both surgeons pushed the development of minimally invasive techniques. Dr Zucherman performed the first percutaneous cervical diskectomy 1987 and first laparoscopic anterior spine surgery in the world in 1992. They had started the San Francisco Combined Spine Fellowship with Stanford University and were prominent faculty members at their alma mater San Francisco Orthopaedic Residency Program. Their body of work had been focused on the improvement of spine surgery with emphasis to develop minimally invasive surgery, internal fixation techniques, prior to X-Stop.

Step 5. The Solution Was Invented

One might think that the money value of an invention constitutes its reward to the man who loves his work. But... I continue to find my greatest pleasure, and so my reward, in the work that precedes what the world calls success   THOMAS A EDISON

In 1997, the X-Stop was invented. The initial sketches of its design were drawn on a paper placemat at a small luncheonette, Straits Café on 3300 Geary Blvd in San Francisco, CA.[9]

Several design features were considered. A feature to separate the spinous processes and limit extension motion between the vertebrae was key. Additionally, the spacer needed a smooth convex profile with no sharp edges that could damage the adjacent bone. Design features to prevent migration were also a priority. Wings on either side of the spacer would prevent migration. These wings could abut the cranial and caudal spinous processes to prevent lateral migration and against the lamina to prevent anterior migration. The congruency of the convex spacer and concave interspinous process space should allow as much bone surface contact as possible to spread bone implant stress concentration. A bullet-nose tissue expander should be included on the insertion tip of the implant for lateral insertion through the interspinous process ligament, preserving the supraspinous ligament and its insertions.

Preserving the supraspinous ligament would prevent posterior migration, prevent overdistraction, increase stability, and possibly allow for cantilever unloading of the middle and anterior columns of the treated motion segment. A small incision would require a small single device or several small components that could be assembled inside the body.

Step 6. Prototypes Were Built and Feasibility Studies Quickly Performed

Success is no accident. It is hard work, perseverance, learning, studying, sacrifice and most of all, love of what you are doing or learning to do   PELE

The earliest prototype for the X-Stop device was a single-component construction of stainless steel. An embodiment of this first prototype is displayed in Figure 22.1. It was created in 1997 with manual machining and finishing processes derived specifically for each of the pilot study patients, based on preoperative X-rays of the interspinous space size.

Cadaveric laboratory sessions were essential to the development of the surgical technique and early feasibility assessments. These early labs brought the surgeons, engineers, and marketers together to collaborate and iterate.

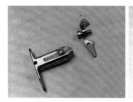 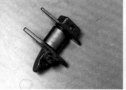 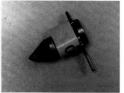

Figure 22.2 Later, multicomponent embodiments of the X-Stop device. The second generation (left) was implanted in nine patients. The fourth and fifth (middle and right) were implanted during X-Stops wide commercial release.

From these labs, key steps in the surgical technique were developed including placing the patient in flexion, accessing the operative level, interspinous ligament dilation, distraction techniques, insertion techniques, and mechanical stability. The first instrumentation set comprised a scalpel, curved dilator, lamina spreaders, and an implant insertion handle. All instruments, with the exception of the insertion handle, were off-the-shelf surgical tools.

The first-generation single-piece design proved too difficult to insert reliably. Altering the design to a two-piece ("keeper wing" and "main body") second-generation implant greatly solved delivery as shown in Figure 22.2, left. This embodiment was implanted in nine patients during a pilot study described later in the chapter.

The third generation of the device was multicomponent as well, implanted in 22 patients during a second pilot study. A critical design flaw caused the device to disassemble and required a revised "welded" version.

The fourth and most widely marketed generation of the device featured the oval-shaped titanium central spacer to further protect the adjacent spinous process bone as shown in Figure 22.2, middle. This was later converted to a fifth generation PEEK spacer after market introduction, shown in Figure 22.2, right.

Step 7. The Pilot Study Was Performed

The sea, once it casts its spell, holds one in its net of wonders forever **JACQUES YVES COUSTEAU**

A pilot study included 10 patients with neurogenic intermittent claudication with lumbar spinal stenosis from focal disease. Only patients with good sitting tolerance were considered proper candidates. Eight of the ten were markedly improved in symptoms, and to the surprise of the team, none of the patients exhibited local pain from the implant.

Interspinous decompression for the treatment of neurogenic claudication due to lumbar spinal stenosis had never been marketed before X-Stop. This is fertile territory for commercialization and a minefield for the risk-averse FDA. Medical literature on the technique served as a provisional predicate for safety and efficacy; however, FDA had no history in its records of a device sold for this purpose, and so it compelled a report of the results of X-Stop's small clinical trial.

FDA accepted the results of the pilot study through its investigational device exemption (IDE). This exemption allows the device to be used in a clinical study in order to collect safety and effectiveness data. Clinical studies are most often conducted to support a premarket approval (PMA). Only a small percentage of 510(k)s require clinical data to support the application. Investigational use also includes clinical evaluation of certain modifications or new intended uses of legally marketed devices. All clinical evaluations of investigational devices, unless exempt, must have an approved IDE before the study is initiated.

Step 8. The Corporate Entity Was Organized for X-Stop Production and Distribution

Great companies are built on great products   ELON MUSK

The X-Stop was first manufactured and marketed by St. Francis Medical Technologies (SFMT). The company was founded in 1997. Mr Henry Klyce served as President and CEO. Mr Burney Winslow was its VP of Engineering. For regulatory purposes, SFMT organized as a specification developer for X-Stop. The product would be distributed under its name but would perform no manufacturing.

Marketing operations were coordinated with education being a critical component. The X-Stop design altered preexisting interspinous technology to meet the specific needs of lumbar spinal stenosis. Hospitals and insurance providers would need to confirm cost/benefit to existing alternatives, and surgeons would need evidence that a quicker surgery did not produce poor decompression results. Furthermore, sales of the X-Stop required FDA approval, after the results of a randomized controlled trial. The device was approved overseas and was being sold in Europe and Japan before U.S. FDA approval.

A capital investment was needed to support these operations. SFMT opened their Series-A Round of investor funding in 2000. USVP was the first outside investor, buying $2 million of shares in the company at a valuation of $8 million.

Step 9. A Level One Randomized Controlled Trial Was Performed

Skeptical scrutiny is the means, in both science and religion, by which deep thoughts can be winnowed from deep nonsense   CARL SAGAN

A total of 191 patients were enrolled in a prospective, randomized, controlled trial. The trial was conducted over a 15-month period from May 2000 to July 2001. A total of 136 X-Stop devices were implanted in 100 of the patients. The trial was conducted by the surgeons and associated medical centers listed in Table 22.1. The X-Stop procedure was intended to be performed under local anesthesia and remote in location from neurologic structures. This was so dissimilar from standard of care laminectomy or laminectomy with fusion that nonoperative treatment including at least one epidural injection was selected as the most meaningful control.

Table 22.1 List of Surgeons and Hospitals That Participated in the X-Stop Randomized Controlled Trial

Principal Investigator(s)	Institution and Location
Dr James Zucherman and Dr Ken Hsu	St Mary's Hospital, San Francisco, California
Dr Charles Hartjen	Greater Baltimore Medical Center, Baltimore, Maryland
Dr Thomas Mehalic	Maine Medical Center, Portland, Maine
Dr Dante Implicito	Hackensack University Medical Center, Paramus, New Jersey
Dr Michael Martin	Tacoma General Hospital, Tacoma, Washington
Dr Donald Johnson	East Cooper Medical Center, Mount Pleasant, South Carolina
Dr Grant Skidmore	East Virginia Medical School, Norfolk, Virginia
Dr Paul Vessa and Dr James Dwyer	Somerset Medical Center, Somerset, New Jersey
Dr Stephen Puccio	Orthopaedic Specialists of Bethlehem, Bethlehem, Pennsylvania
Dr Joseph Cauthen	North Florida Regional Medical Center, Gainesville, Florida
Dr Richard Ozuna	Brigham and Women's Hospital, Boston, Massachusetts

The X-Stop team was able to complete a nine-center level one RCT just 4 years after the implant's invention at Straits Café in 1997. This pace of outreach and engagement was due, in no small part, to Dr Zucherman, Dr Hsu, and Mr Klyce's notoriety in the field of spine surgery. In the 5 years between X-Stop's patient zero in 1996 and the enrollment of the last X-Stop RCT patient in 2001, Dr Zucherman and Dr Hsu presented their work at over 20 conferences. At those conferences, the first users of the X-Stop were cultivated. Mr Klyce's history at the helm of numerous medical device companies selling products to spine surgeons across the country provided SFMT the access they required at each of the nine medical centers.

The results of this trial concluded the efficacy of X-Stop was significantly greater than nonoperative treatment. The results also indicated X-Stop safe and effective for the treatment of neurogenic intermittent claudication patients, compared with nonoperative treatment.

Step 10. X-Stop Was Sold Outside the United States While Waiting for FDA Approval

Patience is not simply the ability to wait – it's how we behave while we're waiting JOYCE MEYER

The X-Stop received CE mark (equivalent to 510 k in Europe) and Japan approval long before FDA PMA. After completion of the successful RCT surgeries in 2001, the X-Stop team submitted applications for FDA marketing approval and European CE marking. Its CE mark was granted in 2002, and its FDA approval, in 2005. In those 3 years, X-Stop was made commercially available in markets outside of the United States (Figure 22.3). A listing of the countries in which the device was commercially available, prior to FDA approval, is included below in Table 22.2.

Step 11. Regulatory Approval Was Granted

A truly strong person does not need the approval of others any more than a lion needs the approval of sheep VERNON HOWARD

X-Stop required a special review panel of outside experts as it was the first device of its kind. The FDA panel meeting resulted in nonapproval recommendation, due to lack of in vivo evidence on the effect of the devices.

Over the next year after the panel voted nonapproval, further evidence was gathered. Using standing MRI, Siddequi, et al showed that the device enlarged the treated spinal canals and did not cause significant kyphosis in single-or double-level applications. A large series of mechanical and

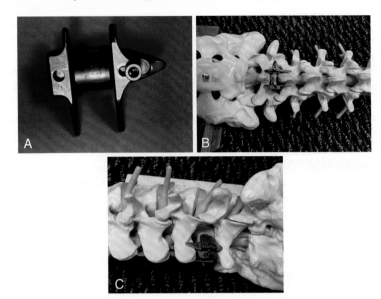

Figure 22.3 The first commercial release of the X-Stop (A) and a demonstration of its placement using a saw bones lumbar spine model (B and C).

Table 22.2 Use of X-Stop in Other Countries Prior to U.S. FDA Approval	
Australia	Netherlands
Austria	New Zealand
Czech Republic	Norway
Denmark	South Africa
Germany	Spain
Greece	Sweden
Israel	Switzerland
Italy	Turkey
Japan	United Kingdom

biomechanical studies were performed before FDA would approve the application. Strength and function mechanical tests were performed at the component and assembly-level of the device.

Biomechanical studies investigating the strength and demands placed on the spinous process were performed. The X-Stop's ability to distract the canal and foramen was quantified.

Standardized multidirectional bending flexibility testing was performed to quantify X-Stop effects on kinematics and stability of the spinal column.

The device was given marketing release in November 2005, about 1 year after the FDA panel meeting. The last patient at 2-year follow-up was in July 2003. The date of the notice of approval sent to SFMT was November 2005, representing a 17-month delay in the regulatory approval process.

It was approved as a class III device through the FDA PMA process. X-Stop received approval to market the following indications and contraindications. The X-Stop was indicated for treatment of patients aged 50 years or older suffering from neurogenic intermittent claudication secondary to a confirmed diagnosis of lumbar spinal stenosis (with X-ray, MRI, and/or CT evidence of thickened ligamentum flavum, narrowed lateral recess, foramen and/or central canal narrowing). The X-Stop is indicated for those patients with moderately impaired physical function who experience relief in flexion from their symptoms of leg/buttock/groin pain, with or without back pain, and have undergone a regimen of at least 6 months of nonoperative treatment. The X-Stop may be implanted at one or two lumbar levels in patients in whom operative treatment is indicated at no more than two levels.

The X-Stop was contraindicated in patients with an allergy to titanium or titanium alloy, spinal anatomy, or disease that would prevent implantation of the device or cause the device to be unstable in situ, such as

- significant instability of the lumbar spine, e.g., isthmic spondylolisthesis or degenerative spondylolisthesis greater than grade 1.0 (on a scale of 1-4);
- an ankylosed segment at the affected level(s);
- acute fracture of the spinous process or pars interarticularis;
- significant scoliosis (Cobb angle greater than 20°).
- Cauda equina syndrome defined as neural compression causing neurogenic bowel or bladder dysfunction;
- diagnosis of severe osteoporosis, defined as bone mineral density (from DEXA scan or some comparable study) in the spine or hip that is more than 2.5 SD below the mean of adult normals in the presence of one or more fragility fractures;
- active systemic infection or infection localized to the site of implantation.

Step 12. Released to the Market

The release date is just one day, but the record is forever   BRUCE SPRINGSTEEN

Through the commercial release, surgeon education and conference presence continued.

Between the years of 2001 and 2006, Dr Zucherman and Dr Hsu both presented at over 75 conferences, bringing X-Stop's interspinous process decompression around the world.

Step 13. X-Stop Was Brought to as Many People as Possible

Life finds its purpose and fulfillment in the expansion of happiness   MAHARISHI MAHESH YOGI

Between the years of 2006 and 2011, the commercialization effort focused on adding to the list of patients who could benefit from X-Stop. A study of lumbar spinal stenosis patients suffering from additional instability (spondylolisthesis) at the operative level showed improvement of symptoms 2 years after surgery. Patient satisfaction was investigated in 2006, and a novel development to the technique involving the use of PMMA augmentation of the spinous processes was reported. A one-year follow-up of scoliosis patients reported good results in 2010. In 2011, both facet cysts and sagittal imbalance were shown to be effectively treated with X-Stop in 6 month and immediate post-op studies.

Step 14. A Successful Exit

Affairs are easier of entrance than of exit; and it is but common prudence to see our way out before we venture in.   AESOP

In September 2006, SFMT announced that it had filed an S1 registration document with the SEC for an initial public offering of its common stock.

In January 2007, Kyphon Inc. acquired SFMT for $525 million in cash, just 13 months after receiving its approval to market the X-Stop. The purchase agreement included additional contingent payments of up to $200 million for a total of $725 million in cash.

In August of that same year, Kyphon completed its payment of more than $200 million as a direct result of its own acquisition by Medtronic.

Step 15. After Concept to Commercialization

Pioneers get slaughtered, and the settlers prosper   DAYMOND JOHN

X-Stop was awarded the *Wall Street Journal's* Technology of the Year Award in 2006. At present, there are more than 60 companies worldwide making different variations of the X- Stop. This "me too" competition combined with a trend away from nonrigid fixation in the spine decreased X-Stop's market share. In 2016, Medtronic pulled the device from the market, citing an inability to support postmarket surveillance activities.

Since the commercialization of the X-Stop, Mr Klyce founded Spartek Medical, Inc, a developer of spinal implants. Mr Winslow served as VP of Research & Development for Spartek, both continuing work with Dr Hsu and Dr Zucherman who served as Clinical Partners for the company. Mr Klyce is listed as an inventor in over 70 patents.

After more than 800 cases of interspinous process spacer surgery, including X-Stop surgery, Dr Hsu and Dr Zucherman continue to practice orthopedic spine surgery in San Francisco at the St. Mary's Spine Center. They have each published more than 100 peer-reviewed journal articles and book chapters in spine surgery.

KEY TAKEAWAY POINTS

- ▶ The innovation for the X-Stop was borne from a clearly defined necessity to treat lumbar spinal stenosis with the use of local anesthesia.

- ▶ Studying the scientific literature simplified the critical requirement to decompress the affected level.

- ▶ X-Stop relied on the historical concept of interspinous process decompression, reducing feasibility risks.

- ▶ Each team member brought specialized skill sets with years of practical experience.

- ▶ Design features were systematically developed to address the primary requirements of nonrigid fixation and being minimally invasive.

- ▶ Major revisions to the design were considered and implemented throughout the premarket and even postmarket process.

- ▶ From these initial patients, the critical requirements of treating lumbar spinal stenosis under local anesthesia were achieved.

- ▶ Conference participation was critical to educate surgeons on an old technique to solve a different problem.

- ▶ A history of relentless participation at medical conferences and business development with medical centers, facilitated X-Stop's rapid outreach and engagement.

- ▶ Outside US sales helped support the growth of the business while the FDA approval was pending.

- ▶ The PMA process took longer than expected and extensive further in vivo, and biomechanical laboratory testing was required in addition to the RCT.

- ▶ Academic conference participation aided in the distribution of X-Stop

- ▶ Expanding the types of patients who would benefit from X-Stop helped distribution.

- ▶ Acquisition cash was released in phases and dependent on market performance.

REFERENCES AND RESOURCES

1. Abrams J, Zucherman J. Interspinous spacers. In: Eck J, Vaccaro A, eds. *Surgical Atlas of Spinal Operations.* New Delhi: Jaypee Brothers Medical Publishers Ltd; 2013.

2. Mavrogenis A, Megaloikonomos P, Panagopoulos G, Maffulli N. Biomechanics in orthopaedics. *J Biomed.* 2017;2:89-93.

3. Gomleksiz C, Sasani M, Oktenoglu T, Ozer AF. A short history of posterior dynamic stabilization. *Adv Orthop.* 2012;2012:629698.

4. Senegas J. Mechanical supplementation by non-rigid fixation in degenerative intervertebral lumbar segments: the Wallis system. *Eur Spine J.* 2002;11(suppl 2):S164-S169.

5. Anderson PA, Tribus CB, Kitchel SH. Treatment of neurogenic claudication by interspinous decompression: application of the X STOP device in patients with lumbar degenerative spondylolisthesis. *J Neurosurg Spine.* 2006;4(6):463-471.

6. Hsu KY, Zucherman JF, Hartjen CA, et al. Quality of life of lumbar stenosis-treated patients in whom the X STOP interspinous device was implanted. *J Neurosurg Spine.* 2006;5(6):500-507.

7. Idler C, Zucherman JF, Yerby S, Hsu KY, Hannibal M, Kondrashov D. A novel technique of intra-spinous process injection of PMMA to augment the strength of an inter-spinous process device such as the X STOP. *Spine.* 2008;33(4):452-456.

8. Rolfe KW, Zucherman JF, Kondrashov DG, Hsu KY, Nosova E. Scoliosis and interspinous decompression with the X-STOP: prospective minimum 1-year outcomes in lumbar spinal stenosis. *Spine J.* 2010;10(11):972-978.

9. Abrams J, Hsu K, Kondrashov D, McDermott T, Zucherman J. Treatment of facet cysts associated with neurogenic intermittent claudication with x-stop. *J Spinal Disord Tech.* 2013;26(4):218-221.

CHAPTER 23

IlluminOss: The World's First Patient-Conforming Polymer Intramedullary Implant

ROBERT A. RABINER

ABOUT THE AUTHOR

Robert A. Rabiner is a medical device entrepreneur and the Founder and Chief Technical Officer of IlluminOss Medical, Inc., located in East Providence, RI. Bob has led successful product and corporate enterprise launches, acquired and integrated new technologies, and directed external partnerships at a number of medical device companies. Prior to founding IlluminOss, he was president of Selva Medical (sold to WL Gore in 2006) and was founder, president, and CEO of OmniSonics Medical Technologies. He has also held executive-level positions at American Cyanamid, United States Healthcare and Hospital Products Ltd., Australia. Bob has been a member of the World Economic Forum's Technology Pioneers Program since 2003 and is one of Fast Company's "Fast 50 Champions of Innovation" for his medical technologies. He is the named inventor on over 78 US-issued patents and over 125 issued patents worldwide and has many additional patent applications pending.

The Background to Intramedullary Fracture Fixation

The first attempts in intramedullary fracture fixation were recorded in the 16th century by Spanish explorers in South America during their battles with the Aztec Indians, who stabilized long bone fractures with wooden bars placed within the intramedullary canal. At the start of the last century, various materials, such as bone, metal, or silver bars, were tried out in the quest to achieve adequate intramedullary stabilization.

The history of modern intramedullary nail (IMN) osteosynthesis began over 70 years ago with Gerhard Küntscher. On November 9, 1939, Küntscher was the first surgeon to treat a patient at the University Clinic at Kiel with a so-called dynamically stable intramedullary osteosynthesis known as intramedullary ("IM") nailing.

In March of 1940, Küntscher introduced the procedure he had developed at the 64th Annual Convention of the German Surgery Association. As this happened during World War II, technical developments, dissemination, and basic medical research on the principles of IMN osteosynthesis were delayed. During this time, most research was strictly limited to the shaft of long bones, but some attempts were made to include fractures close to joints. After the war, basic research and development work could be expanded, and word on Küntscher's principle of intramedullary splinting spread rapidly. The establishment of IMN osteosynthesis was on a roll. Küntscher called the principle he developed an "elastic fixation of the implant inside the intramedullary canal." His process resulted in a stable osteosynthesis in the shaft area, which was successful even without opening the fracture zone; however, it provided no rotational or axial stability.

The use of an intramedullary canal reamer allowed an application of this procedure for fractures at the diametaphyseal transition, as reaming of the intramedullary canal improved its inside shafting. Reaming the intramedullary canal and the associated disruption of endosteal perfusion was considered a major cause for the commonly occurring complication of deep intramedullary infection. Knowledge and relevance of intramedullary canal perfusion led to the idea to combine the proven principle of IM nailing with the benefits of a biological osteosynthesis.

Gerhard Küntscher provided the basic foundation for this concept. His principle of de-tensioning explained why it was wrong to completely immobilize and compress a fracture during surgery in order to achieve a union. The pressure applied to a fracture gap by compression increases the stability but does not promote healing of the bone. This hypothesis, which was derived from Küntscher's basic research, was confirmed in 1987 during a clinical follow-up study series. This study series at the University of Kiel provided clear proof that the rate of post-op deformities was very high; however, there were no nonunions when using IM nailing.

The demand for more biological data on IM nailing was first answered by Klemm and Schellmann in 1971, who under the sponsorship of Küntscher developed a method for intramedullary nail osteosynthesis with locking screw. This technique provided stability against rotational forces and axial loads.

Today's state of IM nailing is marked by an almost unmanageable variety of implants. During recent years, the IM nailing environment has been mainly marked by the general demand for better preservation of the intramedullary canal perfusion, which has led to an increased interest in developing unreamed nails with the smallest diameters possible.

PLASTICS IN MEDICINE

In the 50s, plastics became increasingly interesting for medical researchers. The clinical use of polymers began in the 60s, not only for economic reasons, but primarily for hygienic reasons. The use of sterile disposable products made of plastic resulted in a significant reduction of infections. Earlier, instruments were made of glass and metallic materials and were reused many times. An increasing number of polymers and an increasing demand for medical treatments in the last 40 years have led to the rapid establishment of plastic applications in medicine. The product variety is very extensive and encompasses everything from low-cost disposables to implants for virtually any field of medicine. Common applications are, for example, implants such as artificial heart valves, hip joints or vascular endoprosthetics, disposables such as catheters or tubing systems, or resorbable structures such as sutures and stents. The use of tissue cultures or medication release systems is described in current literature. Meanwhile 45% of all engineered medical products worldwide are made of a wide variety of plastic materials.

IlluminOss Bone Stabilization System

The IlluminOss photodynamic bone stabilization system is a new procedure for minimally invasive intramedullary stabilization of long bones and uses a polymer that is cured inside the medullary canal of the bone.

The system consists of a polyethylene terephthalate (PET) (Dacron) balloon mounted on a flexible 3 mm diameter catheter and a photodynamic monomer that is cured within 200 to 800 seconds using a visible blue light with a wavelength of 436 nm (Figures 23.1 and 23.2).

An approximately 5-mm-wide puncture incision is placed at any point above the long bone, followed by preparation of the bone and opening of the intramedullary canal via broach or burr (Figure 23.3).

A small diameter flexible guidewire is inserted through the pathway created to traverse the intramedullary canal. The guidewire may assist in reduction of the fracture or may work in conjunction with other instrumentation delivered via the guidewire.

Once in place, the catheter from the system should be guided through the bone and placed spanning the fracture site. This is accomplished by the catheter (sheath and obturator) being delivered in a monorail fashion over the guidewire (Figure 23.4).

Next, the closed or open reduction temporary stabilizes the fracture using appropriate clamps or other mechanical assistive means. Once reduced, a balloon implant of a specific length or diameter (as anatomically appropriate) mounted to flexible catheter is introduced into the

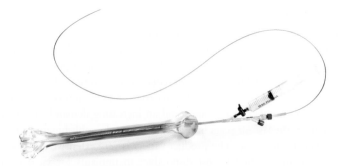

Figure 23.1 Flexible balloon catheter with fiber-optic cable, For balloon inflation, a syringe filled with the monomer is attached to a three-way valve. The balloon then is deployed inside the intramedullary canal, where it conforms to the contour of the canal. (Courtesy of IlluminOss Medical.)

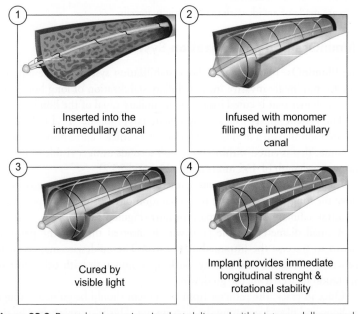

① Inserted into the intramedullary canal

② Infused with monomer filling the intramedullary canal

③ Cured by visible light

④ Implant provides immediate longitudinal strength & rotational stability

Figure 23.2 Procedural overview. Implant delivered within intramedullary canal, infused with monomer, expanding the implant, application of 436 nm light polymerizing the monomer, cured implant. (Courtesy of IlluminOss Medical.)

intramedullary canal via the sheath. Radiopaque markers on the outside of the balloon assist in visibility after implantation.

Once the tear-away sheath has been removed from the balloon, the balloon can be infused with monomer, expanding it to size.

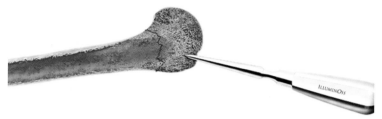

Figure 23.3 Opening of the intramedullary canal to approximately using an awl. The minimally invasive approach and free selection of the incision site helps prevent soft tissue irritation and eliminate the need for a transarticular approach.

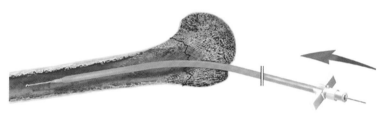

Figure 23.4 Introducing the guide catheter into the intramedullary canal and advancing the system over the fracture site.

The expansion of the balloon causes the implant to conform to the contour of the intramedullary canal, as shown below (Figures 23.5 and 23.6).

Once the balloon is expanded and in position, with the fracture site reduced in a fashion that the surgeon is agreeable to, the polymerization of the implant takes place. This is caused by the activation of the light source to cure the monomer. The visible blue light passes through a fiber-optic cable that is integrated into the balloon to polymerize the liquid monomer within 200 to 800 seconds (depending on implant size).

After the monomer inside the balloon has hardened, the implant can be locked in place by placing pilot-bores at any point of the implant and inserting conventional small fragment screws. Appropriately sized percutaneous locking screws can also be placed at any level of the implant which provides a unique level of customization that other implants have not previously provided to the orthopedic community (Figure 23.7).

This system has been designed to fulfill all the requirements of an ideal system for intramedullary stabilization. Introducing the implant material through a percutaneous minimally invasive approach into the bone will eliminate soft tissue injuries or irritations. As the flexible balloon catheter can be introduced into the bone at any place or position, no transarticular access to the intramedullary canal will be needed.

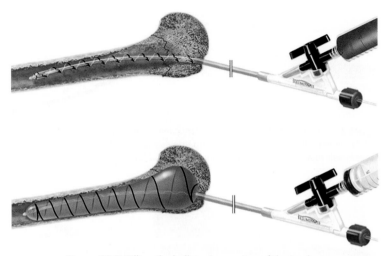

Figure 23.5 Filling the balloon/expansion of the implant.

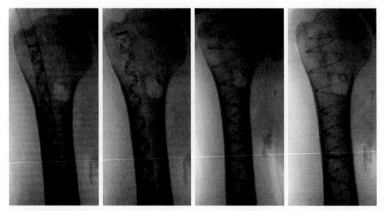

Figure 23.6 Sequential images of the IlluminOss implant delivery within the intramedullary canal: introduced via sheath, sheath removed, expanded within the canal, and polymerized.

As was shown in one of the clinical trials, being able to place and deliver the implant in a more lateral fashion negated significant damage to the rotator cuff, and was one of the keys to getting patients back to daily living activities. The IlluminOss system provides a faster return to a patient's pre-surgical range of motion sooner (Figure 23.8).

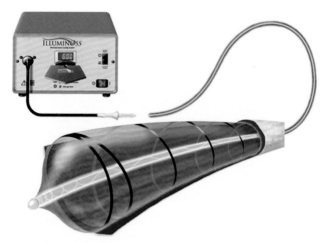

Figure 23.7 The monomer is cured by applying a light source with a visible blue light (436 nm) that passes through a fiber-optic cable into the balloon.

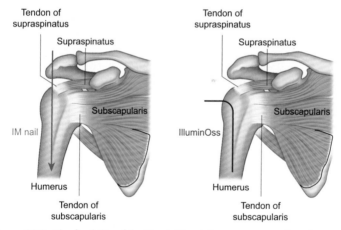

Figure 23.8 The flexibility of the IlluminOss delivery system vs. that of a standard rigid IM nail allows for a more lateral approach, sparing violation of the rotator cuff. The flexibility allows greater optionality in implant delivery location.

Filling the Dacron balloon with liquid monomer creates an increased pressure (albeit minimal) on the inside surface of the intramedullary canal, resulting in maintenance of reliable fracture reduction. As the entire balloon surface conforms to the contour of the intramedullary canal on all

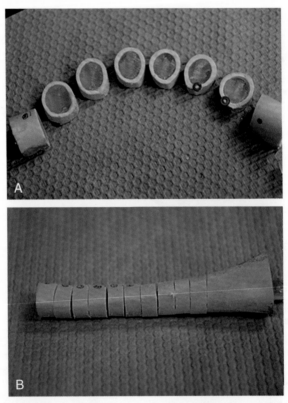

Figure 23.9 A, A sectioned sheep bone filled and cured with the IlluminOss implant. B, Sectioned and displayed sequentially. Illustration of the implants ability to conform and fill intramedullary space.

sides, this eliminates the need of further fracture translation after insertion and curing of the implant (Figures 23.9 and 23.10).

Complete hardening of the liquid monomer by the applied light source within 200 to 800 seconds allows immediate postoperative load bearing of the bone. As the minimally invasive access point can be chosen at any point away from the fracture, post-op complications, like lymph drainage blockage, post-op soft tissue infections, or soft tissue adhesions are minimized.

Owing to the completely liquid state of the monomer, which is maintained until the light source is activated, inflation and deflation of the balloon can be repeated as often as needed without limitations. This

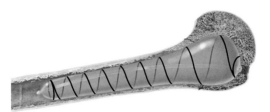

Figure 23.10 The balloon catheter conforms to the contour of the intramedullary canal.

allows the surgeon to correct the balloon position as needed and to control the reduction caused by filling the balloon. X-ray markers around the implant allow better X-ray fluoroscopic estimation of the exact balloon catheter position in every plane. Neither the initially liquid monomer nor the hardened polymer is a radiopaque structure, so consolidation of the fracture can easily be evaluated in all planes during post-op and follow-up X-ray examinations.

Similarly, the delivery of therapeutic radiation is not affected by the implant; beams are not scattered, so more precise delivery of the dosage can be accomplished.

Using the Dacron balloon, which can be formed into virtually any shape, and the aggregate monomer in its liquid state provides the possibility to prepare the implant to be cured in virtually any size, form, and dimension. This combination not only allows the fabrication of an implant that is customized for an individual patient, but also could provide for an extension of indications to include fractures close to joints, or metaphyseal fractures, spinal fractures, maxillofacial reconstruction as well as its use in revision surgery.

Based on the implant material properties and the previously described possibilities of placing locking screws at any place, the device could also be used for nonunions, material failures, or dislocation of preexisting osteosynthesis materials. A combination of intramedullary splinting and supplemental plate osteosynthesis would be a good solution in such cases. The screws for the supplemental plate osteosynthesis also can be placed anywhere along the long bone shaft and driven through the shaft and the IlluminOss implant to increase the holding forces of each implant. Bench testing has shown that the holding power of standard self-tapping orthopedic screws in bone is increased by a factor of approximately 4 times their normal holding power when anchored into an IlluminOss implant (Figure 23.11).

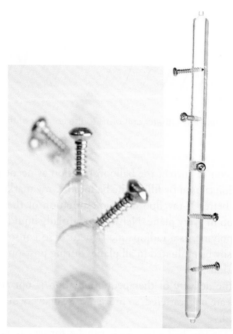

Figure 23.11 Locking possibilities for the hardened IlluminOss implant are provided to the surgeon in any alignment and in any position that they may choose.

Corrections of long bone osteotomy extensions by intramedullary splinting are simpler when using the IlluminOss implant and external distraction with a fixator, as the fixator pins may penetrate the implant at any place on one side of the osteotomy site.

This not only streamlines planning, but also simplifies the completion of an extending corrective osteotomy procedure when using this system.

Material

The photodynamic bone stabilization system consists of an inflatable, thin-walled PET (Dacron) balloon mounted on a small-diameter flexible guiding catheter, a sterile introducer sheath, a sterile dilator, a sterile syringe for infusing the monomer, and the photodynamic monomer (packaged in a light-proof glass container). The balloon catheters are available in various lengths and sizes to accommodate various anatomic locations. Diameters from 4 to 22 mm and lengths from 30 to 320 mm are available (Figure 23.12).

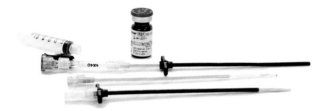

Figure 23.12 Liquid monomer and balloon catheter.

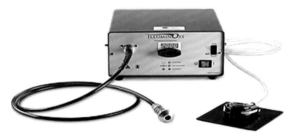

Figure 23.13 Image of the IlluminOss illumination system (system that generates the light to polymerize the monomer in the balloon).

Light Source

In addition, a light source is needed to use this system to cure or polymerize the monomer. Visible blue light with a wavelength of 436 nm is passed via a fiber-optic cable into the balloon to activate the polymerization process (Figures 23.13 and 23.14).

Polymerization

The photoactivation or photoinitiation causes the release of radicals, which transforms the infused monomer in the balloon from a liquid to a solid material. The biocompatible monomer is based on a series of monomer and oligomeric chain compounds that usually consist of acrylate or methacrylate derivatives. Other ingredients include polyurethanes. The photoinitiator is the key for the curing process, as it starts releasing the radicals for the polymerization process and initiates the chain compounding reaction (Figure 23.15).

Light Conduction

Initiation of the polymerization process is initiated by solely the application of the correct frequency and correct intensity of light. It requires an absolutely uninterrupted transfer of light from the light source through the light fiber

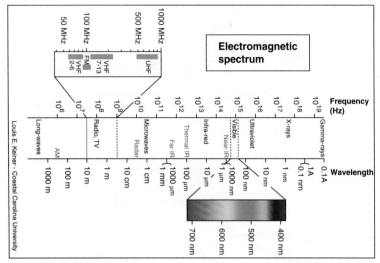

Figure 23.14 Illustration of the light frequency (436 nm) that initiates the polymerization process.

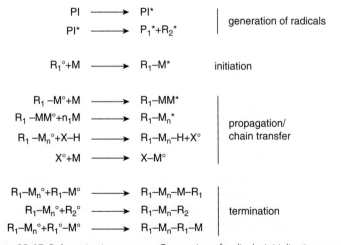

Figure 23.15 Polymerization process: Generation of radicals, initialization process, chain reaction/chain transfer, and termination.

to the internal diameter of the balloon catheter where the polymerization occurs. Other than light, nothing causes the polymerization to occur (neither heat nor radiation will polymerize the monomer), and the improper intensity or frequency of light will not create the desired polymerization effect.

One of the areas of development early on in the project was a means to achieve light delivery over both a long implant length and large implant diameter.

This posed a problem because standard transmission of light through a fiber and the resultant illumination is much like a flashlight, with the light spreading out and diminishing in intensity over distance. The light transmission drop off is guided by the inverse square law, "that a specified physical quantity or intensity is inversely proportional to the **square** of the distance from the source of that physical quantity." The light from a point source can be put in the form:

$$E = \frac{I}{r^2}$$

where E is called "illuminance" and I is called "pointance." This principle is further illustrated below (Figure 23.16).

As the intensity of light delivered from the fiber defines the amount of time that it takes to convert or polymerize the monomer, then a light fiber that had a significant drop off in transmission intensity would be less effective for larger or longer implants.

"Side-fire" technology is a solution to this issue. Side fire is based upon a radial scoring of the optical cladding on the fiber, so as to allow light to emanate along the entire length of the fiber, providing equal intensity along the entire length of the implant being cured. This allows for long and large diameter implants to be cured, as they are receiving equal amounts of optical irradiation along the implant length (Figure 23.17).

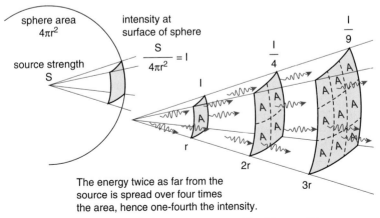

Figure 23.16 The amount of light per unit area reaching 10 mm will be one-fourth as much at 20 mm. (Image from Hyperphysics.)

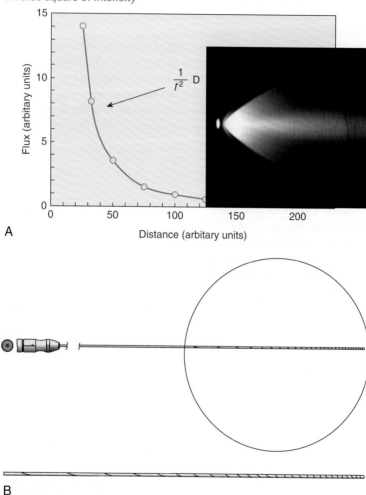

Inverse square of intensity

A

B

Figure 23.17 A and B. Side-fire light transmission technology, allowing for the radial or "side-fire" light transmission along the length of the fiber optic residing within the balloon implant, so as to cure the implant from the inside out, central core outwards, versus from one end to the other.

Using "side-fire" light conduction, the fiber-optic cable is advanced from the light source through the balloon and all the way to the tip of the balloon catheter. After activation of the light source, the light will pass through the fiber-optic cable inside the balloon. The light will radiate from

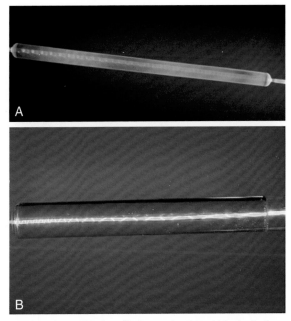

Figure 23.18 A and B. Principles of light conduction within the balloon catheter. Side-fire light conduction through the fiber-optic cable.

the fiber-optic cable to all sides in order to cure the monomer. This allows the polymerization process to take place along the entire implant length and in all directions (Figure 23.18).

Additionally, a means to allow for the visualization of the implant was necessary, as the implant was totally radiolucent, save for four small markers.

The need for radiolucency is important to allow for the appropriate visualization of the implant, the fracture, and its eventual reduction. The surgeon needs complete and accurate visualization of the placement, the inflation, and the positioning of the implant prior to curing.

Traditional means of radiopaque materials, markers and other solutions, inclusive of additives to the monomer were tried, without success. Finally, a liquid metal printing technique was designed, with a spiral helix around the circumference of the implant. This technique provided the needed visualization while at the same time allowing for visibility to the fracture. Additionally, this technique is MRI compatible while at the same time does not scatter radiation delivered for therapeutic treatment (Figures 23.19-23.23).

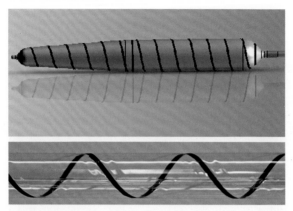

Figure 23.19 Illustration of the spiral radiopaque marker on an implant. Close up of the inked PET balloon /image of the balloon with the inked marking with a greater perspective

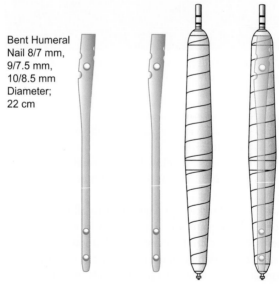

Bent Humeral Nail 8/7 mm, 9/7.5 mm, 10/8.5 mm Diameter; 22 cm

Figure 23.20 Standard nail versus IlluminOss. Smaller diameter: fixed angle and relies upon screws for fixation.

Using the Dacron balloon, and the aggregate monomer in its liquid state toward the creation of a patient customized implant designed toward the treatment of poor quality bone, allows for the surgeon to treat an underserved and rapidly growing patient population.

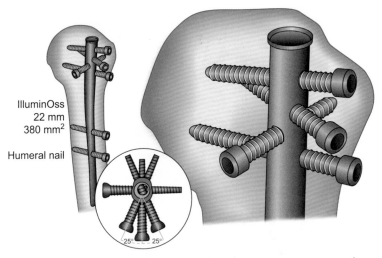

IlluminOss
22 mm
380 mm²

Humeral nail

25°   L   25°

Figure 23.21 IlluminOss supports the bone by volume versus trying to attach osteoporotic bone by means of screws.

- Less soft tissue injury = less postoperative pain
- Better for older patients with poor quaity impaired tissue
- Band aid surgery

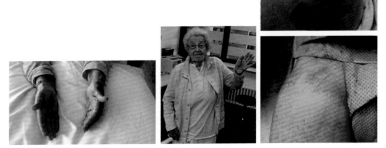

Figure 23.22 Minimally invasive small stitch incision. (Courtesy of Paul Vegt MD, Albert Schweitzer Hospital Dordrecht Netherlands.)

IlluminOss technology provides the medical community the means to prepare an implant to be cured in virtually any size, form, and dimension. This versatility not only allows the fabrication of an implant that is customized for an individual patient, but also provides for an extension of

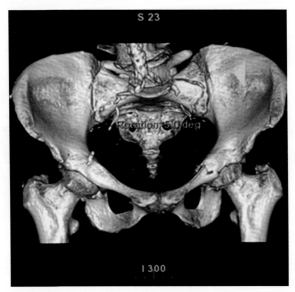

Figure 23.23 Fragility fracture of the pelvis. (Courtesy of L.A.M. Leenders, Department of surgery, Elkerliek Hospital, Helmond, The Netherlands M. Guijt, Traumasurgeon Department of surgery, section Traumatology, Elkerliek Hospital, Helmond, The Netherlands.)

indications, e.g., the secure application of ancillary orthopedic hardware that could otherwise not be held in position by the patient's own bone strength.

Clinical Outcomes

The following section details several case studies of the IlluminOss system, including processes, treatment, and results.

Osteoporotic Pelvic Ring Fracture Repair Using IlluminOss

PATIENT HISTORY AND DIAGNOSIS

We present a case of an 85-year-old female with a ramus superior and inferior fracture of her left pelvic ring due to a fall inside her house. She also sustained a left subcapital humeral fracture. Her history consists of osteoporosis and a right medial column fracture, which was treated with a dynamic hip screw. She was still very active for her age. She was mobile without support inside her house and walked more than 1 km with a rollator outside. Initially she was treated conservatively with physiotherapy. Despite adequate pain medication, she was not able to mobilize. This, in combination with the subcapital humeral fracture, was the reason to choose IlluminOss to stabilize the fracture of the pelvic ring to make mobilization possible.

DISCUSSION

It is generally known that the life expectancy and activity levels of people in developed countries has been increased over the last years and will increase even more in the future. This will also lead to more age-related fractures. Kannus described that the number of osteoporotic pelvic ring fractures in Finland between 1970 and 1997 increased dramatically and will increase even more over the next years. They also describe an increase in the age of the patients, which is likely to increase the injury-induced morbidity. To decrease the incidence and severity of complications, improve the patient's well-being, prevent loss of independence, and decrease the cost and burden of caregiving in these fragile geriatric patients, early mobilization is necessary.

TREATMENT

The operation was performed under general anesthesia due to combined operative treatment of the subcapital humeral fracture. A minimal supra pubic incision was made, so the intramedullary canal of the symphysis could be opened with a sharp awl. The guidewire was introduced and situated across the fracture, following the curve of the pelvic bone over the dome of the acetabulum. After the acetabulum was checked under X-ray guidance, flexible burrs cleared the canal to desired size of 5.5 mm. The introduction sheath was placed over the guidewire and an 8 × 120 mm balloon was inserted. X-ray guidance was used once more to check for proper positioning, before the balloon was filled with liquid monomer. To harden the monomer, the balloon was attached to a light source of 436 nm for 400 seconds; afterward, the light source was disconnected, and the wound was closed in layers. The surgical side was changed to start operative treatment of the subcapital humeral fracture also with IlluminOss.

OUTCOME/POSTPROCEDURE NOTES

The postoperative control X-ray showed a good position of the IlluminOss polymer, and the patient started mobilization with help of a physiotherapist. She was instructed for partial weight bearing of 50% on her left leg. After discharge from the hospital she stayed a few days in a geriatric rehabilitation clinic before she was able to return to her own home. At the first policlinic appointment (after 2 weeks), she was pain free when mobilizing without pain medication and was allowed to start full weight bearing. There were no signs of complications.

CONCLUSION

Owing to the use of IlluminOss, this patient was able to start mobilization on the first postoperative day. From this case, we can conclude that IlluminOss is a good alternative method to stabilize a ramus superior fracture and make early weight bearing mobilization possible by a minimal invasive procedure (Figure 23.24).

IlluminOss: A New, Patient-Conforming, Intramedullary Implant for Treatment of Osteoporotic Fractures

P.A. Vegt MD, PhD
Department of Surgery, section Traumatology, Albert Schweitzer Hospital, Dordrecht, the Netherlands
C.A.S. Berende MD
Department of Surgery, section Traumatology, Amphia Hospital, Breda, the Netherlands
A.J.M. Karthaus MD, PhD
Department of Surgery, section Traumatology, Deventer Hospital, Deventer, the Netherlands
J.P.A.M. Vroemen MD
PhD, Department of Surgery, section Traumatology, Amphia Hospital, Breda, the Netherlands

PATIENT HISTORY AND DIAGNOSIS

A case study is presented of a 77-year-old female, in generally good health and living independently, who suffered a low-energy fall on her left arm, sustaining an AO type 23-A2 extra-articular fracture in her radius.

TREATMENT

The fracture was stabilized with plaster of Paris in preparation for placement of an IlluminOss implant. The implant procedure was performed in a supine position with Chinese finger traction. Anesthesia was administered prior to a closed reduction of the fracture and creation of a 1.5 cm incision over the styloid process of the distal radius. The operator used a straight awl to gain entry to the intramedullary canal and then used a cannulated awl

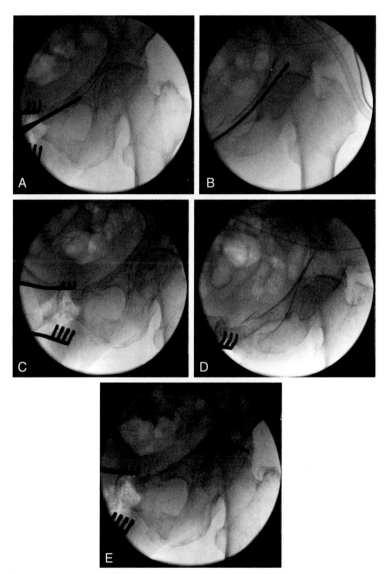

Figure 23.24 A, Cannulated awl introducing 1.2 mm guidewire into the medullary canal. B, Small diameter flexible burrs (4.5 mm-6.5 mm) delivered over the guidewire. C, Tear-away sheath providing access for implant positioning via the radiopaque markers. D, The implant being infused with monomer filling and conforming to the shape of the intramedullary canal. E, Postoperative image; show an expanded and polymerized implant achieving cortical wall contact over it's length.

to introduce a guidewire. Flexible burrs were then used to clean the canal to 5.5 mm. Under X-ray guidance, a balloon catheter was introduced via a sheath and dilator and positioned across fracture site. After proper positioning was confirmed by fluoroscopy, a liquid monomer was infused to inflate the balloon. An optical fiber residing within a lumen in the balloon catheter was then attached to a light source and activated for 400 seconds to deliver visible 436 nm light and harden the monomer, creating the implant in situ. Afterward, the optical fiber and catheter were removed, leaving the implant to stabilize the fracture site.

DISCUSSION

As life expectancy and activity levels among the elderly continue to increase in developed countries, wrist fractures are an increasingly important factor in maintaining quality of life (QOL) and controlling health care costs. A wrist fracture resulting in a nonfunctional wrist joint may cause reduced mobility, loss of work, and eventual loss of independence. Chung et al estimated that internal fixation for distal radius fractures would result in direct costs of $240 million per annum in the United States alone, with higher secondary costs related to prescription drugs, loss of work, and loss of independence.

In the case of a bilateral fracture of the wrist, patients may require assistive living support or interim nursing care. Despite the growing need for effective treatment, there is no gold-standard therapy. Current treatments include splinting, cast immobilization, and surgical treatment with fixation devices—yet treatment protocol remains "controversial" and varies from center to center. New treatment options are urgently needed to help elderly patients recover, rehabilitate, and regain mobility and independence

OUTCOME/POSTPROCEDURE NOTES

The patient was treated on an outpatient basis with a stand-alone IlluminOss implant. She returned home the same day of the procedure with instructions to use her wrist as tolerated and begin physiotherapy. There was no infection, secondary procedure, or delayed union at the fracture site.

CONCLUSION

The IlluminOss system provides a safe, minimally invasive treatment option for fracture fixation. The small incision required for surgical access and the rapid longitudinal and rotational support may contribute to improved recovery time, so patients can return home faster and maintain QOL and independence (Figure 23.25).

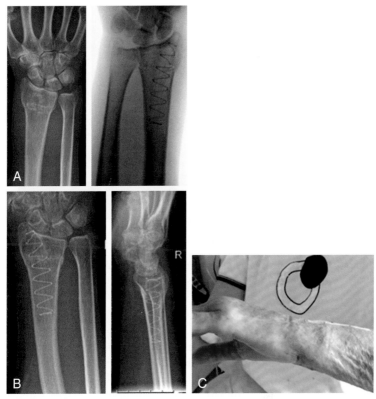

Figure 23.25 A, Preoperative x-ray. AO type 23-A2 extra-articular fracture. B, Postoperative x-ray with IlluminOss implant. C, Postoperative. Patient was discharged on the same day as the surgery without a tourniquet or other heavy bandaging on the wrist.

The IlluminOss Intramedullary Stabilization Device: Potential Benefits over Standard Nail Fixation for Pathologic Humerus Fractures

Jason Hoellwarth, MD; Kurt Weiss, MD; Mark Goodman, MD; Alma Heyl, LAS, RTR, CCRC; Richard McGough, MD (Figure 23.26).

BACKGROUND

Fractures through pathologic humerus lesions occur frequently. This significantly decreases QOL for patients with already short life expectancies. Current treatment of impending or actual pathologic humeral fractures is via either a titanium IMN or cement-plate technique.

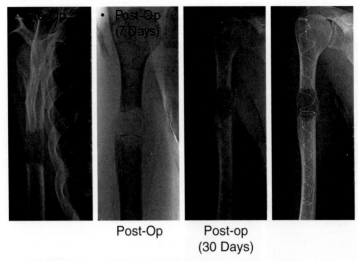

Figure 23.26 Metastatic humerus case from the US clinical trial illustrating an impending fracture and subsequent filling and stabilization with the IlluminOss system.

Drawbacks of IMN are mismatched canal-implant geometry and inability to place proximal screws intra-articularly. Cement plating's downsides are extensive incisions and difficulty with fixing the entire bone. Both also require delaying radiation therapy until wounds heal. The IlluminOss (IO) intramedullary stabilization device, currently under investigation, seeks to solve those issues. Via a 1-cm proximal incision a small diameter flexible catheter delivers a PET balloon to the intramedullary space.

The balloon is inserted past the fracture then filled with a biocompatible liquid polymer that cures through the application of visible light emitted from a fiber-optic catheter. The resultant implant is radiolucent allowing for better visualization of the surgical site. This leads to no wounds in the radiation zone, conforming rigid fixation without intra-articular prominence and a tamponade effect to stem bleeding.

QUESTIONS/PURPOSES

1. Is IO a reliable technique?
2. Is the material adequately durable?
3. Can IO offer QOL benefits compared with IMN such as shorter hospital stays and quicker radiation therapy?
4. What unique benefits, complications, and subsequent solutions exist with IO?

METHODS

Retrospective analysis was performed of all pathologic humerus fractures occurring since 2010 which were managed by IMN or IO stabilization. IMN was exclusive until June 2015 when we added IO in addition. Variables examined were patient age, gender, laterality, tobacco use, chemotherapy, tumor pathology, operative time, estimated blood loss, transfusion need, postoperative hospital stay, time until radiation therapy, and postoperative complications. Patients were followed at least 3 months postoperatively and then annually/as needed or until they died.

RESULTS

We treated 17 patients (18 fractures) with IO and 55 patients (56 fractures) with IMN. There was no statistical difference for age, gender, laterality, or transfusion need. No infections occurred in either group. No IO patients required reoperation whereas 4 (7%) of IMN patients did. Significant differences of IO vs. IMN were as follows: tobacco use (78% vs. 25%, P = .0001); chemotherapy (83% vs. 54%, P = .0286); near-zero blood loss (67% vs. 22%, P = .0024); radiation within 24 hours (73% vs. 3.4%, P = .0001), notably 44% of IO were within 8 hours; operation minutes (59.6 vs. 77.8, P = .020) with 61% of IO taking under 1 hour vs. 25% of IMN (P = .088); and next-day discharge (56% vs. 29%, P = .049) with 28% of IO discharged the same day. One IO failed to polymerize intraoperatively, possibly due to balloon rupture; this was immediately converted to IMN. This was recognized intraoperatively, and the device was exchanged for a conventional IMN immediately, without any clinical sequelae.

CONCLUSIONS

The IlluminOss intramedullary fixation technique has allowed us to change our approach to pathologic humerus fractures. In our early experience, it has proven safe, fast, and reliable. There has been one intraoperative complication which was managed without delay or morbidity, no patients who required return to the operating room, and no infections. No implants broke postoperatively. IO seems to offer significant QOL benefits of rapid radiation and discharge home, often within 1 day and some the same day. Three patients (17%) seem to set a new ideal scenario, coming in from home for scheduled surgery which required less than 1 hour, having radiation therapy immediately afterward, and going home with pain controlled that same day. We have also modified our treatment protocol for renal cell carcinoma, and have omitted preoperative embolization, as the balloon seems to sufficiently tamponade bleeding as to eliminate this necessity. If successful in the future, IO could convert our pathologic humeral fractures, including renal cell cancer, from up to 3 days inpatient (embolization HD1, surgery HD2, discharge HD3) to a single full-service outpatient day.

LEVEL OF EVIDENCE: III

CONCLUSION

The IlluminOss Bone Stabilization System presents a promising and innovative method of stabilizing bone using minimally invasive technology and vastly improving the QOL of patients during treatment and recovery.

CHAPTER 24

Concept to Commercialization: SOMAVAC® Sustained Vacuum System

ESRA ROAN, JOSHUA D. HERWIG

ABOUT THE AUTHORS

Esra Roan, PhD, is the CEO and cofounder of SOMAVAC® Medical Solutions, Inc. Previously, she was an Associate Professor in Biomedical Engineering at the University of Memphis. She has a diverse background in mechanical engineering, spanning 20 years including optomechanics research at Oak Ridge National Laboratory (ORNL) (Oak Ridge, TN) on product development at 3M Precision Optics (Cincinnati, OH). In her academic role, Esra built a soft-tissue and cell mechanics lab at the University of Memphis. She cofounded SOMAVAC Medical Solutions to design and commercialize medical technologies focusing on the post-surgical recovery at home.

Josh Herwig is the CTO and cofounder of SOMAVAC® Medical Solutions, Inc. He is a serial tinkerer with professional experience in design, automation, and manufacturing. He holds a B.S. in Mechanical Engineering from Tennessee Technological University and a M.S. in Biomedical Engineering from the University of Memphis and The University of Tennessee Health Science Center. Josh serves as the CTO and Director of Engineering for SOMAVAC® Medical Solutions and is responsible for current and new product development.

Our goal in this chapter is to present the story of the SOMAVAC® *Sustained Vacuum System* from concept to commercialization. This was created by two highly technical founders with no prior business or medical device development experience and limited resources. The team arrived at the problem statement in 2016, received Food and Drug Administration (FDA) clearance in 2018, and is executing a commercial launch in 2019.

Clinical Problem: The Problem of Fluid Accumulation After Surgeries

A variety of surgical procedures, including orthopedic surgeries, lead to the formation of dead space or flaps among the layers of tissue. This region of undermined tissue leads to the development of fluid that has to be drained. Otherwise, the fluid can build up and lead to the formation of *seroma (in the case of serous fluid)* or *hematoma (in the case of whole blood)*. As such, at the end of a surgical procedure that causes a void or flap, physicians may place one or more closed suction drains (see Figure 24.1) to help drain the fluid and to avoid seroma or hematoma formation. The drains are attached to suction devices, i.e., bulbs or canisters, to generate a negative pressure to encourage removal of the fluid (Figure 24.1). In many indications, patients are discharged home with these closed suction drains, which may then be removed individually when the drainage drops below a certain amount (usually between 25-50 ml/d) or at a predetermined time. The criteria for removal are dependent on the indication. In the case where drains are removed based on the volume, patients are responsible for the maintenance of drains at home with minimal training.

As a researcher and engineer, in my previous role as an academician, I may have read this type of a problem in any scientific text and appreciated the issues relating to inadequate suction provided by the current standard-of-care manual suction devices. There are obvious limitations in the design such as the pressure loss with fluid collection. However, the more nuanced, overlooked aspects of this problem became clear when we were able to have honest conversations with breast cancer survivors who experienced drains. They hated these suction bulbs of the drains as they are cumbersome and nearly impossible to conceal under clothing. This, in turn, prevented them from returning to their jobs or normal activities. In addition, drain maintenance was a major burden on patients and their loved ones during their recovery; this was especially true for mastectomy patients.

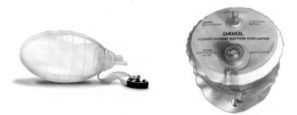

Figure 24.1 Examples of manual suction devices for closed suction drains.

Patient stories motivated our team immensely. We were surprised to find, in this modern age of medicine with robotic surgery and telemedicine, that patients are discharged home with medieval devices and have no way of vocalizing their unnecessary suffering. Our team wanted to bridge the gap between the patient and the health care providers to solve this overlooked problem.

Millions of Patients Are Impacted

Early on we understood the significance of seroma and recovery after surgeries. However, a more detailed review of the problem and the market would be required to launch a company and garner interest leading to funding. This led us to focus on the number of patients who may be directly impacted and found that 750,000 surgeries (mastectomies, breast reconstruction, ventral hernia repairs, abdominoplasties) utilized suction drains outside of a health care facility for reasonably long periods of time exceeding 5 days. Additionally, closed suction drains were utilized in trauma, orthopedic, cardiothoracic, and many other surgical specialties, which collectively added to more than 3 million closed suction drains utilized in the United States annually.

The ultimate size of the market is based not on the price of the current gold-standard device but rather the associated health care cost of the one in five patients who experience seroma complications and require an intervention. This leads to a $1bn burden on the US health care system. We utilize existing research studies to understand rates of seroma, infection, and interventions to build a credible market size based on expenses. For example, in a recent study of hernia repairs, it was shown that complicated seroma led to 2.3 extra visits to the clinic, which increases outpatient resource utilization.[1] In breast reconstructions, persistent seromas can lead to delays in adjuvant therapies and completion of reconstructions.[2]

In summary, the team quickly realized that the commercial potential of solving this problem was immense and turned their attention to solving the problem. It is important to note that the translation of research and clinical information into business models occurred during the accelerator phase, which was instrumental to SOMAVAC® Medical's funding success.

The SOMAVAC® Solution

The SOMAVAC® concept ideation was influenced, and we feel greatly aided by the founding team's limited exposure to medical device design and development but deep experience in mechanical engineering and manufacturing. Initially, like the development of other medical technologies, the team sought a solution that would address the concerns primarily of

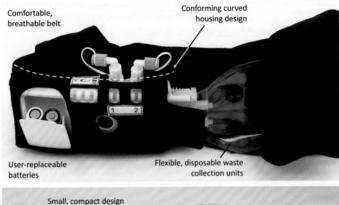

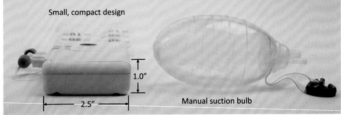

Figure 24.2 The design of the SOMAVAC® *Sustained Vacuum System* (top) was driven primarily by patient experience concerns, while maintaining safety and efficacy. This is evidenced by the contoured housing (left) and overall compactness of the vacuum source (right).

the physician stakeholders—namely the necessity for effective removal of fluid. By following this basic requirement, the team initially created a system resembling the majority of the portable vacuum devices on the market—a large device that utilized a relatively inexpensive air pump to create a vacuum in a rigid canister. Although this solution was easy to envision and could be manufactured rather inexpensively, it failed to address the aspect of patient satisfaction. Taking a patient-focused approach to the problem led the team to create requirements for the device which, while somewhat complicated, and occasionally costlier than the mundane solution, ultimately proved to be novel and highly desirable to the physician but more importantly, the end user—*the patient.* This led the team to create the SOMAVAC® *Sustained Vacuum System* (see Figure 24.2).

One problem, not unique, but especially challenging to the medical device industry centers around vetting the concept. How do I know that I have a solution that meets the needs of the physician, nurse, end user, hospital, and ultimately payor? Unlike most consumer-focused tech start-ups, early-stage medtech companies cannot launch product to the market, gather customer feedback, and rapidly iterate the solution. This problem is especially pernicious in the start-up environment where raising necessary capital is often dependent on de-risking the product-market fit. SOMAVAC® approached this in two ways:

1. Deciding early on that the patient was going to be the driving factor in everything we do. At our core, we believe that if we create a solution that is ultimately desirable by the patient (while obviously meeting the clinical need), we will be successful. This laser-focused approach allowed us to define the goal of iteration as that which led us to a safe, efficacious product, which was the most preferred by the patient. Our user interviews were thus split 70% patient, 30% physician and care providers. This simplified the prototype iteration loop by decreasing the amount of input necessary to create the next prototype, allowing us to move more quickly to the ultimate validation step of market acceptance or rejection.

2. The ultimate validation of solution is market adoption, which could not be assessed without first receiving an FDA clearance. Thus, making FDA submission the driving business concern allowed us to achieve an FDA clearance in less than 2 years from founding the company with an 85-day timeframe from initial submission to clearance notice. We want to stress that, while speed was important, we placed significant resources to support a robust design control system, employing expert advice at every decision point—from material selection to battery performance.

SOMAVAC® was founded by two biomedical engineers with degrees in mechanical and biomedical engineering and backgrounds in manufacturing but lacking consumer product development experience. Because of this, the team was tempted very early on to outsource the entire development of the product to a contract design and development firm who would take the product from napkin sketch to manufacturable product. This was ultimately undesirable because it meant loss of control of the product design process, long lead-times, and increased costs. One important note is that while the SOMAVAC® team decided to keep a large portion of the design in-house, it took a tremendous amount of effort to accomplish this and focus on building the company with seed funding. This was possible because of the unique background of these founders. Early-stage medtech companies should be cautioned to carefully consider whether they have the skills and commitment (read: desire) to follow this path. If sufficient funding can be garnered, a fully outsourced design with design history file support is a very attractive alternative.

For SOMAVAC®, however, the autonomy in the design process was important, and the founders had a desire to build a company focused on tackling hard engineering problems by developing internal resources with a long-term potential, rather than focusing solely on building the business. This had tangible payoffs for the company including a reduction in cost, speedier time to FDA submission, and the development of capabilities within the company.

Regardless of the path chosen, SOMAVAC® identified several personnel key to the engineering development of their device. Whether these resources are internal or external, they should be viewed as the bare minimum requirement for the development of an electromechanical medical device. They are presented below with some critical standards in which they should be highly trained: these are in addition to a general knowledge of relevant FDA/ANSI/AAMI/ISO/IEC regulations, guidances, and standards.

1. Principal Mechanical Engineer (ANSI/AAMI/IEC 60601 family of standards)
2. Principal Electrical Engineer (ANSI/AAMI/IEC 60601 family of standards)
3. Principal Software Engineer (ANSI/AAMI/IEC 62304)
4. Quality Engineer (IEC 13485, ISO 14971)
5. Industrial Designer (this may be a skill possessed by the lead mechanical engineer)
6. Manufacturing Engineer (this resource may be leveraged from the contract manufacturer)

The final step in the development of a medical device is the transfer of the design to the manufacturer. The team identified this as a critical item very early on and selected a contract manufacturer even before choosing a design and development partner.

Regulatory Strategy and Submission

The team placed significant time in understanding the regulatory landscape and drafting a regulatory strategy that was well-aligned with company stage, marketing plans, and funding goals. The latter is key to most early-stage medical device companies as they most likely have access to *seed* funding prior to FDA clearance.

FOCUS ON THE SUBMISSION

As mentioned previously, we understood the importance of FDA clearance on our business and ability to raise funding. This led us to focus all of our attention to complete product development and validation to reach FDA submission milestone. We not only focused our efforts but also our funds that we garnered in achieving this goal of FDA submission timely.

UTILIZE REGULATORY EXPERTS, BUT SPEND YOUR OWN TIME

The accelerator provided basic regulatory introduction, and we were able to interact with regulatory experts very early. We launched our efforts in this area by asking for an initial report that summarizes the FDA guidances, other existing standards that were applicable to our product, and potential list of predicates as we knew our device would undergo the 510(k) clearance process. This can cost anywhere from $1,000 to $5,000, but we believe it is critical for any medtech start-up. Once the report was in place, we as the cofounders studied the details of the guidances, standards, and predicates. This helped us to utilize the regulatory experts as advisors for building a viable strategy. Ultimately, this helped us to minimize costs and expedite submission.

THINK LONG TERM

The commercialization of a new medical technology often involves multiple FDA clearances as new discoveries are made relating to additional indications, features, and performance characteristics. This knowledge led us to also undertake a multitiered approach to our submission strategy. We decided that it was in our best interest to seek clearance for the core technology (continuous negative pressure) and plan for additional submissions as we determined that additional features and indications were justified. We then chose to seek clearance to market SOMAVAC® 100 Sustained Vacuum System and then allow for market adoption and feedback to inform our regulatory strategy as our company grows.

Nothing Can Move Forward Without Funding

One of the cofounders, Dr Roan, spent years growing a research program from start-up funding to securing National Institutes of Health (NIH) funding. Fundamentals between academic and private fund-raising are very similar, but mechanisms are obviously very different. In either case, building trust between the funder and the recipient is key. In academic fund-raising, this is achieved through conference attendances, manuscripts, first submissions, small grants, etc. In private venture funding, there is a chance to meet the investor in person and answer questions directly. The positive or negative feedback is received quickly, and the entrepreneur has the chance to adapt nearly in real time. During this process, it is imperative that the entrepreneur remains authentic and realistic in their explanations of the problem, solution, and projections. This is very challenging in medtech as revenue is multiple years away and projections are very speculative. In our experience, it has been more productive to focus on the team and the problem during the seed funding phase rather than the speculative revenue projections. A thoroughly vetted, adequately large market will to get most investors interested and excited!

There are many entrepreneurs who have great ideas with extremely limited experience in medtech industry. In fund-raising for a medtech venture, this is a significant limitation as the capital needed to support a revenue-generating solution is almost certainly greater than $1 million. We addressed this issue by fund-raising for milestones. This allowed us to build trust with angel investors and diminish wasteful use of funds. We raised as we achieved milestones and priced the next steps carefully.

Raising for milestones was complemented by our *patient* approach with fund-raising, which can be seen in the overall timeline of our growth (Figure 24.3). With the backing of two institutional investors, we were able to "date" our angel investors for long periods of time. In some cases, we closed funding after 1-year of follow-up meetings. For many entrepreneurs, this sounds like a very inefficient process over a long period of time; however, for angel funding (in middle America especially), this is often the case. In addition, SOMAVAC® took any possible opportunity to meet angel investors anywhere in the world without prejudging their potential to invest in medtech ventures. Here, the accelerators and local start-up ecosystem were influential in networking and generating opportunities.

We now find ourselves executing the commercial launch of our flagship product, SOMAVAC® 100, in several indications leading to large flaps. Here the patients suffer significantly during a delicate time of their life after a major surgery. During our interactions with our local medical community, rich with world-class orthopedic device manufacturers (Smith and Nephew, Medtronic, etc.) and institutions (Campbell Clinic, St. Jude, UTHSC), we quickly learned the role of suction drain use in revision joint replacement surgeries, trauma, and oncologic orthopedic resections and how these surgeries lead to large flaps and are at risk for seroma or hematoma formation. Although, the utilization of closed suction drains in some of the orthopedic surgeries is under strong scrutiny,[3-6] we believe that the delivery of sustained vacuum with minimal risk of fluid backflow may provide opportunities to reduce complications. Furthermore, compact and portable nature of our SOMAVAC® 100 system may allow increased mobility of patients in and out of the professional health care setting.

Our goal in this chapter was to present the story of the SOMAVAC® 100 *Sustained Vacuum System* from concept to commercialization. As we approach the commercialization of our system, we are preparing to face new challenges. However, because of our careful disciplined approach, seamless teamwork, and robust support, we believe we are well positioned to execute

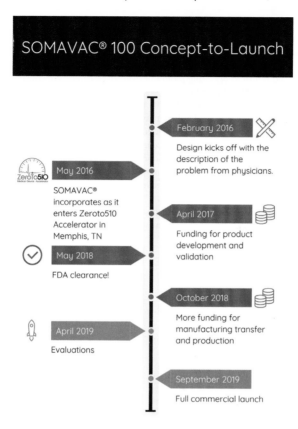

Figure 24.3 Timeline of Concept-to-Launch activities for SOMAVAC® Medical.

our evaluations, limited release, and then launch nationally. We will continue to grow as a company and as individuals as we prepare to launch additional products.

KEY TAKEAWAY POINTS

- ▶ Medtech fund-raising can be slow. A patient approach is likely necessary.
- ▶ It is important to gather information from all stakeholders and iterate thoughtfully rather than making rash design changes based on every suggestion.
- ▶ A sound regulatory strategy including quality management, *well-understood* by the founders, must be part of the early-stage research and development efforts.

REFERENCES AND RESOURCES

1. Wade A, Plymale MA, Davenport DL, et al. Predictors of outpatient resource utilization following ventral and incisional hernia repair. *Surg Endosc.* 2018;32(4):1695-1700.
2. Ollech CJ, Block LM, Afifi AM, Poore SO. Effect of drain placement on infection, seroma, and return to operating room in expander-based breast reconstruction. *Ann Plast Surg.* 2017;79(6):536-540.
3. Esler CN, Blakeway C, Fiddian NJ. The use of a closed-suction drain in total knee arthroplasty: a prospective, randomised study. *J Bone Joint Surg Br.* 2003;85(2):215-217.
4. Lee QJ, Mak WP, Hau WS, et al. Short duration and low suction pressure drain versus no drain following total knee replacement. *J Orthop Surg.* 2015;23(3):278-281.
5. Omonbude D, El Masry MA, O'Connor PJ, et al. Measurement of joint effusion and haematoma formation by ultrasound in assessing the effectiveness of drains after total knee replacement: a prospective randomised study. *J Bone Joint Surg Br.* 2010;92(1):51-55.
6. Patel VP, Walsh M, Sehgal B, et al. Factors associated with prolonged wound drainage after primary total hip and knee arthroplasty. *J Bone Joint Surg Br.* 2007;89(1):33-38.

Glossary

2 × 2 graphic: Graphic that compares key variables to provide a 3-D visual framework, aiding strategic business and marketing decision-making. Target area structured for optimal solutions for this business tool is placement in the upper right-hand quadrant.

510(k): Premarket submission made to FDA to demonstrate that the device to be marketed is at least as safe and effective, that is, substantially equivalent, to a legally marketed device (21 CFR 807.92(a) (3)) that is not subject to PMA. Typically a less rigorous approval process because a product already exist that performs similarly.

Assignment: The transferring of intellectual property rights from one entity to another, whereby the owner of the rights transfers or assigns ownership (of patent rights, for example) to another, much like transferring the title to a vehicle, or a deed to real estate.

Claim: The "claim" in a patent is the description of the elements that make the invention authentic and unique. It describes the parameters within which others are excluded from using or practicing your patent's teachings without the patent holder's permission.

Clinical problem: A clinical issue that has been observed multiple times that represents an inefficient or suboptimal delivery of care.

Concept: An idea for a device or product and the business plan/strategy for how that idea can be commercialized.

Confidentiality agreement: A legally binding contract between two entities that establishes conditions and terms for the exchange, use, and disposition of confidential information or materials.

Confirmation bias: An error of accepting an innovation in its current form despite outside information suggesting the need for reform, typically as a result of personal attachment.

Cost-effective analysis: Projections of the costs required to improve a selected clinical outcome. An analytic tool that includes clinical efficacy outcomes with costs to achieve them, against alternate clinical solutions to compare therapeutic alternatives. Cost-effective clinical outcomes of a novel technology are often compared against the current standard of care.

Customer discovery: Process of engaging potential customers to obtain a deeper understanding of the problem and the relevance of the product concept.

De novo: Submission process if the FDA determines, through means such as a 513(g) or Pre-Submission, that the device is "novel" with no existing classification or predicate device on the market.

Disease burden: The intensity or severity of a disease measured by epidemiology, mortality, morbidity, financial cost, or other indicators.

Distribution channel: The virtual avenue used to transfer goods from the manufacturer to the end user. For example, a distribution channel for automobiles may be from factory to dealership to consumer. It is generally delineated each time the ownership changes hands.

Distribution share: Manufacturer (mfg) A may sell 10 million products at 5,000 retail stores, and mfg B may sell 2 million products at all of the same 5,000 retail. Although, mfg A may have 5 times more market share by units sold, both mfg A and B enjoy an equal amount of distribution share because they have sales presence in the same number of stores.

Due diligence: A comprehensive strategic investigation and appraisal of a technology, investment or business to evaluate and determine commercial potential.

Ethnography/ethnographic research: A systematic approach to gathering information and insights into how the concept/device will be used.

Focus group: A structured data collection process where prospective product consumers can sample the product and provide constructive feedback.

Group purchasing organization (GPO): An organization that provides health care providers savings by leveraging aggregated purchasing volume to negotiate discounted pricing between health care providers and manufacturers, distributors, and other vendors.

Incidence: Occurrence rate of a disease or condition within a population, over a given time, usually annually. Disease incidence indicates the number of newly diagnosed cases.

Innovation: The process of creating a novel solution to an unmet need.

Intellectual property (IP): Creations of the mind, the expression of which may be documented in patents, trademarks, trade dress (a secondary meaning to trademarks), copyrights, trade secrets, know-how, formulas, methodologies, and the like.

Intended use: The description of the primary performance goal of the product.

License: To permit use of intellectual property rights from the owner of the rights to another, whereby the owner of the rights retains ownership. Much like a leasing arrangement for real estate or vehicles. The owner would be licensing (leasing) their patent rights, for example.

Licensee: The entity (or person) that is receiving a license for intellectual property.

Licensor: The entity (or person) that is granting to another the use of at least some part of their intellectual property rights.

Market analysis: A multistep, iterative process to determine the probability of commercial success for a technology within a specific market that involves qualitative and quantitative assessment of the market.

Market opportunity: The potential market size of the segment anticipated to be captured by the technology over time.

Market penetration: The level of sales or adoption of a target market by a specific product or service, also called the penetration rate.

Market position: Is essentially an identity for which an entity is perceived. Think of inexpensive, reliable, consistent chocolate, available anywhere, and what might come to most people's minds? Hershey's? If so, they would hold the number one market position for chocolate products with those attributes. What about a luxury German car? Maybe Mercedes commands the number one market position for high-end, daily driver, luxury cars in Europe, for example? Market position includes a number of factors that together help one differentiate between brands, and even between people.

Market segment: A group or category of customers that share measurable characteristics or traits such as product requirements, needs, or specialization used to define the relevant market.

Market share: The portion of a given market that one manufacturer or entity may control versus their competitors. Usually measured in sales revenue or by number of units distributed to a given market. Example, at retail stores, Apple may receive 40% of revenue, Samsung, 38% of the revenue, and the remaining 22% of revenue market share is held by others.

Market size: Given volume or value of products or service sold to potential acquirers.

Minimum viable product (MVP): A product that embodies the concept but with just enough features to satisfy early adopters.

Observation: The process of mentally or physically recording an aspect of the patient care process, frequently one that occurs in a suboptimal manner.

Pattern recognition: Identifying a key theme or underlying thread of a recurring scenario; this common thread may represent the cause of a clinical problem.

Pivoting: Modifying an innovation or the course of a company as a direct result of feedback or new information.

PMA: Standard FDA process of scientific and regulatory review to evaluate the safety and effectiveness of medical devices. Such devices require a premarket approval (PMA) application under section 515 of the FD&C Act in order to obtain marketing approval.

Predicate device: A device that have been cleared/approved by the FDA for the same intended use.

Prevalence: Rate of the total number of cases existing within a population at a given location within a specific period, usually expressed as a percentage of the population.

Primary market research: A method used to research a market whereby the researcher receives a direct response from people and situations in that market, through in-person interviewing, direct sales results, and real-time experience and the like.

Product category: A category in hardware products may be tools, and a subcategory, hand tools, and a sub, subcategory, hammers. Product categories are normally divided by their uses and their markets.

Product requirements document: Document that describes a new product by identifying overall performance and provides the basis for traceability throughout development.

Provisional patent: A lower-cost, early-filing option that establishes a claim to intellectual property for a period of 12 months and allows the term "patent pending" to be used in connection with the description of the invention; a *nonprovisional* application must be filed within the 12 month period.

Requirement(s): A product trait that provides the basis for validation testing, not to be confused with specifications.

Scope: The overall clinical and economic burden that a problem produces. This commonly occurs in the form of negative patient outcomes or lost health care dollars.

Secondary market research: Methods for performing research that may include online research, virtual scenarios, and extrapolating data.

Specifications: A numerically driven description that describes specific performance and provides the basis for verification testing.

Stakeholder: A user or person who is involved in any way with the product under development.

Total addressable market: The total revenue opportunity that is available for a specific product or service. Includes top-down sizing using industry research and reports, bottom-up sizing from market research, and early selling efforts and value theory, using primary market data that drive conjecture about a buyer's willingness to pay.

Traceability: Traceability is the process that connects product requirements and specifications to verification testing and validation results. Traceability is always performed by evaluating results with the goal of reducing risks and hazards.

Type 1 error: Falsely believing that an unmet need exists when the current state is acceptable, typically resulting from a lack of data, conflict, or bias.

Unmet need: In surgery, an unmet need can be satisfied by the development of a device that performs a new surgical function. An unmet need can also be satisfied by improving an existing device or procedure.

Value analysis: A systematic assessment performed by diverse and experienced teams to confirm the comparative cost and clinical effectiveness of a product under consideration for purchase.

Vetting: An ongoing effort to identify and minimize the risks and reasons not to move forward.

Key Terms

510(k): A 510(k) is a premarket submission made to FDA to demonstrate that the device to be marketed is at least as safe and effective, that is, substantially equivalent, to a legally marketed device that is not subject to PMA. When found acceptable, 510(k) submissions are cleared by the FDA.

513(g) request: Submission used to obtain the FDA's classification and regulatory requirements applicable to a particular device.

Accelerator: Typically a fixed-term, cohort-based program for start-up teams that includes seed investment, connections, mentorship, educational components, and culminates in a public pitch event or demo day to accelerate growth.

Accretive: Accretive is the process of accretion, which is growth or increase by gradual addition, in finance and general nomenclature. An acquisition is considered accretive if it adds to the item's value or corporation's earnings per share. (https://www.investopedia.com/terms/a/accretive.asp)

Acquisition: An acquisition is a corporate action in which a company buys most, if not all, of another firm's ownership stakes to assume control of it. An acquisition occurs when a buying company obtains more than 50% ownership in a target company. (https://www.investopedia.com/terms/a/acquisition.asp)

Alice Corp v. CLS Bank International, 134 S. Ct. 2347 (2014): A United States Supreme Court decision holding abstract ideas without an additional inventive concept are subject-matter patent ineligible.

AMA/Specialty Society Relative Value Scale Update Committee: The American Medical Association (AMA) manages the Specialty Society Relative Value Scale Update Committee (RUC), and its activities are a collaborative venture between the AMA, national medical specialty societies, limited license and allied health provider organizations, and the Centers for Medicare and Medicaid Services (CMS.)

Ambulatory surgical center (ASC): Ambulatory surgery centers—known as ASCs—are modern health care facilities focused on providing same-day surgical care, including diagnostic and preventive procedures. ASCs have transformed the outpatient experience for millions of Americans by providing them with a more convenient alternative to hospital-based outpatient procedures—and done so with a strong track record of quality care and positive patient outcomes.

Anchoring: The act of first proposing a particular number during negotiation, which can strongly affect the outcome of the negotiation.

Angel investor: Individual who invests their own money in an entrepreneurial company in exchange for equity ownership.

Association for Molecular Pathology v. Myriad Genetics, Inc., 133 S. Ct. 2107 (2013): A United States Supreme Court decision holding isolated genes are objects of nature, and therefore, not patentable.

Bilski v. Kappos, 130 S. Ct. 3218 (2010): A United States Supreme Court decision holding that a process must be tied to a particular machine or transform an article into a different state to be patentable.

Brainstorming: The process where any idea is a good idea! Documented brainstorm ideas are the seeds of concepts.

Bundled pricing: Sales strategy to drive sales volume by grouping similar or complimentary products or services together at reduced prices than they would command individually.

Business model: A model of the business that describes, in stylized form, how management intends to both create and deliver value to its customers as well as make a profit.

CAD: Computer-aided design is a tool to assist in concepting-to-scale. It reduces risk of expending financial and development resources prior to product development under design controls.

Capital equipment: Equipment or goods with a minimal cost of $5,000 to $10,000 that support the longer-term strategy of a health care entity. These fixed assets provide long-term operating benefits and depreciate over time.

Cash flow model: This tracks a company's cash inflows and outflows during a specific period. The analysis begins with a starting balance and generates an ending balance after accounting for all cash receipts and paid expenses during the period.

Claim(s): Define, in technical terms, the extent of the protection conferred by a patent.

Clinical data: Detailed information (usually related to safety or effectiveness) about a device that is gathered from use of the device in humans.

Co-development: The creation of new intellectual property in collaboration with another party.

Cold-calling: The process of soliciting interest in a business proposition without the benefit of personal introduction.

Company valuation: The assessed financial measure of a company's net worth, considering cash flow, potential for growth, and other relevant factors.

Computer numerical control machines (CNC machines): Versatile and flexible method of machining components into precise specifications via robotic-type equipment.

Concept development: The overall process of developing solutions that meet product requirements.

Concept generation: The process of refining brainstorm ideas into concepts.

Concepting-to-scale: A particular form of concept development well-suited for products that are small or technically challenging in nature, such as laparoscopic instruments. These concepts must be developed in CAD or to scale so that the result is more likely to meet product requirements and specifications when tested.

Confidence: What you get when you follow the concepting-to-scale process.

Confidential: Adjective used to describe information that has not been disclosed in a patent filing or otherwise previously published.

Coordinate measuring machines (CMM): A type of robotic-type equipment that can measure and verify the machined components against a specification (blueprint).

CPC: Cooperative Patent Classification.

Crowdfunding: A financing method that involves raising small amounts of money from a large number of individuals.

Customer intimacy: A value-creation model archetype whereby the business aims to deliver best total solutions by tailoring its products or services to satisfy unique, or highly targeted, customer needs.

Data locker: A form of secure electronic data storage for documents and materials to be reviewed during a potential investor's due diligence process.

De Novo: The De Novo process provides a pathway to classify novel medical devices for which general controls alone, or general and special controls, provide reasonable assurance of safety and effectiveness for the intended use, but for which there is no legally marketed predicate device. Devices that are classified into class I or class II through a De Novo classification request may be marketed and used as predicates for future premarket notification (510(k)) submissions.

Decision-maker(s): The employee or employees of a company who are authorized to make intellectual property licensing decisions.

Design control: The application of a formal methodology to the conduct of product development activities. It is often mandatory (by regulation) to implement such practice when designing and developing products within regulated industries (eg, medical devices). The development process that follows concept development where feasibility has been proven. ISO 13485 product development practices are employed during this phase.

Design validation: Establishment by objective evidence that product specifications conform to user needs and intended use(s). In simplest terms, these activities answer the question "Did I make the correct product?"

Design verification: Confirmation by examination and provision of objective evidence that output meets input requirements. In simplest terms, these activities answer the question "Did I make the product correctly?"

Development kits: Off-the-shelf (OTS) electronic and software subassemblies that enable timely feasibility studies for electronic devices.

Device classification: FDA-established groupings of generic types of devices based on the level of control necessary to assure the safety and effectiveness of the device. Federal regulations classify devices into three different levels. The class to which a device is assigned determines, among other things, the type of premarketing submission/application required for FDA clearance to market. The generic device types are further defined within a classification using three-letter product codes.

Design for manufacturability (DFM): Fit, Form, and Function of the product designed concurrently with the manufacturability in mind.

Diagnostic related group (DRG): DRG Codes (Diagnosis Related Group) Diagnosis-related group (DRG) is a system to classify hospital cases into one of approximately 500 groups, also referred to as DRGs, expected to have similar hospital resource use.

Differential pricing: Strategy of selling the same product or service to different customers at different prices, based on factors such as sales agreements, volume commitments, delivery requirements, customer segments, and other market segmentation.

Dilutive funding: Any kind of funding where investor receives an ownership stake in the company.

Distribution channels: Channels to deliver a medical device to the target market can include direct sales representatives, independent sales representatives often within a defined territory or region (also called manufacturers' representatives), selling product to a distributor at a reduced price who then resells the product or partnership with a large, well-established company with an aligned and proven sales force.

Distributor: Supply chain entity that purchases, warehouses, and resells life science products to health care facilities and providers, often within a defined territory or region.

EPO: European Patent Office.

Feasibility: A result of concepting where the concept proves feasible in meeting product requirements and specifications.

First contact: The employee of a company with whom an inventor initially communicates.

Freedom to operate: Having the ability, or "clearance", to make, use, sell, or import a product or process without infringing on another's patent.

Gainsharing: Business management strategy being adopted by some health care facilities to increase profitability by motivating health care staff to reduce cost of care through inclusion in financial profit-sharing incentives.

Group purchasing organizations (GPO): Purchasing organization to aggregate the purchasing volume of health care providers such as hospitals, surgery centers, clinics, and home health agencies to realize savings by negotiating discounts from manufacturers, distributors, and other vendors.

Guidance document: Guidance documents represent FDA's current thinking on a topic and describe FDA's interpretation of policy on a regulatory issue. They are not binding nor do they have the effect of law (statutes passed by Congress) or regulation (rules, which have the force of law, adopted by administrative agencies, such as the FDA, that address details of how laws are enforced). Guidance documents are published to provide industry an understanding of FDA's expectations and how the FDA is interpreting and enforcing requirements applicable to medical products. You can use an alternative approach compared with that described in a guidance if the approach satisfies the requirements of the applicable statutes and regulations.

Health maintenance organizations (HMOs): A type of health insurance plan that usually limits coverage to care from doctors who work for or under contract with the HMO. It generally would not cover out-of-network care except in an emergency. An HMO may require its members to live or work in its service area to be eligible for coverage. HMOs often provide integrated care and focus on prevention and wellness.

Healthcare Common Procedure Coding System (HCSPCS): The Healthcare Common Procedure Coding System (HCPCS, often pronounced by its acronym as "hick picks") is a set of health care procedure codes based on the American Medical Association's Current Procedural Terminology (CPT).

Hospital Outpatient Prospective Payment System (HOPPS): The system for payment, known as the Outpatient Prospective Payment System (OPPS), is used when paying for services such as x-rays, emergency department visits, and partial hospitalization services in hospital outpatient departments.

Initial public offering: An initial public offering (IPO) is the first time that the stock of a private company is offered to the public. (https://www.investopedia.com/terms/i/ipo.asp)

Inpatient Prospective Payment System (IPPS): Short-term acute-care hospitals are reimbursed under the inpatient prospective payment system (IPPS) within the Medicare program. The rates are prospectively set based primarily on the diagnosis each year for implementation October 1.

Integrated health care systems: Integrated health care systems are health care organizations that have an HMO component or other integrated method of paying for physician and hospital services without necessarily relying on third-party health insurers.

International Classification of Disease (ICD): The International Classification of Diseases (ICD) is the international "standard diagnostic tool for epidemiology, health management, and clinical purposes." Its full official name is International Statistical Classification of Diseases and Related Health Problems.

Investigational device: Medical device that does not have market authorization.

Investigational device exemption (IDE): Application, that when approved, allows an investigational device to be used in a clinical study in order to collect safety and effectiveness data.

License: A formal grant of legal rights by one party to another, subject to various terms. The chapter specifically discusses *manufacturing licenses*.

Licensee: The receiver of rights granted in a license. In this chapter, also used to describe a party engaged in negotiating to become a licensee.

Licensor: The grantor of rights in a license. In this chapter, also used to describe a party engaged in negotiating to become a licensor.

Liquidity event: When the founders and investors in a company receive cash compensation for the shares they own in the company.

Local coverage determination (LCD): Medicare administrative contractors (MACs) and the Centers for Medicare and Medicaid Services (CMS) sometimes develop policies to limit Medicare coverage of specific items and services. MACs issue local coverage determinations (LCDs) that limit coverage for a particular item or service in their jurisdictions only.

Logic of the business: An argument showing, for a specified business goal, why and how the business will meet that goal.

Manufacturer: Entity that makes, by chemical, physical, biological, or other procedures, any article that meets the definition of "medical device" in the Federal Food, Drug, and Cosmetic (FD&C) Act.

Market authorization: Process of reviewing and assessing information to grant the ability to commercially distribute a medical product in the United States.

Marketing plan: Organizational framework, built on market research, that strategically identifies, defines and quantifies marketing objectives to achieve financial goals and maximize profit potential. The plan describes target markets, outlines marketing strategies and includes the required budget to allocate corporate resources.

Mayo Collaborative Services v. Prometheus Laboratories, Inc., 132 S. Ct. 1289 (2012): A United States Supreme Court decision limiting medical method and diagnostic patent claims.

Medicare administrative contractor (MAC): A medicare administrative contractor (MAC) is a private health care insurer that has been awarded a geographic jurisdiction to process Medicare Part A and Part B (A/B) medical claims or durable medical equipment (DME) claims for Medicare Fee-For-Service (FFS) beneficiaries. CMS relies on a network of MACs to serve as the primary operational contact between the Medicare FFS program and the health care providers enrolled in the program. MACs are multistate, regional contractors responsible for administering both Medicare Part A and Medicare Part B claims.

Merger: A merger is an agreement that unites two existing companies into one new company. (https://www.investopedia.com/terms/m/merger.asp)

Milestone: Steps along the way to completing concept development. Milestones reduce risk by forcing important deliverables during development at specific points in the project plan.

National coverage determination (NCD): NCD is a United States nationwide determination of whether Medicare will pay for an item or service.

New technology add-on payment (NTAP): The new technology add-on payment (NTAP) program used by the Centers for Medicare and Medicaid Services (CMS) to provide additional payment for breakthrough technologies in the Medicare hospital inpatient prospective payment system (IPPS).

Nondilutive funding: Funding, typically a grant, that does not result in an ownership stake in the company.

Nonpracticing entity: An entity that holds a patent for a product or process with no intentions of producing or developing it. May be also known as a patent troll, patent holding company, or patent assertion entity.

Nonprovisional patent application: Establishes an invention's filing date, unless it claims the benefit of an earlier filed application. Filing a nonprovisional application starts the official examination process with the USPTO to determine if the invention is patentable.

Office action: Document written by a patent examiner during the patent application examination process.

Operational excellence: A value-creation model archetype whereby the business seeks to minimize the delivered cost of the products or services it offers to customers.

Patent infringement: Commission of a prohibited act, such as making, using, selling, or importing, with respect to a patented invention without permission from the patent holder.

Payment bundling: Bundled payment, also known as episode-based payment, episode payment, episode-of-care payment, case rate, evidence-based case rate, global bundled payment, global payment, package pricing, or packaged pricing, is defined as the reimbursement of health care providers (such as hospitals and physicians) on the basis of expected costs for clinically defined episodes of care.

PCT: A patent application filed under the Patent Cooperation Treaty (PCT) is an international application.

Pilot launch: A small controlled experiment to measure real-world interest in a new product, confirm assumptions underlying the business model, and pressure test newly created operations.

Pitch deck: A short slide presentation geared toward potential investors that provides an overview of the company, its technology, and the business plan for providing a return on their investment.

Preclinical/nonclinical data: Detailed technical information about a device gathered from bench or animal testing (nonhuman).

Premarket approval (PMA): The FDA process of scientific and regulatory review to evaluate the safety and effectiveness of class III medical devices. PMA is the most stringent type of device marketing application required by FDA. The applicant must receive FDA approval of its PMA application prior to marketing the device. An approved PMA is, in effect, a private license granting the applicant (or owner) permission to market the device. The PMA owner, however, can authorize use of its data by another.

Presubmission meeting: Mechanism available to applicants through which they can request feedback from the FDA, regarding potential or planned medical device applications, as well as address any significant issues that may arise during the course of review of an application.

Private equity: Capital that is not listed on a public exchange. Private equity is composed of funds and investors that directly invest in private companies or that engage in buyouts of public companies, resulting in the delisting of public equity. (https://www.investopedia.com/terms/p/privateequity.asp)

Private pay organizations (PPOs): A type of health plan where participants pay less if they obtain their health services from providers who participate in the plan's network. Doctors, hospitals, and providers outside of the network without a referral cost more.

Process Failure Mode Effect Analysis (PFMEA): Method of accessing the risks involved in order to prevent failures proactively.

Product/service innovation: A value-creation model archetype whereby the business seeks to invent and deliver the best products or services for customers.

Proof-of-concept: The concept(s) that prove feasibility of achieving performance goals.

Prospect: A company that may be a suitable candidate for licensing intellectual property.

Provisional patent application: Establishes an early filing date but does not mature into an issued patent unless a nonprovisional patent application is filed.

Quality management system (QMS): A complete system of managing an organization in accordance with an international regulatory standard specifically established for medical products (ISO13485). A formalized system that documents processes, procedures, and responsibilities for achieving quality policies and objectives. A QMS helps coordinate and direct an organization's activities to meet customer and regulatory requirements and improve its effectiveness and efficiency on a continuous basis.

Quality System (QS) Regulations: FDA requirements related to the methods used in and the facilities and controls used for designing, purchasing, manufacturing, packaging, labeling, storing, installing, and servicing of medical devices. Manufacturing facilities undergo FDA inspections to assure compliance with the QS requirements.

Risk: Risk takes many forms. Four types are project, technical, regulatory, and lastly, risk to the clinician or patient. There are other risks, such as business, market, and financial, but those are not covered here.

Sales plan: The specific strategies, tactics, and methods to achieve sales revenue objectives. The plan is based on defined sales targets, outlines sales tactics anticipated to secure market share, describes measurement metrics to determine performance, and includes a budget for estimated expenses.

SBIR: An acronym for Small Business Innovation Research, a competitive US Government grant program, which provides awards to domestic small businesses to support R&D efforts associated with innovative technologies.

Sepsis: An overwhelming and potentially fatal inflammatory response that develops following severe infection.

Stage-gate funding: In this model, an idea or project is not funded entirely at conception but rather is broken into several discrete stages. It has to meet or exceed measurable, predetermined goals (or "gates") in order to be eligible for funding for the next stage.

Statistical process control (SPC): Method of building the quality of the product into the process through statistical evaluation.

Strategics: A strategic buyer acquires another company in the same business to capture synergies so that the whole becomes greater than the sum of the parts. (https://www.investopedia.com/terms/a/acquisition.asp)

The Patient Protection and Affordable Care Act: The Patient Protection and Affordable Care Act, often shortened to the Affordable Care Act (ACA) or nicknamed Obamacare, is a United States federal statute enacted by the 111th United States Congress and signed into law by President Barack Obama on March 23, 2010. Together with the Health Care and Education Reconciliation Act of 2010 amendment, it represents the US health care system's most significant regulatory overhaul and expansion of coverage since the passage of Medicare and Medicaid in 1965. After the law went into effect, increases in overall health care spending slowed, including premiums for employer-based insurance plans.

Unit economics: The profit contribution directly associated with one unit of the product or service.

USPTO: United States Patent and Trademark Office.

Valuation: Defensible company value critical to secure potential investments. Requires the quantification of the value proposition through market projections, company comparables when possible, the range of potential exit values, and probability of achieving a successful exit.

Value analysis committee (VAC): This multidepartmental committee is tasked with reducing costs in the hospital supply chain. The VAC reviews a wide range of information in making a recommendation on new products, to include clinical outcomes, product quality and comparison, and financial models. New products generally must gain VAC approval to be used in the hospital setting.

Value analysis teams: A systematic, evidence-based process to evaluate current and emerging technologies to reduce/manage expenses by considering alternate products, services, and practices, which meet the clinical and end-user's specifications while maintaining or improving safety and quality of patient care.

Value chain: A description of the value-adding steps leading to a product or solution, going from materials and components to the products and services provided to customers.

Value proposition: Business or marketing statement that identifies measurable and demonstrable benefits provided by a product and the potential to outperform similar products on the market.

Venture capital: A form of funding where professional investment managers utilize money raised from other sources to invest in companies with the goal of receiving a high rate of return over a defined time period.

Waiver: A document companies may require inventors to sign before they will review a solicited invention.

Waterfall model: A linear sequential (noniterative) design approach for development, in which progress flows in one direction downwards (like a waterfall) through the phases of conception, initiation, analysis, design, construction, testing, deployment, and maintenance.

WIPO: World Intellectual Property Organization.

Index

Note: Page numbers followed by "f" indicate figures and "t" indicate tables.

CCS1019